## Hormones and Behaviour

Recent advances in non-invasive sampling techniques have led to an increase in the study of hormones and behaviour. Behaviour is complex but can be explained to a large degree by interactions between various psychological and physiological components, such as the interplay between hormonal and psychological systems. This new textbook from Nick Neave offers a detailed introduction to the fascinating science of behavioural endocrinology from a psychological perspective, examining the relationships between hormones and behaviour in both humans and animals. Neave explains the endocrine system and the ways in which hormones can influence brain structure and function, and presents a series of examples to demonstrate how hormones can influence specific behaviours, including sexual determination and differentiation, neurological differentiation, parental behaviours, aggressive behaviours and cognition. This is an accessible introductory textbook which will appeal to second and third year social science undergraduate students in psychology and biomedicine.

Nick Neave is a Reader in Psychology at Northumbria University.

# Hormones and Behaviour

## A Psychological Approach

NICK NEAVE

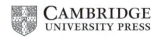
CAMBRIDGE
UNIVERSITY PRESS

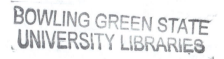

CAMBRIDGE UNIVERSITY PRESS

Cambridge, New York, Melbourne, Madrid, Cape Town, Singapore, São Paulo

Cambridge University Press
The Edinburgh Building, Cambridge CB2 8RU, UK

Published in the United States of America by Cambridge University Press, New York

www.cambridge.org
Information on this title: www.cambridge.org/9780521692014

© Nick Neave 2008

First published 2008

Printed in the United Kingdom at the University Press, Cambridge

*A catalogue record for this publication is available from the British Library*

ISBN   978-0-521-87145-7 hardback
ISBN   978-0-521-69201-4 paperback

# Contents

*List of diagrams*     page vi
*Preface*     vii
*Acknowledgements*     x

1 **Background to psychobiology**     1

2 **Hormones and the endocrine system**     22

3 **Behavioural endocrinology**     48

4 **Neurological effects of hormones**     69

5 **Typical sexual determination/differentiation**     85

6 **Atypical sexual differentiation**     109

7 **Neural differentiation**     135

8 **Reproductive/sexual behaviours**     154

9 **Attachment/parental behaviours**     191

10 **Aggressive/competitive behaviours**     224

11 **Sex steroids and cognition**     248

*References*     283
*Index*     345

# Diagrams

1.1   Organisation of the nervous system                                      *page* 2
1.2   Organisation of the brain                                                        3
1.3   Subdivisions of the telencephalon and diencephalon                               4
2.1   Endocrine activity                                                              24
2.2   Pathways for the synthesis of androgen and estrogen                             27
2.3   Summary of hypothalamic control of pituitary hormones                           32
2.4   Negative feedback loop involving the thyroid hormones                           43

# Preface

In 1996 there was a timid knock at my office door. It was one of our final year undergraduates seeking a tutorial with me to discuss an idea for her dissertation, an empirical piece of research conducted independently by our students under the guidance of a supervisor. The student in question was Meyrav Menaged and (as per instructions) she had come along armed with several research papers that had given her some possible ideas for this important project. The papers were rather outdated, and concerned the possible differences in circulating hormone levels between heterosexuals and homosexuals. I read the papers with interest and not a little scepticism; her proposal sounded worthy of pursuit, but my main reservation was the lack of psychology (she was after all studying a psychology degree). I asked her to reconsider her plan and include something of psychological merit. She seemed fine with that suggestion and off she went. Several days later she returned with a pile of other papers, some addressing cognitive differences between heterosexuals and homosexuals, and others reporting links between circulating testosterone and certain kinds of spatial ability – a project was born. She would focus on cognitive differences taking into account sexual orientation and circulating hormone levels (testosterone).

The first bit was easy for me: I had taught a module on sex differences and was well acquainted with the literature, different theories, 'best' kinds of tasks to use, etc. The latter issue was more of a problem: how the hell were we going to measure testosterone? I had visions of us attempting to extract gallons of blood from some poor unsuspecting undergraduate with little idea of what to do with it afterwards. At that time our University, and my colleagues within our Division had neither the expertise nor the facilities to enable us to do this. I made a few inquiries and came across the name of David Weightman, an endocrinologist in the Medical School of our more prestigious and better-off rival (Newcastle University) across the road. With fingers firmly crossed behind my back I promised my Head of Division (and holder of the purse strings) that we would be sure to get a research paper out of this enterprise and, much as we hated to be seen to be providing funds for our rival, decided to go ahead. I made an appointment to see David and nervously gave him my spiel; while he knew little about psychology, or the supposed cognitive differences between heterosexuals and homosexuals, he knew a hell of a lot about endocrinology, and must have been impressed by our proposal, because he agreed to come on board and provide his expertise. The fact that we would be paying his group around £12 per sample of saliva, from which they assured us they could gain an accurate record of circulating (free) testosterone, was perhaps by the by.

We (or should I say Mey) went ahead and tested a smallish group of male and female homosexuals and heterosexuals on two spatial and two verbal tasks, and impressively managed to persuade them all to drool into a small plastic pot. Mey gathered the results, conducted the statistical analyses, and hey presto we had a story to tell. She got to complete her project, and I (with some assistance from Dave) set to work putting together and submitting my first paper in behavioural endocrinology. After a rather lengthy wait (I think it was the journal rather than the quality of the paper) it was revised, accepted and published, and I had found a new and exciting research avenue. Since those days my understanding of this field has multiplied enormously. I now have two excellent PhD students (Helen Brookes and Sarah Evans), both of whom are routinely extracting saliva from (almost) willing volunteers, and our technician Anthea Milne buys-in testosterone kits and assesses levels of this hormone in our purpose-built Biophysical Analysis Unit. The cost per sample has plummeted (which pleases the purse-strings holder enormously) and now our undergraduate and postgraduate students are able to conduct behavioural endocrinological research (typically on testosterone or cortisol) on an almost routine basis. We have even begun selling our expertise to other institutions. My principal research interests focus on the possible relationships between testosterone and various physical/psychological/behavioural characteristics, and over the last few years I have been able to share my burgeoning knowledge and deliver an option entitled 'Hormones and behaviour' to our final year undergraduates.

My key problem in delivering this option has been the lack of an appropriate textbook. There are two texts addressing behavioural endocrinology on the market – Nelson's *Introduction to Behavioral Endocrinology* and Becker *et al.*'s *Behavioral Endocrinology*. Both in their own way are excellent, but both from the point of view of social science students are not so good, focussing as they do on 'hard' endocrinology, and using examples principally drawn from non-human animals. Over the course of the last few years I have written a set of lecture notes that have addressed behavioural endocrinology from a more psychological point of view, addressing topics and drawing examples that are more pertinent to social scientists, hopefully without diluting the high level of science inherent in such an endeavour. This book, then, is those lecture notes, greatly expanded and offering hopefully a slightly different insight into behavioural endocrinology from what has previously been available.

The first four chapters lay out the science of behavioural endocrinology, chapter 1 providing a basic grounding in neurobiology, essential for any student who has not come from a biological/physiological background (as many social science students have not). Chapter 2 then provides essential coverage of the endocrine system and the key hormones that will be addressed further in this text. Chapter 3 explains what is meant by the term 'behavioural endocrinology' and provides some theoretical and conceptual background before describing the principal ways in which hormone–behaviour relationships can be established. Chapter 4 addresses the neurological effects of hormones. The following three chapters then consider the more psychological/behavioural effects of hormones, chapters 5 and 6 covering typical and atypical sexual determination and differentiation, chapter 7 focussing on neurological differentiation. Thus far the main emphasis in the chapters has been to consider predominantly unidirectional relationships, i.e. the effects of hormones on physiology/behaviour. The final three chapters then begin to bring in more bidirectional relationships and include assessments of the effects of behaviour on neuroendocrine systems. Chapter 8 discusses these more complex hormone/behaviour interactions by assessing reproductive/sexual behaviours, chapter 9 addresses attachment and parental behaviours, and chapter 10 looks at aggressive/competitive behaviours. Last but not least, the final chapter will perhaps be of most interest to psychologists as it considers the possible effects of hormones on cognitive processing. Because of the page limit, and my own particular research experience, this final chapter has had to be limited to the effects of the sex steroids. There is a glaring omission in that I have not been able to consider the glucocorticoids or the thyroid hormones, and should a second edition of this text be possible, then I shall correct this imbalance.

# Acknowledgements

I would like first to express my thanks to those colleagues, PhD students and undergraduate/postgraduate students who have assisted me with various hormones–behaviour research projects over a decade. These are (in alphabetical order): Helen Brookes, Darren Cole, Angela Donaghy, Kirby Eccles, Saskia Ellis, Sarah Evans, Audrey Giles, Colin Hamilton, Sara Heary, Sara Herdman, Paul Hunter, Sarah Laing, Katharine Laughton, John Manning, Meyrav Menaged, Anthea Milne, Brooke Milton, Mary Soulsby, Frances Thorne, Delia Wakelin, Gemma Watson, David Weightman and Sandy Wolfson.

Particular thanks are due to Bernhard Fink from Göttingen, my long-term collaborator, who has ensured that my research interests remain varied and forever evolving.

# 1  Background to psychobiology

Before we can begin to discuss the various types of hormones, how they are formed, how they are secreted, how they act upon the body, and then how they can possibly influence behaviour, it is first necessary to provide a brief background to some basic psychobiological concepts. In this chapter I will describe the general layout of the nervous system, and explain how cells within the body (and especially within the central nervous system) communicate with one another.

## Neuroanatomical directions

Neuroanatomists have devised a three-dimensional system of directional coordinates in order to navigate around the complex machinery of the brain. Instead of terms like 'front' and 'back' or 'top' and 'bottom', which are all relative, they instead employ the following terms that are always taken from the orientation of the spinal cord. There are three main axes: anterior–posterior, dorsal–ventral and medial–lateral. Thus, in most vertebrates that walk on four legs, the front (towards the nose) is called the 'anterior' while the back (towards the tail) is called the 'posterior', though when referring to the brain the terms 'rostral' (towards the front) and 'caudal' (towards the tail) are often used. Towards the surface of the back is referred to as 'dorsal' (think of a shark's dorsal fin) while the aspect towards the chest/stomach is referred to as 'ventral'. Towards the sides is 'lateral' while towards the middle is 'medial'. In addition, something lying above another part is called 'superior', while something lying below another part is called 'inferior'. 'Ipsilateral' refers to structures on the same side of the body or brain, while 'contralateral' refers to structures on the opposite side of the brain or body. This is slightly complicated in humans because we walk on two legs and so the position of our head and brain is altered relative to our spinal cord (Pinel, 2006).

## Organisation of the nervous system

The nervous system is divided into two broad components: the central nervous system (CNS) and the peripheral nervous system (PNS). The CNS consists of the brain and the spinal cord, while the PNS consists of

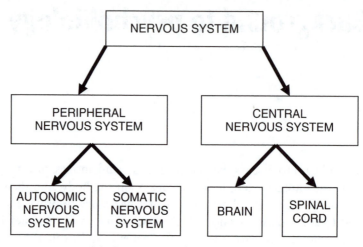

1.1 *Organisation of the nervous system*

the cranial nerves, the spinal nerves, and the peripheral ganglia (ganglion refers to a cluster of nerve cells). A basic way to differentiate these two separate but closely interlocking systems is to think of the CNS as being encased in bone (the skull and the spinal vertebrae), while the elements of the PNS are not. The PNS is further subdivided into the autonomic nervous system (ANS) and the somatic nervous system (SNS) – see diagram 1.1. The ANS acts as the regulator for the internal environment of the body, serving to relay sensory and motor information between the CNS and the internal organs. Thus, neurons (nerve cells) conduct sensory information from the internal organs to the CNS, and transmit motor commands from the CNS back to the internal organs. The SNS serves as the interface between the PNS and the outside world: its nerve cells conduct sensory information from the periphery (the skin, the joints and muscles, the senses, etc.) back into the CNS, while other neurons perform the opposite function by transmitting motor information from the CNS to the skeletal muscles.

## Organisation of the brain

At first glance the human brain appears rather uniform in appearance, a globular lump of grey/white tissue overlaid with blood vessels and formed into a series of bumps and troughs. In fact the brain possesses clear divisions derived from the development of the early neural tube from which the brain forms during gestation (Cowan, 1979). Initially the tissue that will develop into the brain consists of a fluid-filled tube out of which three swellings become prominent; these swellings develop into the forebrain, the midbrain and the hindbrain. Later on in development the forebrain and hindbrain further divide into two parts, and thus the fully formed brain is

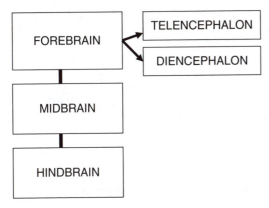

1.2 *Organisation of the brain*

recognised as having five major divisions: telencephalon[1] and diencephalon (which together constitute the forebrain), the midbrain (or mesencephalon) and the hindbrain, see diagram 1.2.

## The forebrain

The telencephalon and diencephalon are subdivided further – see diagram 1.3.

### The telencephalon

The telencephalon comprises three key elements.

### Cerebral cortex

The most notable features of the telencephalon are the two large and roughly symmetrical hemispheres which are in fact separate functional systems interconnected by major fibre pathways called the cerebral commissures. The principal commissure is the corpus callosum (which literally means 'hard body') and this wrist-thick bundle of fibres connects the corresponding regions of cortex, so that for example a specific area of temporal cortex in the left hemisphere is connected to the corresponding region in the right hemisphere. Both hemispheres are covered by a thin layer of tissue called cortex (in Latin this translates as 'bark of a tree'), which is not smooth but deeply convoluted, thus allowing for greatly increased material without an increase in overall brain volume. A deep cleft in the cortex is referred to as a fissure, and a shallow one is called a sulcus (the plural being sulci); each ridge is called a gyrus (plural being gyri). Some two thirds of the

---

[1] The suffix -encephalon is derived from the Greek and means 'in the head'.

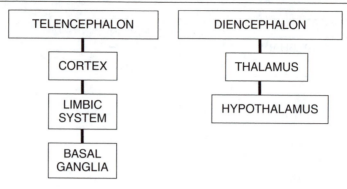

*1.3 Subdivisions of the telencephalon and diencephalon*

surface of the cortex is hidden in these grooves, making the total surface area of an average brain around 2360 cm², with the thickness of the cortex being about 3 mm (Carlson, 2004). Because neurons predominate in the cortex, the cortex has a characteristic hue and is thus referred to as 'grey matter'. Beneath the surface of the cortex run millions of axons that connect the various regions together; as they are covered by a white-coloured protective tissue called myelin this gives rise to the name 'white matter'. The most prominent features of the cortex are the two lateral fissures (the deep grooves which run along each side of the brain), the central sulcus (which runs from the top centre of the brain to join up with the lateral fissures), and the longitudinal fissure (the major gap between the two hemispheres running from front to back). These conveniently clear anatomical divisions are used to help define the different lobes of the brain, and thus the hemispheres are divided into four lobes: frontal, temporal, parietal and occipital.

*Functions of the different lobes*

While the cortex acts as an integrated whole to coordinate behaviour, evidence from anatomical/histological examinations, animal experiments, human cases of localised brain damage, electrical recording and stimulation experiments, and neuroimaging studies, has shown that specific areas of the cortex are responsible for certain aspects of processing. Cytoarchitectonic (cellular architecture) maps have been developed of these subregions based upon differences in cell density, cell shape, size and connectivity. A commonly used map is that produced by the neuroanatomist Korbinian Brodmann in 1909. He used tissue stains to visualise different cell types in different brain regions and described fifty-two distinct regions that are now referred to as 'Brodmann's areas'. While these areas have experienced some modification and further subdivision, experimental and imaging techniques have broadly confirmed their existence and thus we possess specialised brain regions for touch, perception, movement, and even distinct cognitive processes

(Gazzaniga *et al.*, 1998; Kolb and Whishaw, 2001). A basic summary of the key functions of each lobe is provided below:

*Frontal lobes*

These extend from the central sulcus to cover the anterior portion of the brain. They contain primary motor cortex (area 4), premotor cortex (area 6), Broca's area (area 44) and the prefrontal cortex. Each area receives input from the thalamic nuclei, limbic system and hypothalamus, and connections from the other lobes, making it a 'control centre'. A key region of frontal cortex is referred to as 'prefrontal cortex', which forms around a third of the entire cortical mantle, and constitutes a larger proportion of the brain in humans than in other species. A major role of prefrontal cortex concerns working memory – the ability to retain pieces of information for short periods of time. Prefrontal cortex is also involved in higher-order cognitive behaviours such as planning, organisation, the monitoring of recent events, the probable outcome of actions and the emotional value of such actions.

*Temporal lobes*

The temporal lobe comprises all the tissue below the lateral (Sylvian) fissure running backwards to the parietal and occipital cortices. This region is also described by gyri that form it – the superior temporal gyrus, the middle temporal gyrus and the inferior temporal gyrus. The temporal lobe is richly connected to the other lobes, the sensory systems, the limbic system and the basal ganglia, which means that the temporal lobe does not subserve a single unitary function; it seems to have three key functions. First, areas 22, 41 and 42 are concerned with auditory and visual perception, specifically with focussing attention on relevant information and with the perception of speech (left hemisphere), music and faces (right hemisphere). Secondly, the classic case of patient 'H.M.' reported by Scoville and Milner (1957) showed that the hippocampus was critical for the formation of new memories. Finally, the amygdala adjoins the hippocampus and is concerned with emotional control (see later section on the limbic system).

*Parietal lobes*

These lie between the occipital lobe and the central sulcus. Just behind the central sulcus lies the postcentral gyrus (Brodmann's areas 1–3) which houses primary somatosensory cortex, the region of cortex housing the sensory representation of the body. The right hemisphere contains information about the left side of the body and vice versa. Parietal cortex thus integrates sensory and motor information and so spatial navigation and perception are thought to be key functions of this region of the brain. A common feature of damage to the right parietal lobe is 'sensory neglect' – the tendency to ignore the contralateral side of the body and features of the outside world.

*Occipital lobe*

Occipital cortex is primarily concerned with visual perception. It is located at the caudal end of the cortex and comprises primary visual cortex (area 17) and visual association (areas 18 and 19). Area 17 is also referred to as striate (striped) cortex or area V1, and is the main target for the thalamic nuclei that receive input from the visual pathways; this information is relayed to secondary visual cortex (area 18 or V2) and then on to additional areas (area 19, V3, V4 and V5). As in the other cortices, the left half of the visual field is relayed to the right hemisphere, though the map is considerably distorted as much of our visual processing concerns the analysis of information from the central visual field (fovea).

**The Limbic system**

An important group of forebrain structures were defined in the 1930s and their key role was assumed to reflect motivational and emotional processing (Papez, 1937). MacLean (1949) provided further modifications to what was then called 'Papez circuit', and we now refer to it as the limbic ('ring-shaped') system which includes the amygdala, hippocampus, cingulate cortex, fornix, mammillary bodies and septum. The amygdala (means 'almond-shaped') lie at the front end of each of the temporal lobes and are not single structures but in fact consist of around a dozen interconnected nuclei (Aggleton, 1993). Bilateral removal of the amygdala in monkeys leads to profound impairments in social and emotional behaviours, while bilateral amygdala damage in humans leads to similar deficits in emotional processing, with fear and anger being particularly affected (Broks *et al.*, 1998; Scott *et al.*, 1997). The hippocampus ('seahorse') is a bilateral structure located within the temporal lobes. Many studies involving both experimental animals, human cases of brain damage, and brain functioning in undamaged humans have clearly demonstrated that the hippocampus is crucial for what is called 'declarative memory', i.e. memory for explicit facts and episodes (Squire, 1992; Squire *et al.*, 1992).

Lying above the corpus callosum is a large region of cortex formed within the cingulate gyrus; it encircles part of the thalamus (and shares dense interconnections with the various thalamic nuclei) and is referred to as cingulate cortex. Evidence from experimental animal and human case studies demonstrates that damage to cingulate cortex leads to a profound disturbance in the experience and expression of emotion: generally the individual seems completely unresponsive to affective situations or stimuli (Damasio and Van Hoesen, 1983). The fornix ('arch') is a fibre pathway connecting the hippocampus to the mammillary ('breast-shaped') bodies which are part of the hypothalamus, and the septum.

## The basal ganglia

The third element of the telencephalon is a collection of individual nuclei that together are involved in the control of voluntary movements. The principal structures of this system include the caudate ('tailed') nucleus and the putamen ('shell'), which are collectively referred to as the striatum ('striped structure'), and the globus pallidus ('pale globe').

## The diencephalon

The diencephalon contains two key elements: the thalamus and the hypothalamus. The thalamus is not a single structure but is a two-lobed collection of separate but interconnected nuclei. Most of these nuclei receive input from the sensory systems, process it, and then transmit the information to the appropriate sensory processing areas in the neocortex. The thalamus thus seems to act as a kind of sensory relay centre and can thus influence almost the whole of the brain. Some of the thalamic nuclei may also play a key role in certain aspects of learning and memory. The hypothalamus lies underneath the thalamus at the base of the brain. It too is not a single structure but comprises twenty-two small nuclei, the fibre pathways that pass through it, and the pituitary gland attached to the hypothalamus via the pituitary stalk. This array of nuclei control the autonomic nervous system and the endocrine system. Almost all aspects of basic motivations and survival behaviours (such as fighting, escape, mating, feeding, etc.) are coordinated from here. I shall describe the form and functions of the hypothalamus and pituitary gland in more detail in the next chapter.

## The midbrain

The mesencephalon consists of two major parts: the tectum ('roof') and the tegmentum ('covering'). The tectum contains two main structures, the superior colliculus and the inferior colliculus, which appear as four bumps ('colliculus' is Latin for 'mound') on the surface of the brain stem. The inferior colliculus forms part of the auditory system, and the superior colliculus forms part of the visual system, appearing to be important in visual reflexes and reactions to moving stimuli. The tegmentum lies beneath the tectum and it includes portions of the reticular formation, a set of more than ninety interconnected nuclei in the brain stem which play a role in sensory processing, attention, arousal, sleep, muscle tone, movement and reflexes. Two key structures of the tegmentum are the red nucleus and the substantia nigra ('black substance') which are important components of the motor system as they connect to parts of the basal ganglia.

## The hindbrain

The hindbrain contains the cerebellum ('little brain'), a two-lobed structure lying directly underneath the cerebral hemispheres and connected to the brain stem. This important structure receives information from the sensory systems and from the muscles and the vestibular system and it coordinates this information, making our movements smooth. Damage to the cerebellum (which occurs in cerebral palsy) leads to impairments in walking, balance, posture and the performance of skilled motor activities. The hindbrain also houses the pons ('bridge'), a bulge on the brain stem which contains part of the reticular formation and seems to play an important role in sleep and arousal. Finally, a key structure is the medulla oblongata ('oblong marrow') which lies at the end of the brain stem bordering the top of the spinal cord. It also contains part of the reticular formation and contains nuclei that control vital functions such as control of breathing and skeletal muscle tone.

## Communication systems

The body has evolved three different communication systems: the nervous system, the endocrine system and the immune system, each of which has its own type of specialised chemical messenger. The nerve cells (or neurons) use neurotransmitters (but also use certain hormones), endocrine glands use hormones, and the immune system uses cytokines. The three systems are very closely interlinked: the nervous system controls the release of hormones (this process will be described in detail in the next chapter) and can influence the release of cytokines by the immune system. Hormones in turn can influence nervous system activity (neuroendocrinology) and have close links with the immune system (neuroimmunology).

As described by Gard (1998), possibly the most simple form of communication between cells is for one cell to release a chemical into the extracellular fluid; this chemical can then influence the activity of nearby cells. Such a system of course is not very efficient as it is non-specific, and large amounts of the chemical may have to be released to ensure that the nearby cell can be influenced. Nature seems to have solved this problem by ensuring that cells develop specialised outgrowths towards one another, and that only certain regions of the cells can secrete the chemicals. This process in fact describes how neurons within the central nervous system communicate, and it is referred to as 'neurocrine' communication (and will be described in detail in subsequent sections). In a variation of this type of cell, some neurons release hormones which act within the central nervous system – this is called 'neuroendocrine' communication (and is described in the next chapter). The problem with the neurocrine system is that a single neuron is only able to communicate with a fairly limited number of cells within a short distance.

In order for a cell to communicate with more widely dispersed cells, then, another system is required.

Some cells thus release their chemicals into the bloodstream and are thereby able to influence cells all over the body. However, this system has certain drawbacks in that only molecules under a certain molecular size can be transported through the vascular system; the secretory cells must be linked to the vascular system via the capillaries; and the secreted chemicals may be constantly being depleted by blood arriving from other areas of the body. This means that only a small fraction of the secreted chemical can reach the target cell. These problems have been solved by the fact that cells producing a chemical clump together and form glands; they can thus produce larger amounts of the chemical (in this case a hormone). In addition the chemicals that they secrete are very potent and thus only small amounts are required. This is in fact how the endocrine system works. Note that the endocrine glands also release chemicals which act on adjacent cells (just like neurons). This is referred to as 'paracrine' communication.

## Cells of the nervous system

The nervous system consists of two different types of cell.

### Glia

These are by far the most prominent in terms of quantity, outnumbering the neurons by around ten to one. For many years it was assumed that all they did was act as support workers to the much more important neurons. Hence, the different types of glial cells – oligodendrocytes, Schwann[2] cells, astrocytes, and microglia – provide the neurons with nutrition, clear waste products from them and hold them in place; the word 'glial' in fact means 'glue' and often these cells are collectively referred to as 'neuroglia' (literally meaning 'nerve glue'). In fact the status of these humble cells is rapidly rising as research is beginning to demonstrate that they also serve important roles in transmitting and receiving information from neurons, and in establishing and maintaining the connections (synapses) between neurons.

### Neurons

According to Williams and Herrup (1988) the adult human brain contains around 100 billion neurons which combine to form consciousness, sensory experience and controlled behaviours. Neurons have a high metabolic rate and must be constantly supplied with oxygen and glucose or they will die.

---

[2] Named after German physiologist Theodor Schwann (1810–82).

Unlike other cells of the body, neurons are not replaced when they die and we are born with as many as we will ever have. The role played by the various support cells described previously is thus very important. The neurons are specialised cells that receive and transmit information; they vary in size and shape but all consist of the same basic structures:

## Cell body (soma)

The soma contains the machinery which serves to maintain the normal functioning of the cell, and also houses the nucleus which contains the genes housed in twenty-three pairs of chromosomes (thus a genetically 'normal' human will posses forty-six chromosomes). In twenty-two of the chromosomes (referred to as autosomal chromosomes) genes form matched pairs (one inherited from the mother and one from the father). These matched pairs of genes are referred to as alleles. The twenty-third pair of chromosomes are the sex chromosomes – the X and Y chromosomes, designated thus because they roughly resemble these shapes. These special chromosomes determine an individual's sex: normal females possess a pair of Xs, while normal males possess one X and one Y. Since the female always has two X chromosomes her eggs will always carry an X, but a male's sperm can carry either an X or a Y; thus the offspring can be XX (female) or XY (male). Alternatives to this normal pattern of sex chromosomes, and how they affect sex determination, will be discussed in detail in chapter 6.

Each chromosome is a very long molecule of deoxyribonucleic acid (DNA) with many genes along its length, providing a set of instructions for constructing an organism, these instructions being referred to as the 'genome'. The discovery that DNA consists of two helical spirals which can 'unzip' to make copies of itself is attributed to Francis Crick and James Watson in 1953.[3] However, significant credit should also be given to Rosalind Franklin, Maurice Wilkins and Linus Pauling whose research enabled the now famous pair to make the conceptual leap and hence take the bulk of the credit. We now understand that the strands of DNA are composed of a sequence of nucleotide bases attached to a chain of phosphate and deoxyribose. The bases are: adenine (A), cytosine (C), guanine (G) and thymine (T), and they are always linked in a particular fashion (A with T; G with C). Genetic information is copied and transmitted when the two strands became 'unzipped' and collect new complementary bases forming two double-stranded molecules of DNA, each identical to the original.

To assist in the copying process there is another substance in each cell called RNA (ribonucleic acid) composed of adenine, guanine, uracil and cytosine. The number of bases can vary from a thousand to a million, with a sequence of three bases (called a 'codon') along the strand making up a gene.

---

[3] Crick announced the 'secret of life' not to a scientific conference but to the more humble clientele of the Eagle pub in Cambridge!

Each group of three bases represents a simple code for an amino acid, which then forms part of a protein molecule, which in turn defines the structure of cells and tissues. It is estimated that 3 billion base pairs make up the human genome, with less than 5% being genes, the function of the rest remaining unknown at present. Each individual has a different arrangement of these letters in the genetic code, and so it is highly unlikely that two individuals will be exactly identical (unless they are identical twins, of course). All organisms encode their genetic material using DNA and so similar genes for similar things are found in very diverse organisms.

The bulk of the cell consists of cytoplasm, a jelly-like substance containing important structures referred to as organelles ('little organs') which carry out important biochemical functions. One type, called mitochondria, extracts energy from the breakdown of nutrients and provides the cell with its energy source adenosine triphosphate (ATP). Another type is the endoplasmic reticulum which acts as a storage reservoir for chemicals important for the functioning of the neuron; it also transports these chemicals through the cytoplasm. A special type of endoplasmic reticulum called the Golgi[4] apparatus packages up the products of secretory cells (such as hormones) ready for these secretions to be transported and released from the cell. The Golgi apparatus also manufactures complex molecules and enzymes to break down substances no longer required by the cell.

**Plasma membrane**

Separating the cytoplasm from the external environment is the plasma membrane, a double-layered structure consisting of lipid molecules. Small uncharged molecules such as water, oxygen and carbon dioxide move freely across this membrane, but charged ions such as sodium, potassium, calcium and chloride can only pass through specialised openings in the membrane called protein channels. The protein channels can also detect substances outside of the cell (such as hormones) and relay information about the these substances to the cell's interior.

**Dendrites**

Emerging from the soma are a collection of branch-like structures referred to appropriately enough as dendrites ('dendron' being the Greek word for tree). The dendrites are the information-receiving parts of the neuron as they relay neurochemical information between different neurons across a tiny gap called a synapse. The surface of the dendrites is lined with receptors, and the greater the surface area of a dendrite, then the more information can be received; some dendrites possess short outgrowths called dendritic spines that increase the surface area available for synaptic communication.

---

[4] Named after the Italian histologist Camillo Golgi (1843–1926).

## Axon

A key section of a neuron is the axon, a long tube emerging from the soma with small dendritic-like branches at the end called terminal buttons (or presynaptic terminals). The axon forms the information-sending part of the neuron, and its role is to conduct an action potential (a brief electrochemical event) from the area surrounding the dendrites towards the terminal buttons. Axons can be very long (the largest one in the human body stretches from the big toe to the base of the brain). Axons that bring information into the CNS from the senses are referred to as afferent axons. Axons that transmit information away from the CNS towards the muscles and glands are referred to as efferent axons. In the CNS axons are covered with an insulating substance called myelin, a mixture of fat and protein produced by the oligodendrocytes (in the PNS the same function is provided by Schwann cells). Like the insulating plastic surrounding the bare wires of an electrical cable, the myelin forms a sheath around the axon, which not only protects the axon, but also insulates it and ensures that action potentials can be very fast (conduction of an action potential within a myelinated axon is around 120 m/sec as opposed to around 35 m/sec in an unmyelinated axon). Unlike an electrical cable, however, the myelin sheath is not continuous, but consists of segments each around 1 mm in length with a tiny gap in between.[5]

## Synapse

In the late 1800s the histologist Santiago Ramón y Cajal demonstrated that neurons do not physically touch one another – they are separated by a gap called a synapse. When the action potential reaches the terminal buttons they secrete molecules of a specialised chemical (a neurotransmitter) across the synapse towards the dendrites of adjacent neurons. These neurotransmitter molecules (the various types will be discussed in a later section) bind to specialised receptors in the dendrites and determine whether or not the adjacent neurons will transmit a postsynaptic potential or not.

## Electrical events within a neuron

Human neurons are so small that measuring their electrical activity would be extremely difficult. Researchers have therefore tested the much larger axons from the squid in order to investigate the electrical activity within a neuron. In order to measure any electrical charge within the axon, a standard experimental paradigm is to place the axon into a tank of sea water (in which it can survive for several days) and insert a microelectrode into the axon.

[5] This gap (and the myelin) was discovered in 1878 by French pathologist Louis Ranvier (1835–1922), and so the gaps are called 'nodes of Ranvier'.

Another electrode is inserted into the water in order to measure its electrical state. Using this technique, researchers have discovered that the inside of the axon is negatively charged with respect to the outside: a figure of $-70$ mV is routinely described. Provided that the axon is not stimulated in any way, this resting potential will not change, but if another stimulating electrode is placed into the axon and a brief positive electrical charge applied, we see a dramatic change in the internal state of the axon. Remember that the inside of the axon is negative, so when a positive charge is applied, for a brief period of time the inside suddenly becomes more positive (this is referred to as depolarisation).

Now, it is not the case that every brief positive charge will trigger an action potential; in fact each neuron appears to have what is called a 'threshold of excitation' (this threshold may differ between neurons), a point beyond which an action potential will be instigated and the neuron is said to 'fire', and below which an action potential will not be instigated. Thus, only the application of a positive charge (or several charges) of sufficient strength will 'break' the threshold and trigger an action potential. Should the threshold be broken then an action potential must occur at the same electrical level. So, action potentials stay the same strength irrespective of the stimulus that led to them being instigated, i.e. a larger stimulus does not cause a bigger action potential, neurons either fire or they do not, and this is called the 'all or none law'. Once an action potential has been triggered, then the electrical potential within the axon quickly drops back to its resting state. In fact, though, there is a slight temporary overshoot such that the potential assumes a lower state then its previous resting state – i.e. it might drop to $-80$ mV, thus making the neuron slightly less likely to fire for a short while.

## Chemical events within a neuron

In order to understand how a resting potential is established and how an action potential is created following appropriate stimulation, we need to understand the internal and external environment of the axon. In essence, the electrical charge results from the balance between two opposing forces of diffusion and electrostatic pressure. Put simply, diffusion refers to the simple physical fact that, left to their own devices, molecules will distribute themselves evenly throughout the medium in which they reside (in this case the inside and outside of a neuron). Where there are no forces to prevent diffusion, molecules move from regions of high concentration to regions of low concentration (e.g. sugar dissolved in water will initially form a residue at the bottom, but over time will become evenly distributed throughout). Electrostatic pressure refers to the fact that when certain substances called electrolytes are dissolved in water they split into particles called ions, each ion having a different electrical charge (positive ions are referred to as cations, while negative ions are called anions). Ions with the same electrical charge

(− − or + +) repel one another, while particles possessing a different electrical charge (− + or + −) will attract one another. So, diffusion is steadily moving molecules from regions of high concentration to those of low concentration, while electrostatic pressure is constantly shifting ions around as they attract and repel one another.

Inside the axon (intracellular) and outside the axon (extracellular) reside different types of ions: organic ions (A−) are created by the cell's metabolic processes and are only found inside the axon; potassium ions (K+) are found predominantly inside the axon; chloride ions (Cl−) are found predominantly outside the axon; and sodium ions (Na+) are found predominantly outside the axon. Like the membrane of the soma, the axon membrane is selectively permeable for some of the ions (K+, Cl− and Na+) but the organic ions are imprisoned within the axon. Diffusion is trying to force K+ out of the membrane, but as the external environment has a positive electrical charge electrostatic pressure is forcing the K+ ions back in. A similar situation in the opposite direction operates for Cl− outside of the axon. Things are different for Na+: while diffusion is pushing the molecules into the axon, the negative charge inside the axon is also attracting the Na+. Why then is the inside of the axon not filled with Na+? The answer lies with an electrochemical process called the sodium–potassium pump generated by energy in the form of ATP provided by the mitochondria. This system acts constantly to expel Na+ from the inside of the axon while at the same time it draws in K+ molecules from the outside through specialised openings in the membrane called sodium–potassium transporters. As it draws in two K+ molecules for every three Na+ it expels, the net result is an interior rich in K+ and an exterior rich in Na+. In a resting neuron there is thus an uneasy balance between the ions, with dramatic changes possible if the balance is upset in any way – this is what indeed happens during an action potential.

## The action potential

During the resting phase, sodium and potassium are being steadily interchanged between the interior and exterior of the axon via the transporters. Within the membrane is another type of opening called a voltage-dependent ion channel. Each channel is acutely responsive to the electrical state of the membrane, the sodium ones being more sensitive then the potassium ones. Both types remain closed during the resting state. As soon as the threshold of excitation is breached (depolarisation) the voltage-dependent sodium channels in the membrane are the first to open, and sodium pours into the interior of the axon. Owing to this huge influx of positive ions, the interior of the axon briefly changes from a negative state of around −70 mV to a positive state of around +40 mV. The less sensitive potassium voltage channels now begin to open and potassium begins to leave the interior of the axon. After around 1 m/sec the sodium channels become blocked and thus no more sodium can enter. This is called the 'absolute refractory period' and it is a period when another action potential cannot be triggered. During this period potassium continues to leave the axon and the inside of the axon begins to hyperpolarise, i.e. its potential becomes more negative, and drops back towards its resting state. Once the resting state of the axon has been approached the potassium channels close, no more potassium can leave the axon and the sodium channels are reset. This is called the 'relative refractory period' and here the axon can be stimulated to fire, but only if a stronger stimulation than normal is applied. As previously stated, the axon actually overshoots its resting state and for a very brief period becomes more negative; this is due to the accumulation of potassium ions outside of the membrane (the negative organic ions outnumber the positive potassium ones). As soon as the potassium ions diffuse away from the exterior, the normal balance of the axon is restored and the whole process can begin again. The entire action potential takes around 4 m/sec.

## Conduction of the action potential

If an investigator were to record from a series of microelectrodes placed at regular intervals along the length of the squid axon and apply a depolarising electrical stimulus at one end, we would 'see' the action potential travelling along the axon. In an unmyelinated axon, each point along the axon membrane generates the action potential, i.e. with potassium ions being expelled and sodium ions being allowed in causing depolarisation in adjacent areas. The next area of membrane is depolarised, reaches its threshold, and generates another action potential. In this manner the action potential passes down the axon like a wave.

In myelinated axons the process is slightly different. Recall that these structures are partially covered with an insulating layer of myelin, separated by small unmyelinated gaps (nodes of Ranvier). Here the processes of sodium–potassium exchange can thus only occur at the nodes of Ranvier. The action potential travels down the axon, behaving exactly like an electrical charge passing along a household cable, gradually reducing in strength. In household electrical cables this does not create much of a problem as such cables are typically not very lengthy – it does cause problems in undersea cables which may be thousands of miles long! Similarly, in the axon, while the strength of the action potential diminishes, it still retains enough charge to trigger another action potential at the next node of Ranvier. By means of such 'cable properties' the action potential appears to 'jump' from one node to the next all along the axon. This is referred to as 'saltatory conduction'. One advantage of saltatory conduction is that the impulse can travel much faster in a myelinated axon; such neurons convey sensory information in to the CNS and motor commands out to the muscles, and this means that the individual can react very quickly to key environmental stimuli.

## Communication between neurons

As there was clearly a gap between neurons, precisely how they could influence one another was the cause of much scientific speculation, some arguing for an electrical explanation and others for a chemical explanation. In the early 1900s a young researcher, Thomas Elliott, was conducting experiments with the newly isolated hormone adrenaline, and found that it acted as a stimulant on the muscles – by accelerating heartbeat for example. In 1904 Elliott concluded that adrenaline was being released by the sympathetic ganglia whenever they were appropriately stimulated to do so. His studies led his professor, John Langley, to the formulation of the concept of specific receptors which bind neurotransmitters (or drugs) onto a cell, thereby either initiating biological effects or inhibiting cellular functions, a concept which forms the cornerstone of modern pharmacological research. Support for these ideas came in the 1920s from Otto Loewi. In his studies the vagus nerve in a frog's heart was repeatedly stimulated (this causes heart rate to decrease). Fluid from this decelerated heart was then collected and injected into a second heart, which then also began to slow down. The experiment was repeated but this time involved the stimulation of the accelerator nerve (this speeds up heartbeat). When fluid from the accelerated heart was duly injected into another heart it too was stimulated. Synaptic transmission was thus convincingly shown to be chemical in nature.

Through such elegant experiments we now understand a great deal more about the chemical events at the synapse, and these are as follows. Chemicals that serve as neurotransmitters are synthesised within the terminal buttons by the Golgi apparatus in the soma. Transmitter substances are synthesised from precursor molecules derived from the diet, so for example a common type of neurotransmitter acetylcholine is synthesised from choline found in cauliflower and milk. Neurotransmitters are then stored in spherical packets called 'synaptic vesicles', which are then transported to the end of the terminal button where they collect in the 'release zone' and attach themselves to the presynaptic membrane. The release zone contains voltage-dependent calcium channels, and so when an action potential reaches the terminal button it depolarises the presynaptic membrane, opening the calcium channels. The influx of calcium opens specialised channels in the membrane called 'fusion pores' which allow the neurotransmitter stored within the vesicles to be released into the synaptic cleft. This whole process is called 'exocytosis' and lasts around 1–2 m/sec.

The molecules of neurotransmitter then diffuse across the synaptic cleft to the postsynaptic membrane (the dendrites of the adjacent neurons) where they attach to binding sites of specialised protein receptors. A molecule of neurotransmitter fits into the binding site rather like a key in a lock, and so receptors can only 'accept' specific neurotransmitter molecules (though each neurotransmitter can attach to several different types of receptor, each with different characteristics). As neurotransmitters are common chemicals there are many natural and artificial substances (drugs, poisons) that can mimic the effects of neurotransmitters as they fit the same binding sites. Any chemical that attaches to a binding site is called a ligand.

When a neurotransmitter has attached to a receptor, transmitter-dependent ion channels are opened in the postsynaptic membrane, allowing specific ions to enter the cell and thus change the membrane potential. There are two ways in which the arrival of the neurotransmitter at the receptor can trigger the opening of the ion channels: a simple direct method and a longer, more complex method. The simple method is referred to as 'ionotropic' and such events are very rapid as the arrival of the neurotransmitter at the receptor instantly opens the ion channels. As the ion channels are only opened for a very brief time an ionotropic event is also short-lived. This mechanism is seen particularly in the sensory and motor neurons to ensure that we can detect and respond quickly enough to certain environmental cues – possible dangers, etc. The slower, longer-lasting effect is referred to as 'metabotropic' and this involves a more complex sequence of events with two possible actions. Metabotropic receptors are positioned adjacent to G proteins, which are also attached to the synaptic membrane. When the neurotransmitter arrives, the G protein is activated: an alpha subunit breaks away from the G protein and binds to the ion channel, thereby causing it to open. Alternatively, the arrival of the neurotransmitter causes the receptor to stimulate the G protein: the alpha subunit breaks away and then activates an additional enzyme, which then produces a 'second messenger' (a common one is called cyclic AMP) which attaches to the ion channels and opens them. Not surprisingly these metabotropic events take longer to initiate, but last longer.

## Neurotransmitters

Because neurotransmitters can have two types of effect – depolarisation (EPSP) or hyperpolarisation (IPSP) – one would expect that two types of neurotransmitter would exist: excitatory and inhibitory. However, while some are exclusively excitatory or inhibitory, others can produce either effect depending upon the nature of the postsynaptic receptors. According to McGeer et al. (1987) we can divide neurotransmitters into the following general types:

### Acetylcholine (ACh)

Acetylcholine consists of choline (derived from the breakdown of lipids) and acetate (also called acetic acid). This neurotransmitter is released at cholinergic synapses in skeletal muscles, where it has an excitatory effect. It is also found in those regions of the brain that subserve learning and memory, and also plays a role in governing the stages of sleep. In the peripheral nervous system cholinergic synapses are found in the ganglia of the autonomic nervous system, and at target organs, where they have an inhibitory effect. There are two kinds of ACh receptors, one ionotropic and one metabotropic. Nicotinic receptors are ionotropic and are found principally in muscle fibres but are also located in the CNS. Muscarinic receptors are metabotropic and are found principally in the CNS.

## The Monoamines

These types of neurotransmitter are separated into catecholamines and indoleamines and are produced by a small group of cell bodies located in the brain stem. These groups then give rise to a widespread system of axons distributed throughout the brain. These neurons appear to act in a modulatory fashion, influencing a whole range of brain functions. The catecholamines consist of dopamine, adrenaline (also referred to epinephrine) and noradrenaline (also referred to norepinephrine).

### Dopamine

Dopaminergic neurons produce both EPSPs and IPSPs, depending on the nature of the postsynaptic receptor. Dopamine is derived from the amino acid tyrosine, which itself is converted from dietary sources of phenylalanine. At least five types of dopamine receptors have been identified so far: $D_1$–$D_5$, each with differing properties. There are several important dopaminergic systems within the CNS which are involved in movement, the reward value of stimuli, planning, learning and memory.

### Adrenaline/noradrenaline

These are hormones produced by the adrenal glands which are located just above the kidneys (I will describe these hormones more fully in chapter 2). Noradrenaline is actually created within dopamine-containing synaptic vesicles; the presence of an enzyme dopamine β-hydroxylase converts dopamine into noradrenaline. Thus 'adrenergic' neurons convert a neurotransmitter into a hormone, which then acts like a neurotransmitter! (I will discuss this confusing fact later.) In the CNS, adrenergic synapses have been shown to be involved in alertness, vigilance and wakefulness, and they produce IPSPs. Such neurons are also found in the target organs of the sympathetic nervous system where they have excitatory effects. There are several types of adrenergic receptors. In the CNS there are α1, α2, β1 and β2 adrenergic receptors. These receptors are coupled to G proteins (guanylyl nucleotide binding proteins) that generate the secondary messenger cyclic AMP.

## Indoleamines

The indoleamines consist of serotonin and the hormone melatonin (see next chapter). Serotonin (5-hydroxtryptamine to give it its proper name) is derived from the amino acid tryptophan (found in chocolate, meat, eggs, etc.). Most 'serotonergic' synapses produce inhibitory potentials and serotonin appears to play a key role in the regulation of mood, eating, pain, sleep and dreaming, and arousal. Thus far, nine different types of serotonergic receptors have been discovered.

## Amino acids

All the transmitters described so far are all synthesised within neurons, but some neurons use ready-made basic amino acids as transmitter substances. Thus far about eight such amino acids have been identified, and two key ones are as follows:

## Glutamate

This is present in the brain in high concentrations and it was initially assumed to play a generalised role in energy metabolism but was not initially thought to act like a neurotransmitter. Molecular biologists have since discovered that two major families of glutamate receptors exist: ionotropic and metabotropic (Watkins and Jane, 2006). The most common ionotropic receptors are those for NMDA (N-methyl-D-aspartic acid) and AMPA ($\alpha$-amino-3-hydroxy-5-methylisoxazole-4-propionic acid), both of which are widely distributed throughout the nervous system, and crucially involved in the synaptic changes (referred to as 'long-term potentiation') underlying learning and memory (see chapter 4).

## GABA (gamma-aminobutyric acid)

This is produced from glutamic acid by the actions of an enzyme called glutamic acid decarboxylase (GAD). It is an inhibitory substance and is widely distributed throughout the brain and spine. Some investigators believe that it is the widespread presence of GABA in the brain that prevents epilepsy. If all of the neurons in the brain were excitatory then, once one fired, a chain reaction would be produced (as in an epileptic seizure) unless other neurons acted to 'damp down' the spread of excitation. Two GABA receptors have been identified – the ionotropic $GABA_A$ and the metabotropic $GABA_B$. The $GABA_A$ receptors contain binding sites for at least three different substances, one being of course GABA, the second being benzodiazepines and the third being for alcohol and barbiturates, both of which have inhibitory effects.

## Peptides

Neurons in the CNS not only release neurotransmitters and amino acids but in addition also release a large variety of peptides (amino acids linked by peptide bonds). One of the most important classes of peptides are the endogenous opiates discovered by Pert *et al.* (1974). They found that the reason why drugs such as morphine and heroin are so addictive is that they act on the naturally occurring opioid synapses that are normally stimulated by the brain's own substances. These natural opiates are called enkephalins and appear to be important for pain relief and pleasure.

## Neurotransmitter pathways

Neurotransmitters are not randomly spaced throughout the brain but instead occur in specific well-delineated pathways. Neuroanatomical tracing studies which can map out neurotransmitter pathways have routinely been conducted in the rat; we can only assume (though not be certain) that similar pathways are operating in the human brain. The cholinergic system has been identified as comprising several major pathways; one originates in the basal forebrain and sends axons to the neocortex; a second originates in the medial septum and sends projections to the limbic system, lateral hypothalamus, olfactory bulb and cingulate cortex. Two closely linked regions in the pedunculopontine tegmental nucleus (PPT) and laterodorsal tegmental nucleus (LTN) send fibres to the thalamus, tectum, cerebellum and hindbrain nuclei. Dopaminergic pathways comprise two main routes originating in the substantia nigra and ventral tegmental area. They project to numerous sites within the limbic system, midbrain, thalamus, olfactory nucleus and neocortex. Noradrenergic pathways originate in the locus coeruleus and form two key pathways – the dorsal bundle projects to the tectum and thalamus while the ventral bundle projects to the hypothalamus, limbic system, olfactory bulb and neocortex. Serotonergic pathways originate in the Raphe nuclei. The ascending dorsal pathway projects to the cortex, caudate nucleus, thalamus, hypothalamus and limbic system; additional pathways project to the cerebellum and spinal cord (cited in Carlson, 2004). As we will see, there is a close relationship between these neurotransmitter pathways and receptors for certain hormones.

## Pharmacology of synapses

Many natural substances affect the functioning of the synapses, principally because natural selection has tended to preserve substances that are effective – the same neurotransmitter chemicals are found in animals and plants because they are so well suited for conveying information. Effective drugs either increase or decrease the effects of a neurotransmitter; a drug that blocks the effects of a neurotransmitter is called an antagonist, while a drug that mimics or increases its effects is called an agonist. Whether a drug is an agonist or an antagonist is determined by its affinity (the strength of its binding to the receptor) and its efficacy (how well it activates the receptor). An antagonist drug will bind strongly to the receptor but fail to activate it, thereby blocking the action of the neurotransmitter. An agonist will bind tightly to the receptor and will activate it strongly. This gives the impression that all drugs will have exactly the same effects on everyone but clearly this is not so. There are distinct individual differences in drug responsiveness, and these are determined by the fact that different receptors are found in different numbers and sensitivities determined by genetic and environmental factors. For example someone may have a large number of dopamine $D_4$ receptors and few $D_1$ or $D_2$ receptors but someone else may have more of the latter and fewer of the former.

# 2 Hormones and the endocrine system

The term 'hormone' derives from the Greek verb 'ormoa' (meaning 'I excite', or 'I arouse') and was first introduced by the physiologist Ernest Henry Starling in his now-famous 1905 Croonian lecture entitled 'The chemical correlation of the functions of the body'. The scientific definition of this term was long overdue as the realisation that certain substances must be travelling around the body and influencing both physiology and behaviour was not limited to a small number of scientific minds. Any humble farmer could describe in detail the powerful effects of castration upon a young male animal; rather more discomfiting was the common knowledge that castration also had the same kinds of physical and behavioural effects on young human males, as numerous eunuchs and castrati singers were able to testify (see chapter 3).

A series of eminent scientists had indeed been on the verge of formally discovering and describing hormone action (though it would be several years before an actual hormone was discovered). In 1855, Claude Bernard coined the term 'internal secretion', a phrase he had used to describe the release of glucose from glycogen. Until Starling's talk however, this term had been used in a rather ad hoc manner to describe the passage of any molecule from tissues into blood, and thus the specific meaning that he originally envisaged had been somewhat lost (Henderson, 2005). While the effects of abrupt hormone removal via castration had been described for centuries, the opposite effects – namely the apparent rejuvenating effects of secretions from the testes – were also noted, and enthusiastically advocated by Charles Brown-Séquard. This famous physiologist, initially known for his research into the functioning of the sympathetic nervous system, injected himself with testicular extracts from young guinea pigs, and instigated the 'science' of 'organotherapy' to publicise his ideas. In this he could probably be considered a visionary, as his rationale that 'if we could safely introduce the principle of the internal secretion of a gland taken from a living animal into the blood of men suffering from the lack of that secretion, important therapeutic effects would thereby be obtained' (Brown-Séquard, 1893) clearly presaged more modern ideas concerning the benefits of hormone replacement therapies. In his endeavours Brown-Séquard was actually following a long tradition. For example, the ancient Hindus and Chinese recommended the administration of testicular extracts to cure male sexual dysfunction. A little later, Albertus Magnus prescribed pig testicles ground in wine, and the powdered womb of a hare in wine, to cure male impotence and female infertility respectively (Medvei, 1993).

Some saw organotherapy as little more than pseudoscience practised by quacks and charlatans (perhaps not helped by Brown-Séquard's assertions that ground guinea pig testicles, diluted and injected into the anus, could cure numerous diseases, including cancer!). Others, however, saw potentially important medical advances, and this led to a flurry of research activities involving gland extracts. In 1893 George Oliver obtained secretions from the adrenal glands and injected them into his son and showed that they narrowed the brachial artery (he assumed that this would lead to a rise in blood pressure but couldn't actually measure this). Oliver took a sample of his adrenal extracts to the Professor of Physiology at University College London, Edward Schäfer, now accredited as one of the founding fathers of endocrinology (Borell, 1978). Schäfer was initially sceptical, but tried out the extracts on dogs and found that they did indeed cause a rise in blood pressure. He went on to demonstrate conclusively that extracts from the adrenal medulla led to a rise in blood pressure, while extracts from the thyroid gland caused a drop in blood pressure. He also applied the term 'ductless glands' to the organs which release 'internal secretions', and described the role of insulin in the pancreas before this hormone had been discovered (Schäfer, 1895).

Taking over the professorship from Schäfer at UCL on his departure to Edinburgh was the aforementioned Starling, who, along with his brother-in-law William Bayliss, began to investigate the innervation of the pancreas and duodenum. Contrary to the results of Ivan Pavlov showing that the pancreas was solely stimulated by the vagus nerve when acid entered the duodenum, Bayliss and Starling demonstrated that pancreatic secretions could be elicited following the addition of acid, in the absence of nerve impulses. They reasoned that another mechanism must thus be involved and assumed that the introduction of acid into the duodenum must cause the release of some substance into the bloodstream. They carefully isolated duodenal mucosa, filtered it and injected it into a dog, causing pancreatic secretion within seconds (Bayliss and Starling, 1902). This new substance was termed 'secretin' and was soon found to be universal in its effects, i.e. secretin from one species injected into another would produce the same physiological reactions.

In the Croonian lecture series of 1905 Starling reviewed current endocrinological knowledge and of course gave us the term 'hormone'. Rapid progress then ensued, with researchers investigating additional organs and systems; Artur Biedl's textbook of endocrinology was first published in 1910; journals (*Endocrinology* began in the USA in 1917) and endocrine societies dedicated to Schäfer's 'new physiology' began to form across the world (Wilson, 2005). Thanks to Schäfer's rigorous demands that endocrinology be an experimental science, its respectability within physiology grew, while the more extreme claims of organotherapy diminished. During the 1920s researchers began to identify tissues that produced hormones, developed bioassays to identify the hormones, prepared active extracts, and identified the structure and synthesis of the various hormones (Borell, 1978; Wilson, 2005).

## What are hormones?

The term 'endocrine' denotes the 'internal secretion of a biologically active substance', and the endocrine system uses hormones to convey its information. A standard definition of a 'true' hormone is 'a substance released by an endocrine gland and transported through the bloodstream to another tissue, where it acts to regulate functions of the target tissue' (Baxter, 1997).

A more quantitative definition has been provided by Brown (1994), who provided five ways in which to define a hormone. First, a hormone is a chemical messenger which is effective in minute quantities. Second, a hormone is synthesised within ductless glands. Third, a hormone is secreted into the circulatory system and transported around the body in the blood. Fourth, a hormone acts upon receptors in specific target cells, located distantly from the organ of synthesis. Finally, a hormone exerts a specific biochemical or physiological regulatory effect on the target cell.

Despite these fairly clear guidelines, other authors have questioned such simplistic definitions and have even questioned what constitutes a hormone. For example Martin (1985) points out that not all physiological regulators are hormones, and that some hormones (especially neurohormones) are not synthesised in endocrine glands, while others are synthesised in various loca-

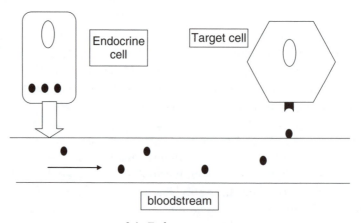

2.1 *Endocrine activity*

tions (e.g. insulin, estrogens). Peptides such as somatostatin are referred to as hormones when synthesised by endocrine glands, but when they are produced by neurons in the brain they are called neuropeptides! In addition, hormones may serve a variety of non-endocrine functions, i.e. they can activate the cell adjacent to their release organ (paracrine function), they can influence the same cells that release them (autocrine function), and pheromones released into the environment by the sweat glands can then influence another individual of the same species (exocrine function).

A number of hormones do not just act on specific cells but can influence a variety of cells in numerous locations throughout the body (growth hormone being an obvious example). Hormones can also not just have a specific action at a target cell, but also have generalised effects; or, by interacting with different cell receptors, have different functions in different target cells. So, the precise definition of what a hormone is can be rather vague. Just to add to this confusion there also seems to be some disparity in how different authors have classified hormones.

Gard (1998) defined hormones by their chemical make-up: chemically there are two classes of hormones, the first class being predominantly composed of amino acids and peptides. There are synthesised and stored as inactive molecules which are then cleaved to release an active hormone. The second class consists of the steroid hormones, which have a characteristic four-ringed chemical base. This terminology is also used by Brown (1994), who simply refers to 'steroid' or 'non-steroid' hormones based on the fact that the endocrine glands secreting steroid hormones (adrenal cortex and gonads) develop from different embryonic tissue from the glands secreting non-steroid hormones. A slightly more complex description is provided by Lingappa and Mellon (2001). They still define two classes of hormones but describe the first class as being stored within membrane vesicles for later release, while those in the second class are secreted immediately. The former contains the polypeptide hormones while the latter contains the steroids (derived from cholesterol) and the eicosanoids (derived from fatty acids). Other authors differentiate between neurohormones (substances like oxytocin and vasopressin that are produced and secreted within a modified nerve cell), pheromones, parahormones (substances such as histamine and the prostoglandins which act like a 'true' hormone but are not secreted within an endocrine gland), prohormones (hormone precursors), growth factors, cytokines and vitamins (Brown, 1994).

For simplicity I shall adopt the chemical description as described by Baxter (1997), who explains that hormones are derived from the major classes of common compounds utilised by the body.

## Amino acids

These hormones are modified from a single amino acid and they include the catecholamines, the indoleamines and the thyroid hormones. As described in chapter 1, the catecholamines consist of adrenaline and noradrenaline (also respectively called epinephrine and norepinephrine) which are synthesised from dopamine via tyrosine; in the CNS and PNS they act as neurotransmitters but are also secreted by the adrenal medulla and act as hormones. Also, as described previously, the indoleamines consist of serotonin, synthesised from tryptophan in the CNS, and melatonin, also derived from tryptophan via serotonin in the pineal gland. The thyroid hormones consist of thyroxine ($T_4$) and triiodothyronine ($T_3$) and are derived when iodine combines with tyrosine in the thyroid gland.

## Peptide hormones

These hormones are synthesised from basic amino acids and consist of chains of these acids varying in length from 3 to 100+. They are categorised according to their size into small peptides, large peptides and polypeptides. Small peptide hormones include: oxytocin, vasopressin, thyrotropin-releasing hormone, angiotensin, somatostatin and luteinising hormone-releasing hormone. Large peptide hormones include: secretin, calcitonin, gastrins, glucagon and adrenocorticotropic hormone. Polypeptide (or protein) hormones include: insulin, parathyroid hormone and growth hormone.

## Steroid hormones

Steroid hormones have a characteristic chemical structure consisting of three six-carbon rings plus one five-carbon ring, and are manufactured within the gonads and adrenal glands via the conversion of pregnenolone from cholesterol derived from the diet. All steroids are fat soluble and pass easily through cell membranes. In the blood the steroids exist in a free (unbound form) which is biologically active, or bound to serum proteins such as albumin and sex-hormone-binding globulin (SHBG). For example around 38% of testosterone is bound to albumin, 60% to SHBG, and thus only around 2% circulates in the 'free' form, though some of the bound form may also split from the protein and enter target tissues (Braunstein, 1997). There are several types.

### Androgens

Specific enzymes convert pregnenolone into various types of androgens, which are then converted into other types via further enzyme action. The key androgens are testosterone (T), dehydroepiandrosterone (DHEA), androstenedione and 5α-dihydrotestosterone (DHT), though the first androgen to be isolated and characterised was androsterone, a somewhat tricky procedure conducted by Adolf Butenant in 1931 which involved 25,000 litres of male urine. It was assumed that this was the principal male hormone until 1935, when Ernst Laquer and colleagues (using tons of bulls testicles to isolate 5 mg) showed that the testes secrete testosterone (Tausk, 1984). Testosterone is the principal circulating androgen, more than 95% of this steroid being produced by the 350–500 million Leydig cells in the testes. These secrete around 5000 µg per day leading to plasma concentrations of around 700 ng/100 ml (Norman and Litwack, 1987). The remainder is produced by the adrenal cortex of the adrenal glands. Testosterone (but not DHT) can be converted into estradiol via the enzyme aromatase (this process being called aromatisation). DHT is converted from testosterone via the enzyme 5α-reductase. See diagram 2.2.

Human males display three major peaks in testosterone production, one during mid-gestation (between weeks 10 and 18), another beginning around week 8 after birth lasting 4–5 months, and then a final surge during puberty. The androgens initially induce the differentiation and maturation of the male reproductive system, and then during and after puberty produce and maintain male secondary sexual characteristics (e.g. antlers in animals, beard growth and muscular development in humans), increase organ size and skeletal muscle mass, and influence courtship, dominance and sexual behaviours (Rommerts, 2004). The effects of androgens in the CNS remain complex and poorly understood, as testosterone may have specific effects, but also from the result of its conversion to DHT and also estradiol (these issues will be further addressed in subsequent chapters). Testosterone is also a potent androgen in women, but levels are around a tenth of those in males; testosterone production shows considerable variability in females in that an increase of 20–30% is seen around the middle of the menstrual cycle (Judd and Yen, 1973). Around 50% of circulating testosterone comes from the ovarian production of the testosterone precursor androstenedione, the remainder

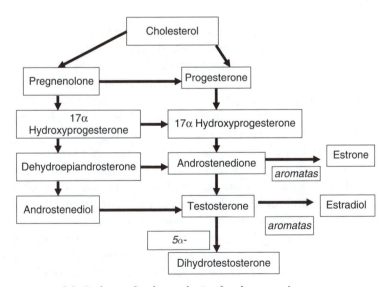

2.2  *Pathways for the synthesis of androgen and estrogen*

coming from adrenal activity. As women age, then levels of androstenedione decline, with a reduction in levels after the menopause to around half those of women of reproductive age (Miller, 2001).

## Estrogens and progestins

In females the two most important steroid hormones are 17β-estradiol and progesterone, though their metabolites estrone and estriol also play important roles in various reproductive processes. In the ovaries in non-pregnant females, the follicles principally secrete estradiol and estrone; during pregnancy estriol is the principal estrogen secreted by the placenta. Progesterone (the principal progestin and named for its progestational role in maintaining pregnancy) is produced by the follicles in non-pregnant females, and by the corpus luteum in pregnant females. Secretion and plasma concentrations of these steroids are greatly determined by the menstrual cycle, for example levels of estradiol range from around 6 ng/100 ml in the early follicular phase to 60 ng/100 ml in the late follicular phase (Norman and Litwack, 1987). In general the estrogens stimulate the development of the internal reproductive structures and later promote female secondary sexual characteristics (e.g. breast development, fat deposition), and promote water retention, calcium metabolism, the stages of pregnancy, and certain reproductive and maternal behaviours. In contrast to the estrogens, it was assumed that the biological actions of progesterone are mainly restricted to the reproductive tract and the mammary tissue (Norman and Litwack, 1987); however a recent review (Wagner, 2006) describes evidence for the important role of progesterone in modifying neural tissue underlying certain sexual behaviours and perhaps cognition (see later chapters).

## Corticoids

Two types of corticoids are produced and secreted in the adrenal glands. The glucocorticoids consist of corticosterone and cortisol (sometimes referred to as hydrocortisone), and were originally named because of their principal role in glucose metabolism. However, they have additional wide-ranging physiological effects as they increase glycerol and free fatty acid release from cells; increase muscle lactate release; inhibit glycogen breakdown; alter carbohydrate metabolism; reduce calcium absorption; suppress the immune system; and influence heart rate (Findling et al., 1997). As they easily enter neural tissue their excess or deficiency may have a direct influence on CNS functioning and thus influence cognition and behaviour (see later chapters). Cortisol synthesis and release follows a clear diurnal pattern, as levels drop in the late evening and then rise sharply before waking to then show a steady decline throughout the day. Transient increases in cortisol secretion are associated with food ingestion and exercise. Cortisol is secreted in an unbound state, but on entering the circulation 75% is bound to corticosteroid-binding globulin (CBG), 15% to albumin, with the remaining 10% circulating in a free form (Findling *et al.*, 1997). The second type of corticoid are the mineralocorticoids, which consist of aldosterone and 11-deoxycorticosterone (DOC). They principally act to maintain blood pressure and water and salt balance in the body by helping the kidneys retain sodium and excrete potassium. When aldosterone production falls below a certain point, the kidneys are not able to regulate salt and water balance, causing blood volume and blood pressure to drop. Aldosterone binds weakly to CBG and circulates mostly bound to albumin (50–70%), the remainder circulating in the free form. DOC is almost completely bound to CBG, with less than 5% circulating in a free form (Don *et al.*, 1997).

## Neurosteroids

The steroid hormones that have previously been described are released by endocrine glands, circulate through the bloodstream (in bound or free form) and enter target cells where they act as transcription factors in the regulation of gene expression, such effects occurring within minutes/hours (see later section for more details on how hormones work). However, ever since the almost immediate anaesthetic effects of intraperitoneal injections of progesterone in rats was described (Selye, 1942), researchers have considered possible non-genomic effects of steroids. There is now increasing evidence that some steroids are produced directly within the brain (via cholesterol-pregnenolone) and these have been termed 'neurosteroids' (Baulieu, 1998). Thus far, two key neurosteroids have been identified – progesterone and dehydroepiandrosterone (DHEA), which are both converted to androstenedione and thence to testosterone and estradiol by actions previously described (diagram 2.2). It is thought that the neuroactive steroids alter neuronal excitability via the cell surface, through interaction with neurotransmitter receptors (principally $GABA_A$, though all other receptors could be involved) and these modulatory effects occur within milliseconds/seconds (Falkenstein *et al.*, 2000; Rupprecht, 2003; Rupprecht and Holsboer, 1999). Owing to their pharmacological properties there is intense speculation that such hormones may play important roles in modulating neuronal, and thence behavioural-/cognitive functions, and form novel therapeutic agents for tackling age-related cognitive decline and anxiety disorders. However, the evidence is complicated by large species differences in neurosteroid metabolism and location of action, and evidence of behavioural effects of the neurosteroids in humans remains sparse (Falkenstein *et al.*, 2000). Wehling (1997) pointed out that any model of steroid hormone action must address both rapid (non-genomic) and delayed (genomic) effects of steroids and the possible interactions between them.

## Lipids

These hormone-like substances are not produced within endocrine glands but are derived from lipids such as linoleic acid, and phospholipids such as arachidonic acid. A key class of lipids are the eicosanoids, which include the prostoglandins. These derivatives of the fatty acids seem to act in a paracrine or autocrine fashion and are produced by most cells, promptly released, and cleared rapidly from the circulation. It was assumed that they acted by binding to cell surface receptors but it has since been discovered that some interact with nuclear receptors (see later section on mechanisms of hormone action). Eicosanoids can regulate hormone release and mediate hormone action, e.g. prostaglandin E inhibits the release of growth hormone from the pituitary (Baxter, 1997).

## Other substances

Other substances that we will come across in our discussions concerning hormones and their possible role in behaviour are as follows. 'Prohormones' are the precursors to 'true' hormones and can consist of modified molecules, or molecules that have split to form a particular hormone. A key prohormone is proopiomelanocortin (POMC), a large molecule which is composed of different sections, each section capable of producing a different hormone. One section forms beta-lipoprotein, which in turn is the precursor for the hormone/neurotransmitter beta-endorphin (an endogenous opiate). Other sections can be synthesised into melanocyte-stimulating hormone (MSH) and adrenocorticotropic hormone (ACTH), both of which are located within the pituitary gland. In fact, testosterone also acts as a prohormone because it serves as the precursor for both dihydrotestosterone (DHT) and estradiol. As stated in a previous section, 'Pheromones' are chemicals produced by exocrine glands that are secreted into the environment, where they act on individuals of the same species. They were originally called 'ectohormones', because they act like hormones but on a different individual from the one that produced them (Brown, 1994). Pheromone secretion is regulated by the steroid hormones.

## The endocrine glands

### Hypothalamus and pituitary

As these structures share dense connections, and together form the critical endocrine control centre, they will be described together. They are located at the base of the brain underneath the thalamus, within the region referred to as the diencephalon in the forebrain (see chapter 1). They form a coordinated system that has a strong influence over the function of certain endocrine glands as well as controlling a range of physiological activities. We shall see later in this chapter that these structures provide an excellent example of neuroendocrinology (brain–endocrine interactions) in action, as through these structures the CNS regulates the endocrine system, and, in turn, endocrine activity influences CNS activity (Aron *et al.*, 1997).

The hypothalamus consists of several interconnected nuclei which contain modified neurons that release neurohormones (hormones that act within the nervous system) into the pituitary gland. These hormones can be divided into those which are then secreted directly into the circulation by the posterior pituitary, and those that are secreted into the anterior pituitary gland (hypophyseotropic hormones), thereby regulating the secretion of its hormones. The hormones secreted into the anterior pituitary gland are referred to as 'releasing' hormones because they stimulate the release of the anterior pituitary hormones. Most are thus excitatory, though some have inhibitory actions. The excitatory ones are as follows.

## Corticotropin-releasing hormone (CRH)

This is synthesised within the anterior portion of the paraventricular nuclei of the hypothalamus (Pva) and it stimulates the secretion of adrenocorticotropic hormone (ACTH).

## Gonadotropin-releasing hormone (GnRH)

This is synthesised within the preoptic area of the anterior hypothalamus and it controls the release of luteinising hormone (LH) and follicle-stimulating hormone (FSH). There seems to be some debate as to whether there is a single GnRH that triggers both LH and FSH release, or whether in fact there are two kinds of GnRH, one controlling the release of LH and the other (as yet unidentified) which controls the release of FSH. Evidence for the 'single GnRH theory' comes mainly from studies demonstrating that the pulsatile release of GnRH does indeed stimulate LH and FSH release in a number of species, including humans. Evidence for the 'two GnRH theory' stresses that FSH release does occur in the complete absence of LH release, and vice versa in many animal species, but perhaps not in humans (Brown, 1994). This raises the issue (and this will be raised again in subsequent chapters) that direct comparisons between human and non-human species with regard to hormone action may not be possible.

## Growth hormone-releasing hormone (GH-RH)

This is secreted within the ventromedial nucleus (VMN) and the arcuate nucleus (ARC) of the hypothalamus and it stimulates growth hormone (GH) secretion.

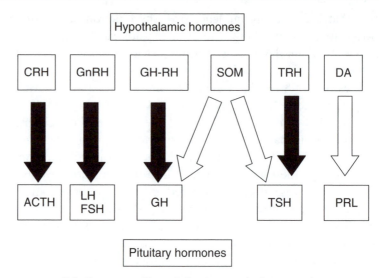

2.3  *Summary of hypothalamic control of pituitary hormones (Filled arrows indicate a stimulatory effect whilst open arrows indicate an inhibitory effect)*

### *Thyrotropin-releasing hormone (TRH)*

This is synthesised mainly in the paraventricular (PVN) and anterior par-aventricular nuclei (Pva) of the hypothalamus. The function of this hormone is to stimulate cells in the anterior pituitary gland to produce and release thyroid-stimulating hormone (TSH).

The inhibitory hormones secreted into the anterior pituitary are as follows.

### *Dopamine (DA)*

These neurons are located in the arcuate nucleus, and it acts as a primary pro-lactin-inhibitory hormone.

### *Somatostatin (SOM)*

This is also referred to as growth hormone-inhibiting hormone (GH-IH), is secreted by the periventricular region and mainly acts to inhibit the secretion of growth hormone (GH) and thyroid-stimulating hormone (TSH), though it also has inhibitory effects on insulin, glucagon and secretin production.

As previously stated, the hypothalamus also manufactures two hormones that are synthesised in the supraoptic nuclei and in the lateral and superior par-aventricular nuclei; these are then transported to the posterior pituitary for release. Antidiuretic hormone (also referred to as arginine vasopressin) acts to regulate water balance, raises blood pressure by acting as a vasoconstrictor, and may also serve a role in memory enhancement. Oxytocin stimulates uterine contractions and milk ejection from the mammary glands, and may influence various reproductive and sexual functions (e.g. orgasm, parental behaviours, and attachment bonds – see chapters 8 and 9).

## The pituitary

The pituitary gland is also called the 'hypophysis' and is attached to the hypothalamus by the hypophyseal stalk (called the 'infundibulum') which conveys the axons from the hypothalamic secretary cells and blood vessels. The pituitary is often referred to as 'the master gland' as it produces a range of hormones which influence the other endocrine glands; in fact this term should really be applied to the hypothalamus which directly controls the pituitary. It lies directly beneath the hypothalamus and consists of three separate regions: the anterior pituitary (pars distalis), the intermediate lobe (pars intermedia), and the posterior pituitary (pars nervosa). The anterior pituitary is formed from an embryonic structure called Rathke's pouch,[1] and along with the intermediate lobe they form a true endocrine gland. These structures are collectively referred to as the 'adenohypophysis'. The posterior pituitary forms during embryonic development as part of the ventral hypothalamus and the third ventricle. It shares dense projections with the supraoptic and paraventricular nuclei of the hypothalamus, and is referred to as the 'neurohypophysis'.

The powerful role played by the pituitary in many aspects of growth and development had been suspected for many years. Several scientists, for example, had noted that the actions of the pituitary and the gonads appeared to be linked in some way. Julius Tandler noted that the pituitary became enlarged in males and females following removal of the gonads (gonadectomy). Harvey Williams Cushing conducted successful operations in which he removed pituitary adenomas (benign tumours) and thereby 'cured' the condition that has since been named after him (Cushing's disease). The pituitary tumours lead to an over-production of adrenocorticotropic hormone which stimulates the adrenal gland to secrete higher levels of cortisol, thereby producing the characteristic symptoms of the disorder (moon-face, upper body fat deposition, skin problems, fatigue, etc.). The anterior pituitary produces six main hormones (they can be classified into three groups) in response to the releasing hormones secreted by the hypothalamus. These hormones are referred to as 'tropic' (from the Greek word for 'nourishment') because they stimulate various physiological processes. The three groups are as follows.

### Corticotropin-related peptides

These include adrenocorticotropic hormone (ACTH), the release of which is triggered by CRH. In turn ACTH stimulates the synthesis and release of the glucocorticoids, mineralocorticoids and androgenic steroids from the adrenal glands. ACTH is stimulated by CRH in a pulsatile fashion (it is not

---

[1] Named after the anatomist Martin Rathke (1793–1860), who discovered it in 1839.

stimulated constantly but rather follows a clearly defined pattern in response to internal and external events). ACTH thus shows a diurnal (daily) rhythm with a clear peak evident before waking and then a gradual decline as the day progresses. This diurnal rhythm in ACTH is reflected in the daily pattern of cortisol release (which is higher in the morning); a change in ACTH leads to a corresponding alteration in cortisol. External stressful events such as pain, exposure to a cold temperature, hypoxia (oxygen deficiency) and hypoglycaemia (low blood glucose levels) can also trigger ACTH release

### Somatomammotropins

These include growth hormone (GH, also referred to as somatotropin) and prolactin (PRL – also called luteotropin). Growth hormone acts to promote linear growth and much of its action is mediated by insulin-like growth factor (IGF-1). These substances working in tandem enhance amino acid uptake and mRNA transcription and translation, thereby increasing protein synthesis. Fatty acids are released from adipose (fat) tissue and thus fat is burned up instead of proteins. Young adults going through so-called 'growth spurts' may secrete 32.5 nmol/d in comparison to adults who may secrete only 18.6 nmol/d (Aron et al., 1997). During pregnancy (in combination with other hormones) prolactin promotes additional breast development, and following parturition (birth) it initiates milk synthesis. It also has functions related to growth, metabolism, and reproductive and parental behaviours. Basal levels of PRL vary considerably in adults but mean values of 13 ng/ml in females and 5 ng/ml in males have been reported (Aron et al., 1997).

### Glycoproteins

These include thyroid-stimulating hormone (TSH, also referred to as thyrotropin), luteinizing hormone (LH), and follicle-stimulating hormone (FSH). TSH attaches to receptors in the thyroid gland and stimulates the uptake of iodide and the release of the thyroid hormones $T_3$ and $T_4$. TSH circulates in the blood in an unbound state and its secretion comes under the control of both excitatory and inhibitory control from the hypothalamus (TRH is excitatory and somatostatin is inhibitory) but is also modulated by inhibitory feedback from the circulating thyroid hormones. Injections of $T_3$ and $T_4$ into the bloodstream lead to small increases in serum levels of these hormones but they cause substantial changes in the TSH response to TRH (Aron et al., 1997). Both LH and FSH are glycoprotein gonadotropins secreted by the same cells; both hormones bind to receptors in the ovaries and testes and regulate the function of the gonads by stimulating sex steroid production and the development of the gametes. Thus, in females LH stimulates the production of estrogen and progesterone, and a characteristic surge in LH is seen during the menstrual cycle which acts as a trigger for ovulation.

Should the ovum be fertilised, then continued LH secretion stimulates the corpus luteum to produce progesterone.

### The hypothalamic–pituitary relationship

The relationship between the hypothalamus and the pituitary gland appears initially straightforward, with substances from the hypothalamus causing the release of hormones from the pituitary (which in turn trigger hormone release from the endocrine glands). However, according to Brown (1994) the picture is more complex for the following reasons. First, there is not a simple one-to-one relationship between hypothalamic and pituitary hormones. Some hypothalamic hormones trigger the release of one pituitary hormone but some have a more wide-ranging effect: for example, TRH triggers not only the release of TSH, but also the release of prolactin. Second, the picture provided thus far is that of a 'one-way street' with hormones flowing in one direction; however, pituitary hormones can be transported back into the hypothalamus (by various means), where they can act as neuromodulators and modify neural activity. Third, several 'hypothalamic' hormones are released from non-hypothalamic brain cells and do not pass to the pituitary but rather to other brain regions. For example GnRH and TRH also project to the limbic system and act as neuropeptides to modify neural excitability and neurotransmitter release (Moss, 1979). Fourth, the pituitary hormones are not solely influenced by hypothalamic hormones but are also regulated by neurotransmitters such as dopamine and GABA. Finally, the hypothalamic hormones do not just act alone on the pituitary but sometimes act in conjunction with other hormones (especially the gonadal steroid hormones); for example, estrogen and progesterone also regulate prolactin, FSH and LH release

### Pineal gland

This pea-sized structure had been noticed by the Greeks. Galen named it the 'conarium' owing to its pine cone shape, and it was subsequently referred to as the 'glandula pinealis'. It is located at the top of the midbrain, above the third ventricle and just in front of the cerebellum, in-between the two hemispheres within a groove where the thalamic nuclei join. It contains secretary cells called 'pinealocytes' that produce melatonin (N-acetyl-5-methoxytryptamine), named after its effects in lightening the colour of frog skin melanopores, and its resemblance to serotonin (Macchi and Bruce, 2004). It is synthesised from serotonin via the amino acid tryptophan and is secreted into the cerebrospinal fluid and bloodstream, regulated by the sympathetic nervous system in response to changing light levels: as light levels fall melatonin secretion increases; as levels rise, secretion ceases. In humans there is thus a close relationship between rising levels of melatonin and sleepiness (Barrenetxe et al., 2004). Numerous myths have grown up around the function of this structure. Philosopher and mathematician René Descartes believed, for example, that it was the physical location of the soul, though Thomas Wharton in the 1600s provided the first accurate description of the pineal gland, and poured cold water on Descartes' theory (Medvei, 1993). Modern practitioners of yoga refer to the pineal gland as the 'third eye chakra' (based upon its established retinal connections) and ascribe various mystical properties to it (based upon nothing in particular).

Much of our (admittedly limited) understanding of the pineal gland comes from work by biochemist Julius Axelrod. He and his colleagues showed that the rates of synthesis and release of melatonin follow the body's circadian rhythm, driven by the suprachiasmatic nucleus (SCN) within the hypothalamus. Light information from the retina is conveyed to the SCN, which then triggers the release of melatonin from the pineal gland. The melatonin then acts back on various neural systems (including the SCN) and influences physiological processes and behaviours which show seasonal variations. In addition, melatonin can also suppress libido by inhibiting secretion of luteinising hormone and follicle-stimulating hormone from the anterior pituitary gland. As melatonin is also metabolised in the liver, levels of its metabolite 6-sulfatoxymelatonin can be assessed in urine, and this can provide a simple and reliable measure in humans (Barrenetxe *et al.*, 2004). Increasing attention is being focussed on the antioxidant properties of melatonin, and in its role in the control of energy balance (and hence possible links with obesity), insomnia, reproductive functions and psychiatric disorders (Macchi and Bruce, 2004).

## Thyroid gland

This large bilateral structure is found in the neck and consists of many spherical follicles, which produce thyroid hormones in direct response to thyrotropin-releasing hormone released by the anterior pituitary. The thyroid gland produces various iodinated substances dependent upon dietary levels of iodate, which enters the body in food or water. In the stomach this is converted to iodide and taken up by the thyroid gland to manufacture its hormones. Low levels of dietary iodine result in reduced thyroid function and hypertrophy manifested as swellings in the neck (goitre). Two key thyroid hormones are 3,5,3'-triiodothryonine (normally referred to as $T_3$) and the much more abundant 3,5,3'-tetraiodothyronine (also called thyroxine or $T_4$). Around 100 nmol of $T_4$ and 5 nmol of $T_3$ are secreted daily by the thyroid gland, but about 35–40% of the $T_4$ produced each day is deiodinated to produce $T_3$ (Chopra and Sabatino, 2000). As such a large percentage of $T_4$ is converted to the much more potent $T_3$ some authors have questioned whether $T_4$ has any intrinsic biological activity and might in fact be simply a prohormone. Chopra *et al.* (1973) did demonstrate, however, that in the absence of normal serum $T_4$ concentrations a normal serum level of $T_3$ was insufficient to maintain normal thyroid functioning (euthyroidism), and thus $T_4$ may well have some biological/hormonal activity.

These hormones are transported in blood bound to carrier proteins (the principal one being thyroxine-binding globulin: TBG) and while only 0.04% and 0.4% of $T_4$ and $T_3$ respectively are 'free', their physiological effects are profound. Their key functions are to regulate body metabolism and control the development of the brain and nervous system, and sexual maturation, and they also play a role in temperature regulation (Greenspan, 1997). Within the thyroid gland, the C-cells also secrete calcitonin, which reduces blood calcium levels. Small glands embedded within the thyroid glands (parathyroid glands) secrete parathyroid hormone (PTH), which is also important in calcium regulation.

This gland holds a particularly important position within the history of endocrinology, as it was the first endocrine gland in which it was established that normal secretions are associated with good health, and that hypo- and hypersecretion would lead to poor physical and mental health. In 1850, surgeon Thomas Blizzard Curling had reported several cases in which he suspected a relationship between defective cerebral development and the lack of thyroid glands, leading to profound intellectual impairment ('cretinism'). In 1873, William Withey Gull[2] delivered the classic description of symptoms associated with a gradually failing thyroid gland. He noted an increase in fatigue, bodily and facial puffiness, facial discolourations, and dry skin. In other cases autopsies showed corresponding brain degeneration. In 1891 an endocrinological landmark was reached when Victor Horsley and George Murray successfully treated hypothyroidism (an underactive thyroid condition referred to as 'myxoedema') with extracts of animal thyroid glands. Robert James Graves provided careful observations of several patients exhibiting characteristic physical symptoms (accelerated heart beat, bulging eyes, weakness, excessive sweating, etc.) associated with an overactive thyroid gland and now this condition bears his name ('Graves' disease').

## Pancreas

This in fact consists of two functionally distinct organs – the major digestive organ (the exocrine pancreas) and the endocrine pancreas, the major source of insulin, glucagon, somatostatin and pancreatic polypeptide. The hormones of the endocrine pancreas are vital for the modulation of cellular nutrition (food adsorption, cellular storage, nutrient metabolism, etc.) and its dysfunction has a major impact on nutrient balance and physical health (Karam, 1997). The endocrine pancreas has a long medical history, with its dysfunction being related to acute physical conditions – most notably diabetes mellitus. In the

---

[2] In various conspiracy theories Gull (1816–90) is named as Jack the Ripper, despite the fact that he was in his seventies and had suffered a series of strokes!

second century AD Aretaeos of Cappadocia provided the first clinical description of diabetes mellitus, noting the thirst cravings, sexual dysfunction, excessive production of urine, nausea and restlessness; other scholars noted that the urine of sufferers of the so-called 'pissing evil' tasted sweet and that symptoms could be exacerbated by sweet foods (Medvei, 1993). In the 1800s Paul Langerhans conducted microscopical analysis of the pancreas and discovered the characteristic clear cells that now bear his name (the 'islets of Langerhans') but did not ascribe any specific function to them. It was not until 1900 that Eugène Lindsay Opie finally confirmed the association between failure of the islets and the subsequent occurrence of diabetes.

We now understand that the islets of Langerhans contain four different types of cells which secrete different peptide hormones. Of key importance are the B (or β) cells which secrete a protein called insulin. In normal adults the pancreas secretes around 40–50 units of insulin per day, with the basal levels being around 69 pmol/L in someone who is fasting, rising to ten times this amount (690 pmol/L) following ingestion of a standard meal (Karam, 1997). There is a close correspondence between insulin and glucose – as glucose rises and falls, so does insulin. This powerful hormone directly or indirectly affects the function of almost all bodily tissues, though key effects are in the liver (where is promotes glycogen synthesis and storage), muscles (where it promotes protein synthesis) and adipose tissue (where it promotes fat storage in the form of triglycerides). Insulin acts to assist the entry of glucose into the cells, where it is used as the primary fuel. In type I diabetes the pancreas is unable to produce insulin, and thus the liver, muscles and fat tissue cannot take up absorbed nutrients, and continue to secrete glucose into the bloodstream from their stored reserves (hyperglycaemia).

Type II diabetes is a term applied to a variety of milder conditions in which the pancreas can still make some insulin, but this is insufficient, or the insulin that is produced does not work properly (known as insulin resistance). In both types the key symptoms are similar – excessive thirst, weakness, blurred vision, peripheral nerve damage (neuropathy) and excessive urination (only type I usually). In direct contrast to insulin (promotes energy storage), glucagon makes energy available to the tissues (stimulating the breakdown of stored glycogen), with the liver representing the major target of glucagon action.

## Adrenal glands

The adrenal glands were first described in detail by Italian anatomist Eustachius.[3] They are located on the top of the kidneys and consist of two distinct structures. The adrenal cortex comprises around 90% of the total volume of the adrenal glands and consists of three distinct zones. The zona

---

[3] Bartolomeo Eustachius (c. 1500–14, died in 1574) also discovered the tube in the inner ear which now bears his name (Eustachian tube).

glomerulosa acts independently of the other zones and produces only aldosterone. The zona fasciculata and the zona reticularis produce cortisol, androgens and small amounts of estrogens, and both work in conjunction under the control of ACTH (described in a previous section). Alterations in the secretion of this substance thus have a major impact on the structure and function of these zones. The adrenal medulla releases three monoamine hormones, adrenaline, noradrenaline and dopamine; it also releases a class of protein hormones – the enkephalins.

The clinical symptoms of adrenal insufficiency leading to hypocortisolism have long been noted. In 1855 Thomas Addison was the first to recognise a disorder of the adrenal glands that now bears his name (Addison's disease). Initially he was interested in skin diseases and noted the abnormal skin pigmentation in patients with dysfunctional adrenal glands but did not initially connect the two. This disorder is characterised by atrophy of the adrenal cortex, at the time principally caused by infectious diseases such as tuberculosis, and key symptoms include abnormal pigmentation of the skin on the face and neck, weakness, fatigue, nausea, weight loss, low blood pressure, dehydration and gastrointestinal upsets.

The opposite condition of hypercortisolism takes the name Cushing's syndrome, after neurosurgeon Harvey Williams Cushing who noted connections between tumours of the pituitary gland (known as pituitary adenomas) and symptoms of chronic glucocorticoid excess. The tumours themselves secrete ACTH and this in turn leads to the hypersecretion of the glucocorticoids (principally cortisol). Key symptoms include obesity, high blood pressure, gonadal dysfunction, glucose intolerance, acne and hirsutism on the face, and the skin bruises easily. Another disorder of the adrenal glands – congenital adrenal hyperplasia – will be discussed in chapter 6.

## Gonads

These manufacture the sex cells (gametes). They also produce hormones required for gamete development, the development of secondary sexual characteristics and the mediation of sexual behaviours. The gonads are regulated by tropic hormones from the anterior pituitary. The sexes have different forms of gonads but all produce three types of sex steroid hormones – androgens, estrogens and progestins.

### Female ovaries

These are paired nodular structures comprising a covering of columnar cells called the germinal epithelium, which encloses a dense connective layer (the tunica albuginea); the remainder of the ovaries consists of an outer cortical layer and an inner medullary layer. The cortical layer contains follicles that house the developing ova, and also cells responsible for manufacturing the ovarian hormones (principally estrogens, androgens, progesterone and their precursors). The ovaries are attached to the uterus and lie in close proximity to the oviducts and fallopian tubes below the kidneys (Goldfien and Monroe, 1997). A normal pattern of menstruation (endocrinological and physiological changes that are associated with the cyclical process of ovulation) is governed by interactions between the hypothalamus, anterior pituitary and ovaries, though the latter appears to be responsible for regulating these cyclical changes and for determining the length of the cycle. Most women between the onset of puberty and the onset of the menopause (cessation of the menstrual cycle) are regularly affected by the endocrinological and physiological changes associated with the menstrual cycle, and on average the cycle ranges between twenty-five and thirty-five days, with the average being around twenty-eight days (Goldfien and Monroe, 1997). However, the female menstrual cycle is often depicted as a standardised diagram with the mean levels of the various hormones plotted as a series of curves. Alliende (2002) pointed out that much of the available information concerning these mean levels is derived from primate studies, or from women experiencing ovulatory pathology. There are actually few hormonal studies of 'normal' healthy women undergoing spontaneous menstrual cycles, free from contraception. In her study of twenty-five women aged around thirty, data from a total of eighty-two cycles were investigated, and considerable individual variation was noted, with hormone profiles deviating considerably from the standard curves reported.

For convenience the cycle is normally split into three stages: menses (days 1–5), follicular (days 6–14) and luteal (days 15–28). During the follicular phase rising levels of FSH (and small amounts of LH) cause the follicles to mature, and as they do so they release estrogen which thickens the lining of the uterus and alters the composition of the cervical mucus. When estrogen levels reach a certain point this triggers the pituitary to secrete high levels of LH (via stimulation from the hypothalamus), which causes a follicle to release an egg (ovulation).[4] During the luteal phase the ruptured follicle becomes the corpus luteum, and this secretes some estrogen and more progesterone which are necessary for maintaining a pregnancy (should the egg be fertilised). If the egg remains unfertilised, levels of all hormones fall and the uterus lining is discarded during menses.

## Male testes

These are bilateral endocrine glands housed externally in the scrotum, which not only acts as protection (scant though this is!) but also acts to maintain the testes at a constant temperature around 3.6°F below that of the abdomen. The primary hormone-producing units consist of millions of Leydig cells (also

[4] Many contraceptive pills contain estrogens, progestins, or combinations of both, and essentially work by blocking the LH surge and thus prevent the release of the egg. They also alter the cervical mucus and the lining of the uterus to make conception and implantation less likely.

called interstitial cells) that principally produce testosterone but also smaller amounts of dihydrotestosterone, dehydroepiandrosterone, estradiol, estrone, progesterone and androstenedione (Braunstein, 1997). Testosterone production is not constant but shows a conspicuous circadian cycle; for example, Rowe *et al.* (1974) sampled plasma from seven male volunteers over the course of twenty-four hours and found that testosterone levels rose throughout the night to peak around 6 a.m., and then gradually decline during the day to reach a low around 10 p.m. Other authors have confirmed this rhythm but have noted wide individual variations (reviewed in Nieschlag, 1974). Whether this testosterone rhythm is due to alterations in FSH or LH from the anterior pituitary remains debatable. Studies have failed to find a daily cycle of LH secretion (e.g. Alford *et al.*, 1973) but do report a cycle in plasma FSH so this may be the crucial factor, or it may simply augment a lesser influence of LH (e.g. Faiman and Winter, 1971). In addition to this general daily cycle, testosterone concentrations also fluctuate in a pulsatile fashion, with a surge being noted every 90 minutes or so (Veldhuis *et al.*, 1987), and show a seasonal pattern, with higher serum levels being found in the autumn months and lower levels in the summer months (Dabbs, 1990a; Nieschlag, 1974).

## Mechanisms of hormone action

Hormones can be divided into two groups depending upon how they function at their target cells. The first group cannot enter cells but instead interact with receptors at the surface of the cell, and generate a secondary messenger (such as G protein) that then regulates the generation or inhibition of cyclic AMP or cyclic GMP (see chapter 1). These molecules bind to other proteins which alter cell metabolism, or which can influence gene expression. All polypeptide hormones, as well as monoamines and prostoglandins, work in this fashion (Lazar, 2002). The second group includes hormones that can enter cells, bind to intracellular receptors and form a 'hormone-receptor complex' which penetrates the cell nucleus and attaches to 'accceptor sites' on the chromosome. This then triggers the synthesis of messenger RNA corresponding to a gene on an effector site; the messenger RNA then leaves the nucleus and migrates to the endoplasmic reticulum which then synthesises the protein encoded by the activated gene (McEwen, 1976). For example, in response to estradiol the oviduct in the hen responds by making a protein called ovalbumin which is secreted into the growing eggs. Thyroid and steroid hormones, various fatty acids and the eicosanoids work in this fashion. It should be noted that while overall hormone concentration is important, of potentially equal importance is the receptivity of the cells to a hormone. A high hormone concentration will have little effect if cells lack receptivity, an excellent example of this being androgen insensitivity syndrome (AIS) which will be further described in chapter 6.

## Hormone regulation

Hormone concentrations are determined by production rates, the effectiveness of delivery to its target tissues, and how easily the hormone molecules become degraded on their way to, or at, their target. Such processes are finely regulated, with hormone production being the most carefully controlled at the synthesis and release stages. Most classes of hormones have short half-lives (thyroid hormones are an exception to this) and so this is an effective means of preventing any excessive responses. Responses are also blunted by negative feedback: for example, when blood levels of calcium decrease, parathyroid hormone is released which raises calcium concentration in the blood; when an optimal level has been reached parathyroid hormone release stops. (This is very similar to the way in which a thermostat works.) Similarly, TRH triggers the release of TSH, which in turn triggers the release of the thyroid hormones. As levels of these hormones increase a negative feedback loop is initiated such that both TRH and TSH secretion is reduced. Levels of thyroid hormones then drop accordingly, see diagram 2.4.

However, such feedback loops are not always so simple. For example, in response to an environmental stimulus the hypothalamus releases gonadotropin-releasing hormone (GnRH) which stimulates the release of the gonadotropins from the anterior pituitary. These in turn stimulate steroid production in the gonads, but the release of steroids feeds back to the hypothalamus to prevent further GnRH production, as well as stopping production of the gonadotropins from the anterior pituitary.

Positive feedback also occurs: when a rapid endocrine response is required, feedback may increase hormone production – for example, in states of chronic stress glucocorticoids are released continuously and this only stops when the source of the stress is removed. Just to complicate matters further, there are two other processes which can influence hormone action. First, 'up-regulation' refers to the fact that hormones can affect their own receptor levels; for example increases of prolactin in the blood stimulate the production of more prolactin receptors. Secondly 'down-regulation' refers to the opposite process; for example high concentrations of insulin reduce the number of insulin receptors.

Hormones can thus influence all organs and tissues of the body and are vital from the early stages of foetal development; for example, hypothyroidism at this stage results in gross developmental and intellectual impairments. Hormones are important for cell growth (e.g. LH and FSH on the ovaries and testes; growth hormone in general) but also for the inhibition of cell growth (e.g. glucocorticoids inhibit growth in several types of cell). Hormones regulate chemical metabolism, the cardiovascular and renal systems, mineral and water metabolism, skeletal functions, reproductive functions, the immune system, and – perhaps most importantly for the

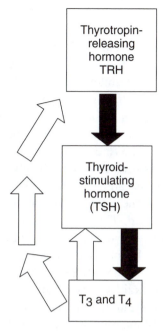

2.4 *Negative feedback loop involving the thyroid hormones (Filled arrows indicate a stimulatory effect, whilst open arrows indicate an inhibitory effect)*

considerations of this text – the central nervous system and its impact on behaviour.

## Measuring hormones

In order to begin to assess possible hormone–behaviour interactions, it is of course vital that the researcher is able accurately to measure levels of certain hormones. Some basic techniques are as follows.

### Bioassay

This involves weighing endocrine glands, or measuring the physical characteristics that result from endocrine action. For example, as TSH stimulates growth of the thyroid gland, weighing this gland can provide a broad measure of circulating TSH levels. Similarly, the size of a cock's comb is directly related to testosterone levels and thus serves as a marker for circulating testosterone levels. As biochemical techniques improved, bioassays became more scientific as researchers could take extractions from certain glands and then measure the effect of the substance by injecting it into an animal deprived of the gland in question (Beach, 1981). This method of course involves the sacrifice of numerous animals and only provides a rough measure of hormone levels.

### Radioimmunoassay

Technical advances led to the development of methods by which hormones can be accurately measured from bodily samples in living animals/humans, the most common being the radioimmunoassay (or RIA). The basic idea behind the RIA is that of competitive binding. In a typical procedure, a blood or saliva sample containing an unknown amount of a hormone is added to a known amount of antibody for that hormone (hormone molecules will bind to their specific antibody on a one-to-one basis) and a small, known amount of the same hormone that has been radioactively labelled. The hormone in the sample will compete with its radioactively labelled counterpart for binding sites on the antibody, and as there are insufficient binding sites some hormone molecules will be left stranded. The unbound hormone is removed from the sample and the amount of radioactively labelled hormone bound to the antibody is measured. The more hormone molecules in the original sample the less the radioactively labelled molecules will be able to bind with the antibody, and thus the lower will be the radioactivity reading of the sample. The level of the hormone in the original sample can then be calculated by comparing the results to what is called a 'standard curve' (Riad-Fahmy et al., 1981).

RIAs have been developed for the detection of specific hormones; they are highly accurate and very sensitive, though there can be various problems associated with them (Brown, 1994). Analysis from some participant groups, for example, may require particular care, especially when hormone levels may be very low (say in children and females) but slightly different types of assays can be utilised that address such problems (Granger et al., 1999; Shirtcliff et al., 2002). In the past, researchers have had to require participants to provide urinary or faecal samples from which to asses hormone levels via RIA. While such methods are easy and non-invasive they do require a certain commitment on the part of the volunteer, and cause a certain degree of embarrassment for all concerned. Such techniques are particularly useful for obtaining levels of certain hormones (or their metabolites) which are eliminated in the urine, e.g. cortisol, the gonadotropins, melatonin, etc. For example, urinary detection of the LH surge just prior to ovulation now forms a simple commercially available test by which women can assess their potential fertility. Similarly, detection of the presence of human chorionic gonadotropin in the urine forms the basis of the pregnancy test, also now relatively cheap and easy to conduct in the home.

For behavioural purposes such samples would need to be taken once or twice per day and provide a window into the average secretion over a number of hours, but not the possible brief surges or reductions over a shorter time period. When the behaviour of interest is perhaps of short duration then such techniques are too general to be of much use (Ellison, 1988). Blood samples then provide the researcher with the opportunity to gain a rapid measure of a hormone before, during, or after a brief behavioural response (bound measures are quantified but free levels can also be calculated), and such methods have a long clinical history and a set of well-established protocols. However, this is invasive and painful, and requires an appropriately trained technician to be on hand, and it is not always appropriate in non-clinical settings, in children or in overly nervous participants.

## Salivary analyses

Salivary measures (for steroid hormones in particular) are now increasingly popular as they are relatively cheap, and easy to collect, store and analyse (Dabbs, 1993; Ellison, 1988; Lipson and Ellison, 1989). Such sampling can be conducted out of the laboratory with the minimum of training and so is particularly useful for certain behavioural situations and non-clinical settings (e.g. schoolchildren, the elderly, sporting events, etc.). Moreover, the hormonal concentrations in saliva reflect the biologically active or 'free' fraction of the hormone in circulation, which, unlike the 'bound' hormones circulating in the blood, is able to cross the blood–brain barrier and influence the CNS (Vermeulen *et al.*, 1999). There is a strong relationship between free and bound levels (Vittek *et al.*, 1985), and the assumption has been that the biological activity of a given hormone is better correlated with the free version rather than the bound version.

This is the so-called 'Free Hormone Hypothesis' (Mendel, 1989), and while this hypothesis seems to work nicely for testosterone, it is not quite so clearcut for estrogen. The hypothesis also may not be correct as regards cortisol. Levine *et al.* (2007) have recently pointed out that corticosteroid-binding globulin (CBG) itself may have a biological role, binding directly to membrane receptors in the CNS, and cortisol bound to albumin ought to be considered free as the bond is a weak one. As different ways of calculating free cortisol are typically used, and these result in diverse readings (especially when diurnal factors are taken into account), these authors recommend care when using salivary sampling with this hormone. They suggest that the most accurate method is to use 'calculated free cortisol' derived from blood plasma.

In a standard session participants would wait at least 30 minutes after eating, as certain foods such as dairy products, eggs and black coffee can artificially raise steroid hormone measurements (Ellison, 1988; Whembolua *et al.*, 2006). They are then asked to rinse out their mouths with cold water to remove possible contaminants from food and blood, and then after a short delay drool into a small plastic or glass container (readings are equivalent from either: Lipson and Ellison, 1989), perhaps using a small straw. Sometimes it is necessary to provide a stimulant in the form of chewing gum or lemon juice; the choice here may be important as Lipson and Ellison (1989) reported that certain hormone values may be influenced by the choice of stimulant – readings of testosterone and androstenedione for example being lowered by around 20% when stimulated by sugarless chewing gum. One stimulant (Wrigley's Doublemint gum) was also found to increase measured levels of progesterone by around 50% compared to unstimulated values! The presence of certain substances in such stimulants may thus cause aberrant values of certain hormones to be recorded – obviously a potentially major problem when assessing hormone–behaviour relationships.

The use of cotton-absorbent material provided to participants to chew and then deposit in a container is less 'messy' and more socially acceptable than drooling, but cotton can also affect the results of immunoassays, especially for testosterone, DHEA, progesterone and estradiol (Shirtcliff *et al.*, 2001). In our laboratory we play it safe and simply ask participants to provide an unstimulated sample (not always easy!). Samples are then typically frozen until assayed, though samples stored at room temperature appear to produce highly correlated readings with those stored immediately on extraction. However over time samples stored at room temperature can produce significantly higher readings (Lipson and Ellison, 1989). For practical and health and safety reasons we always try to get our samples safely tucked away in the freezer as soon as possible after sampling.

It is also important to consider additional factors when perhaps considering the comparison of values within and between laboratories. Dabbs *et al.* (1995a) reported a multicentre evaluation of salivary testosterone measurements. They sent identical saliva samples from males and females to various laboratories who had a reputation for conducting such assays (though each used its own preferred method). Significant differences in the reported values for both males and females were revealed, with mean values in the range 240–410 pmol/L and 48–101 pmol/L respectively (Dabbs *et al.*, 1995a). The authors suggest that such large variations are probably due to the fact that radioimmunoassay results are very sensitive to changes in the reagents and operating procedures utilised, even within the same laboratory. It thus makes good sense to assay all of one's samples using the same technique, preferably by the same person (not always possible), to minimise possible variation. It may also be very difficult to compare mean values between different centres, though Dabbs *et al.* (1995a) did note that laboratories are in good agreement on the relative ordering of the individual samples, i.e. someone with the lowest value reported from one laboratory was also reported as having the lowest value from a different laboratory.

An additional important factor to consider is the date/time at which samples are collected. Most hormones of interest in behavioural endocrinology (testosterone being a notable example) show considerable variability. Because there is a strong diurnal change, with morning levels of testosterone being higher than evening levels (Dabbs, 1990a, 1990b), it is prudent to take such samples within a fairly narrow time window, preferably in the morning. Cortisol is a particular problem here, as there is a well-established rise in this hormone in the first hour after awakening (Pruessner *et al.*, 1997). Studies need to control not only for time of day effects, but also time of waking when considering potential links between cortisol and behaviour. For example, one of my research students was assessing possible relationships between cortisol and personality in males and females. She carefully ensured that all were tested at around the same time of day, and intriguingly found a strong sex difference in cortisol levels – males having higher levels. This was puzzling as we were not aware that such sex differences should exist. Thankfully, she had made a note of when the participants had woken and found that the males woke around an hour later than the females, and were thus in the 'higher' phase of the normal cortisol peak. When this factor was controlled for in the analysis, the previous sex difference disappeared.

Similarly, testosterone varies across the seasons (Dabbs, 1990a; Nieschlag, 1974) and so when assessing possible changes in differing groups over a wider time course, then one should also consider seasonal factors and perhaps ensure that all groups are tested at roughly the same time(s) during the year. In women, testosterone levels vary across the menstrual cycle, increasing towards the middle (Vermeulen and Verdonck, 1976). Use of the contraceptive pill can also suppress testosterone levels (Bancroft et al., 1980) and thus menstrual cycle phase/contraceptive pill use should be controlled for when assessing testosterone–behaviour relationships in females. Finally, just to make life increasingly complex, Moffat and Hampson (1996) first measured handedness in forty male and forty female volunteers and then sampled their testosterone levels via saliva, carefully controlling for time of day and season. Somewhat surprisingly, right-handers demonstrated significantly higher testosterone levels than left-handers, this being seen in both sexes. The precise physiological cause of this apparent difference remains to be explained but handedness thus appears to be yet another potential confound to consider.

# 3  **Behavioural endocrinology**

## Background

At its simplest level, behavioural endocrinology can be described as the scientific study of the relationships between hormones and behaviour. While the existence of hormones remained speculative, our scientific forebears certainly suspected that certain physical and behavioural characteristics were the result of some imbalance/irregularity of particular substances within the body. As we have seen in the previous chapter, such observations were normally medical in nature, i.e. certain physical ailments appeared to display characteristic symptoms, and the course of a particular ailment seemed to follow a set clinical pattern. Folk remedies were in place (with varying degrees of success), and, whilst understanding remained basic at best, and with sophisticated analytic techniques being several hundred years away, scientists used their powers of observation and deduction, and made some remarkable observations.

For example, goitre is an enlargement of the thyroid gland caused by a lack of iodine (recall from chapter 2 that the thyroid cannot manufacture its hormones $T_3$ and $T_4$ without sufficient dietary iodine). If a person's diet is low in iodine, the pituitary keeps sending TSH to the thyroid, and the gland swells, leading to an enlarged throat. The Chinese and the Romans had observed that entire districts could be afflicted by goitre (now referred to as 'endemic goitre' but once commonly called 'Derbyshire neck' after the common occurrence of this condition in the Peak District of Derbyshire). They suspected that poisoned water could be the culprit (it is actually caused by people growing and eating vegetables in soil which is iodine deficient) and recommended seaweed as a curative; with some fair degree of success as seaweed is indeed a good source of iodine.

In the 1500s Paracelsus was the first to link outbreaks of endemic goitre with cretinism and congenital idiocy, based upon his first-hand observations in Salzburg. The term 'cretin' is now used as a less than politically correct insult, but during the 1800s and 1900s was an accepted medical term used to describe the stunted physical growth and intellectual deficiencies of those suffering from congenital hypothyroidism (underfunctioning thyroid glands). It was not until 1811 that iodine was finally discovered by Bernard Courtois. He was washing seaweed with vitriol (sulphuric acid) to generate potash (a form of potassium carbonate used for many generations as a fertiliser and in the manufacture of glass and soap) and created vivid violet-coloured fumes. With the help of some chemist associates, Courtois condensed the fumes into crystals and thus iodine was born (from the Greek word 'ioeides', meaning 'violet coloured'). Iodine was then used as a highly successful treatment for goitre, and since then iodine has been a common additive in table salt, and endemic goitre has all but disappeared in industrial societies.

## John Hunter (1728–93)

The true scientific beginnings of behavioural endocrinology can be traced back to Hunter's experimental studies. While many others had made accurate and important observations, and proposed various theories concerning the possible physical and behavioural effects of blood-borne secretions, Hunter improved things by bringing his extensive grasp of anatomy and physiology to the questions at hand. He was the first experimentally to manipulate the endocrine glands and their secretions; he observed for example that unilateral ovariectomy (removal of a single ovary) did not interfere with the breeding ability of female pigs. He also discovered that both male and female pigeons secreted 'milk' for their offspring, and described the crop sac as being like the udder of a cow (Medvei, 1993). It was not until the 1930s that prolactin was established as being the hormone responsible for milk production in mammals, and crop sac secretions in birds.

Hunter was keenly interested in the development of secondary sexual characteristics, and, while he was not the first to speculate on the role of the ovaries and testes in sexual differentiation, he was the first to manipulate this scientifically. Young male and female chickens are physically similar until puberty, when the male develops prominent secondary sexual characteristics (larger comb and wattle, onset of crowing, etc.). One key feature is the spur (the spiky outgrowth protruding from the back of the leg, used for aggressive encounters). In female birds the spur remains small, but in males it grows significantly at puberty and becomes an active weapon in inter-male aggressive encounters. Hunter successfully transplanted a hen's spur onto a cock bird and observed that the spur grew to resemble that of a normal male.

Like the good scientist that he was, Hunter also reversed the procedure and showed that a male spur transplanted onto a female failed to develop. Following on from that remarkable success, Hunter then attempted more complex procedures: gonadal removal and transplantation, during which he also noticed a seasonal effect on testis size – testes removed from sparrows in the breeding season were significantly larger than those removed at other times. Testes were thus transplanted from males into females and Hunter noted that the female birds then began to exhibit male characteristics, and he speculated that the effects of the newly transplanted organ were to influence the mind of the female bird – a radical concept at the time, and one which could truly be argued as announcing the birth of behavioural endocrinology.

### Adolph Berthold (1803–61)

While Hunter demonstrated surgical skill *par excellence* and perhaps a little good fortune as well, he did not progress to establishing clear theoretical mechanisms underlying these hormone–behaviour relationships. This was left to Berthold, who is now often described as the founding father of behavioural endocrinology. In 1849 Berthold published his now-famous paper in which he described an experiment comparing the effects of removal alone, versus the removal and subsequent reimplantation of testes in male birds. He took four young birds and removed the testes in one pair, in the other pair he removed the testes but subsequently reimplanted the organs back into the abdomen. While the castrated pair failed to show normal male physical development (atrophy of the comb being particularly noted), the 'transplant' pair developed as normal. He subsequently established that testes removed from one bird and implanted into a different male also had the same effects – i.e. normal secondary sexual development. Berthold realised that as the nerve supply had been disconnected in the transplanted males, their testes (whether their own or those from another male) must be secreting some substance(s) via the bloodstream which must be responsible for an immature male developing into a normal adult rooster (Beach, 1981).

From then, a steady stream of technological and theoretical advances ensured that suspected links between internal secretions and physical behaviours became stronger and stronger. In 1917 Stockard and Papanicolau were the first to describe the estrous cycle in female guinea pigs and demonstrated that the differing stages of the ovarian follicle were correlated with different kinds of cell in the vaginal mucosa.[1] Previously, research questions were dominated by medical/clinical questions, but increasingly psychologists, psychiatrists and neuroscientists have been able to ask more behavioural-type questions, in part as a result of the increasing ease of conducting painless hormonal assessments in a non-clinical setting (see chapter 2). The journal *Hormones and Behavior* was established in 1969 with its prime focus being on experimental animal studies, and in 1975 *Psychoneuroendocrinology* made its first appearance. This aptly named (though tricky to spell) journal was aimed specifically at researchers from multidisciplinary backgrounds who were keen to ask, and attempt to answer, questions addressing links between hormonal, psychological, immunological, psychiatric and neurological functioning. While it

---

[1] This discovery led to the 'Pap test' in 1943 (named after Papanicolau), now a routine screening tool for discovering abnormalities in the cells of the cervix.

continues to publish research derived from animal models, much of its focus is now on human behavioural studies.

## Hormones, brain and behaviour

In 1959, Charles Phoenix and colleagues reported the results from a series of landmark experiments concerning the effects of testosterone administration on sexual development in guinea pigs (we shall examine this research in more detail in chapter 5). Whilst these pioneering authors did not explicitly investigate the brain, in their concluding paragraph they set the stage for the future of behavioural endocrinology by stating that 'behavior may be treated as a dependent variable and therefore … we may speak of shaping the behavior by hormone administration just as the psychologist speaks of shaping behavior by manipulating the environment. An assumption seldom made explicit is that modification of behavior follows an alteration in the structure or function of the neural correlates of the behavior' (Phoenix *et al.*, 1959: 381).

So, it sounds fairly straightforward then: hormones shape behaviours by altering neural circuitry and we can simply monitor hormone levels and then associate these levels with various different behaviours (and perhaps with associated changes in neural circuitry). There is a tendency amongst students in behavioural endocrinology (and very commonly amongst the media who are reporting the outcomes of hormone–behaviour studies) to assume that hormones *cause* direct behavioural alterations. This is a simple mistake to make because it is often easier to conceptualise hormone–behaviour relationships in this one-way linear fashion, rather than try to think about such relationships in a more multidirectional sense. In addition, previous studies in animals have in fact demonstrated fairly simple unidirectional hormone–behaviour links: for example, male boars secrete musky pheromones ('boar-taint') in their saliva which contain testosterone-derived chemicals called 16-androstenes. If females come into contact with such chemicals they immediately adopt a mating stance (this is called lordosis), triggered by their own hormones in response to the male pheromones. In this instance hormones thus instigate (or release) a behaviour.

However, it must be emphasised that in many cases (and perhaps especially so for humans) hormones do not produce such easy to conceptualise unidirectional effects; they only influence neural (and hence behavioural) systems such that specific stimuli may be more likely to elicit specific responses in the appropriate behavioural or social context. For example, placing a group of male students into a bland laboratory room and dosing them with high doses of testosterone may have no appreciable effect on their sexual behaviours. If however you conducted the same study within the confines of a table-dancing club then the outcome might be rather different!

Forgive me for labouring the point, but it is a rather crucial one that for the most part hormones do not *cause* behaviours to change. It is more likely that they change the likelihood that a particular behaviour will occur within an appropriate social/environmental context. A recent example has been provided by Maney *et al.* (2006). They note that in seasonally breeding birds, a surge in gonadal steroid acts to coordinate social/reproductive behaviours to maximise reproductive success. In female white-throated sparrows, their behavioural responses to male song change according to their reproductive state: during their fertile period they respond with a characteristic courtship display called 'copulation solicitation display' (CSD); during non-fertile phases, however, they do not perform the CSD even if presented with the same song that during the fertile phase would elicit a CSD. This plasticity has been attributed to changes in circulating estradiol, as administration of estradiol to females in a non-breeding state leads to CSD behaviours in response to male song within several days (Kern and King, 1972). Maney and colleagues investigated the effects of estradiol treatment on the cortical areas that are responsive to male signing, exposure to male song triggering gene expression which underlies the behavioural responses. Non-breeding female birds were isolated, and male songs or neutral tones were played to them, while their behavioural responses were noted; half of the sample received estradiol implants, while the remainder received inert implants. Hearing tones led to no behavioural changes in either group, but in those receiving estradiol treatment exposure to male songs led to characteristic CSD behaviours. The estradiol-treated group also showed changes in their song-response regions indicating alterations in gene expression.

However, we remain a fair way from coming to firm conclusions about hormone–behaviour relationships for the following reasons.

## Complexity of the interrelationships

There is a highly complex set of interrelationships between hormones, the brain and any behaviour. For example, assume that we place an animal in a situation where it is suddenly faced with one of its natural predators. What we assume then happens is as follows: when the animal perceives this significant and potentially dangerous event in its environment, the threat is detected by the sensory nerves (visual, olfactory, auditory), and a relay of neurons acting by neurochemical processes (see chapter 1) transmit this information to the higher cortical centres, which recognise the stimulus as a threat. Neurotransmitters are promptly released and induce the hypothalamus to release its hormones, which in turn stimulate the anterior pituitary gland, which then induces the endocrine (adrenal) glands to secrete glucocorticoids. The release of these stress hormones leads to longer-term increases in arousal, and bodily readiness to adopt the 'fight or flight' response – to stand up to the threat or to flee quickly – but also influences emotional and learning processes. A negative feedback loop is also initiated so that further hormone release is reduced. So here we have a very complex interplay between hormones, brain and behaviour and we remain in the early stages of explaining such interactions.

A major problem for behavioural endocrinologists is the 'chicken and egg' problem, i.e. do hormones influence behaviour by directly affecting neural responses, or does behaving in a particular manner influence hormone production? An interesting example comes from clasping behaviour in amphibians. Male frogs and toads grab on to females during copulation to ensure that the male fertilises the eggs that are released by the female. This is referred to as 'amplexus', or 'amplectic clasping' (Moore *et al.*, 2005). Gobbetti and Zerani (1999) sacrificed some unfortunate male water frogs during the very act of amplexus and noted that they had higher circulating levels of plasma testosterone than males sacrificed when not embracing a female. This seems simple then – higher levels of testosterone trigger this clasping behaviour. However, other researchers have noted that the very act of amplexus can produce significant increases in gonadotropins (which then act to increase circulating testosterone) and so differences in hormone levels between clasping frogs and non-clasping frogs may be the *result* rather than the *cause* of the behaviour (Ishii and Itoh, 1992).

It is also possible that some hormone–behaviour relationships may be bidirectional, i.e. the behaviour in question and its hormonal underpinnings may be mutually reinforcing. A good example here is that of the association between testosterone and competitive encounters (see chapter 10): higher testosterone levels may increase such encounters, which in turn may lead to a further increase in testosterone and so on. These bidirectional examples remain thus far sadly neglected in the research literature, which tends to focus on unidirectional examples (van Anders and Watson, 2006a). At present, teasing apart these separate (yet obviously interrelated) mechanisms, especially in humans, remains very difficult and the cause of much debate.

## What do we mean by 'behaviour'?

Before we look at how hormones might possibly shape behaviour, we need first to examine just what we mean by 'behaviour', and how we can explain it. Nikolaas (Niko) Tinbergen was an ethologist[2] who asked the question 'why does an animal behave as it does?' (Tinbergen, 1951). He understood that this rather simple question covers a uniquely complex set of problems, and proposed that behaviour could be explained on four different levels of analysis.

(a) **Causation**: How is the behaviour triggered? What is the nature of the external stimulus or internal state of the animal that triggers a behavioural response?

---

[2] Ethologists study the scientific basis of behaviour in an animal's natural surroundings.

**(b) Function**: What function(s) does the behaviour serve? How does the behaviour affect the survival and reproduction of the individual performing the behaviour? This entails an understanding of the functions of the sense organs, the nervous system, hormones and muscles, the interrelationships between them, and then how they are coordinated to achieve the behaviour.

**(c) Development (ontogeny)**: How does behaviour change as the animal grows and develops? This needs to encapsulate maturational and developmental aspects, in terms both of physiology but also of learning and experience.

**(d) Evolution**: How does the behaviour compare with other animal species that are related in evolutionary terms?[3]

To illustrate these levels, Tinbergen used the example of instinctive aggressive behaviours in male three-spined sticklebacks. If a lone male is introduced to an 'opponent' in the form of a mirror then it will respond aggressively to its own reflection. The function of such behaviour is obvious in terms of territorial/resource defence. As male sticklebacks do not 'fight' when they are on their own, the introduction of a perceived 'intruder' (actually a reflection of itself) is clearly the stimulus that invokes the response. The nature of the stimulus is vital as the male does not respond aggressively to every stimulus he is exposed to (clearly this would be futile); instead he is selective about what to respond aggressively to. Male sticklebacks who are reproductively capable have an intense red patch on their throat and belly (juvenile males and females do not possess this characteristic) and it is this 'sign stimulus' to which the male is responding (this is the 'cause' of the behavioural response). Tinbergen showed this in simple experiments in which he first exposed lone males to models of male sticklebacks differing in size, shape and colour markings. The males responded specifically to the red colouration and paid little attention to the other physical features. In addition, however, movement was found to be a key factor, as a dummy invoked stronger aggressive responses when it was presented in a specific 'threat' orientation – so the combination of these two stimuli (colour and posture) triggers (or releases) a specific behavioural response (cited in Tinbergen, 1951: 28, 37–8).

This of course only represents a single behavioural response to a single stimulus. Tinbergen considered the reproductive behavioural repertoire of the stickleback in a wider context, and speculated on the interplay between internal and external factors. He noted that in spring the days gradually increase in length (external stimulus) and this triggers an increase in reproductive motivations (internal factors) in adult males. The males migrate to shallower water (behavioural response) where the temperature is higher; this

---

[3] The study of evolutionary relatedness is called phylogenetics.

alteration in temperature combined with an appropriate visual stimulus of a suitable territory (external stimuli) releases various territorial behaviours – specifically nest building and aggressive responses to strangers (behavioural responses to specific stimuli). So, external factors lead to the initiation of innate behaviours, but the internal state of the individual is also very important. Aggressive responses are only shown by males who themselves are in reproductive condition – juvenile males do not respond aggressively to such stimuli (the developmental aspect). In addition, the same stimulus (an intruder) may evoke a slightly different aggressive behavioural response (chasing, biting, threatening, etc.), perhaps dependent upon external characteristics (size or behaviour of the intruder) or perhaps upon internal factors (motivation). Tinbergen speculated that sex hormones might be a key internal factor acting in conjunction with the nervous system to influence a behavioural response to a specific external stimulus.

If we look at such simple innate behaviours closely, we can visualise an individual's behaviour as consisting of three components: a sensory system (input); the central nervous system (behavioural integration); and an effector system (output). An appropriate input (a male intruder bearing a red belly and displaying a threat posture) is registered by the sensory apparatus and this information is conveyed to the CNS where it is integrated/processed. Neurochemical and hormonal events, most likely working in combination, then trigger appropriate behavioural responses in the output system (threaten, chase, etc.). As we shall see in later chapters, the involvement of hormones at all three levels is likely to be pronounced. Hormones may influence the sensory system such that certain stimuli are more (or less) likely to be perceived – the salience of the stimulus is thus altered. Hormones may influence the integrative system such that certain kinds of information are preferentially processed, or processed faster. Finally, hormones may influence the effector system such that certain responses or behaviour patterns are attenuated (e.g. improvement in reaction times). It is in fact probable that hormones, in conjunction with neurotransmitters, act on all three levels simultaneously but perhaps with different emphases.

To measure behavioural changes one must first attempt to quantify the behaviour in question; significant progress has been made in animals, though such quantification remains much more problematical in humans. In animal studies (either in the 'field' or in the laboratory) a specific behaviour can be broken down into distinct units which can be easily coded by the observer; for example the sexual behaviour of the male rat has been broken down into a series of discrete behavioural units (Brown and McFarland, 1979) which we will address more fully in chapter 8. Various quantifiable measures such as latency to begin a behaviour, duration of the behaviour and frequency of the behaviour can be recorded. Obviously, such measures are carefully detailed in 'normal' animals and then the same units of behaviour can be assessed in hormonally manipulated individuals.

## Differential hormonal action

Based upon the experiments of Phoenix *et al.* (1959), Beach (1975) argued that hormones exert their effects on behaviour in two principal ways.

### Organisational

During prenatal (or early postnatal) development, hormones sculpt the neural/behavioural machinery that underlies a behavioural response. Such effects are referred to as 'organisational' and, according to Arnold and Breedlove (1985), they are distinguished by five key characteristics. First, such effects are permanent and irreversible. Second, they generally occur during specific stages of early development – generally before birth or shortly after. Third, such effects can only occur during 'critical' or 'sensitive' periods (though their effects may only become apparent at a later time), and once such stages have passed then hormones can no longer exert permanent effects. Fourth, such effects must lead to permanent structural changes in the brain, or at least to long-term physiological changes such as alterations in neuronal responsiveness. Finally, such effects are assumed to be asymmetric with regard to the sexes (at least where sex steroids are concerned).

Thus, in mammals at least, androgens are required for masculinisation, but estrogens are not required for feminisation (rather a lack of androgens is important). Numerous studies have now demonstrated that the prenatal hormonal environment can have a profound effect upon the development of bodily structures, neuroanatomy, physiology and certain kinds of sexually dimorphic behaviours. Phoenix *et al.* (1959) demonstrated that pregnant guinea pigs injected with testosterone propionate (a very potent anabolic steroid) produced daughters who were physically and behaviourally masculinised/defeminised. Goy and Phoenix (1971) also showed that female rhesus monkeys exposed prenatally to the same substance engaged in the typically male rough and tumble play at a greater frequency than untreated females.

### Activational

At a later point in development the same neural/behavioural machinery is temporarily modified by fluctuations in hormone levels. As described by Arnold and Breedlove (1985), their distinguishing characteristics are fivefold. First, they are impermanent – hormone-sensitive behaviour is displayed only as long as the hormone is present. Second, such effects occur in adulthood. Third, they have no developmental or temporal constraints, though it is assumed that activational effects cannot occur until associated neural circuits have already been organised. Fourth, such effects may not involve large-scale neurological changes but rather more subtle changes, perhaps in neurological wiring, or neurotransmitter production, release or sensitivity. Lastly, activational effects are assumed to be symmetrical, such that androgens are required for the activation of male-typical behaviours, and estrogens are required for the activation of female-typical behaviours.

We can thus see that organisational/activational effects can be used to explain the influence of hormones on the three behavioural levels of sensory input, CNS integration and motor output. For example, Diamond *et al.* (1972) showed that perceptual capabilities of human females (the sensory level) were influenced by alterations in circulating hormones during their menstrual cycle. During menstruation, when levels of ovarian hormones drop dramatically, women showed poorer visual discrimination than males and women who were taking a contraceptive pill (which acts to maintain hormone levels at a steady rate). More recently, other authors have also demonstrated that gonadal steroids appear to increase the salience of certain sociosexual signals (e.g. Penton-Voak *et al.*, 1999; Lacreuse and Herndon, 2003; Feinberg *et al.*, 2005). Others have shown physical changes in certain sensory modalities in response to hormonal fluctuation (e.g. McFadden, 2000; Caruso *et al.*, 2003).

At the level of integration, numerous reports have demonstrated that alteration in hormone levels (particularly sex steroids) during development causes permanent alterations in central nervous system structures. For example, in some bird species only the males sing; their songs are learned, and controlled by a distinct set of brain regions. These brain regions show clear sexual dimorphism in that they are much larger in males, and these differences are assumed to reflect the action of testosterone or its metabolites, as these areas contain numerous androgen receptors. Nottebohm and Arnold (1976) reported that castrated male canaries showed a reduction in the volume of their singing centres, while females receiving androgen implants showed increased volume in certain regions. However, Arnold (1980) compared the volumes of these brain regions in zebra finches and, contrary to expectation, found that castrated males showed an increase in volume (not limited to the song areas) and no effect of androgen administration in females! At the level of the response, adult male frogs and toads produce stereotyped 'advertisement calls' to attract nearby females and intimidate potential male rivals (Moore *et al.*, 2005). At puberty, a surge in androgen levels alters the male larynx such that it develops more muscle fibres, especially the 'fast twitch' variety, which is vital for successful call production (Sassoon *et al.*, 1987).

## Measuring organisational effects

In the previous chapter I have described how circulating hormone levels can be reliably and accurately measured by radioimmunoassays. Obviously such techniques provide a very useful (though by no means foolproof) mechanism by which potential activational effects can be considered. If we are to compare organisational and activational effects, or try to tease out the relative contribution of each to a particular behaviour, then we need some means by which we can ascertain organisational effects. Recall that such effects are assumed to take place very early in development, either during foetal development or during the first few weeks/months of postnatal life. But how can we possibly determine the hormonal milieu at such times, bearing in mind that for the majority of human studies (our key focus) we are dealing with adults? As yet we do not have a definitive solution to this problem as of course we are trying to determine what happened to an individual during very early stages of its development, perhaps many years in the past. However, we do have at our disposal a set of indirect (or proxy) markers which, it has been argued, enable us to peer back in time to when organisational effects were taking place, and allow us to make an educated guess about the individual's hormonal environment at that time.

*Dermatoglyphic measures*

One possible such measure concerns dermatoglyphic[4] characteristics. These are the skin patterns on the hands and feet, caused by height and shape differences in the dermal ridges. Measurements can easily be taken via fingerprinting (or dactylography to give it its proper name) and they form an important identification tool, because, as noted by Francis Galton in his 1892 book *Fingerprints*, they remain unchanged throughout life and show characteristic individual differences in the key patterns (named whorls, radials and ulnar loops). Human dermatoglyphic traits are determined early in foetal life before four months of age, and their development is preceded by the formation of localised eminences called volar pads which appear at around six weeks of age (Babler, 1987).

A key feature of human ridge counts is that they show asymmetry in that the right hand has a higher ridge count then the left (Holt, 1968); they show sex differences in that males have a higher ridge count than females (but females show a higher count on their left hand (Penrose, 1967; Kimura and Carson, 1995). It has also been suggested that ridge count reflects the rate of embryonic growth, and certain features may be related to variation in sex steroid hormones. For example, Jamison *et al.* (1993) took hand prints and saliva samples in thirty-nine adult males and reported significant relationships between testosterone levels and certain dermatoglyphic characteristics. Of course, as these physical characteristics are determined well before birth, just because they correlate with adult levels of testosterone does not mean that we can draw direct inferences about the prenatal hormonal milieu from their analysis. Ridge count asymmetries have however been associated with cognitive patterns (Kimura and Carson, 1995) and sexual orientation (Hall and Kimura, 1994), but such evidence is controversial (see Forastieri *et al.*, 2002 for example), perhaps because the methodology is tricky, time-consuming, and open to subjective interpretation.

---

[4] In Greek 'derma' means skin and 'glyphein' means carvings.

*Finger length ratio*

A second (and rather more straightforward to utilise) method concerns the ratio between the second and fourth finger digits (2D:4D). More than a hundred years ago, a very entertaining paper concerning various customs and superstitions associated with the hand was presented to the Anthropological Society of Washington by Frank Baker, Professor of Anatomy at the University of Georgetown. Following some fascinating tales, and a debunking of palmistry, he concluded by discussing the comparative lengths of the digits, and noted that the second (index) finger is usually shorter than the fourth (ring) finger. He did not report a difference between the sexes, but did note that measuring differences between the fingers could be problematical, especially if just done by eye (Baker, 1888). In the 1870s, Ecker had also focussed on the distribution of finger length ratios and had noted that there were three manifestations of 2D versus 4D: $2 > 4$, $2 = 4$ and $2 < 4$ (cited in Phelps, 1952). Some years later George (1930) noted a sex difference in the distribution of finger length ratios in that males were more likely to show the $2 < 4$ pattern (i.e. a longer ring finger relative to the index finger), while females were more likely to show the opposite pattern ($2 > 4$). Phelps (1952) confirmed this sex difference, noting that such differences were observed in foetuses, and then appeared to be stable throughout life.

The hormonal significance of these morphological differences remained unaddressed until John Manning's seminal book *Digit Ratio*. In this he reviewed evidence for sex and population differences in 2D:4D and provided a theoretical basis for such differences based on differential prenatal hormone exposure (Manning, 2002). The central assertion is that prenatal testosterone stimulates growth in the fourth finger while estrogens promote growth in the second finger. A low 2D:4D ratio (fourth finger longer than the second) is thus associated with a uterine environment higher in testosterone (a 'masculine' 2D:4D) while a high 2D:4D ratio (second finger longer than the fourth) is thus associated with a uterine environment higher in estrogens (a 'feminine' 2D:4D ratio). The term 'higher' here can be misleading as it is possible that the observed morphological differences do not result from raised hormone levels, but rather an increase in receptor sensitivity to the hormones (or perhaps a combination of both).

There are several lines of evidence in support of this assertion. First, androgens and estrogens promote skeletal growth and maturation, with androgenic and estrogenic receptors being present in bone tissue. In particular testosterone (either acting alone, or after being aromatised to an estrogen) promotes greater bone length and mass (Kung, 2003); higher circulating androgen levels, and higher androgen receptor expression at specific skeletal sites, thus contribute to adult sex differences in skeletal morphology (Kasperk *et al.*, 1997). As relative finger lengths are determined before birth, possibly around weeks 13–14 post-conception (Garn *et al.*, 1975), and sex differences in finger length ratios are seen in children as young as two years old (Manning, 2002) and do not change at puberty (Manning *et al.*, 1998), this suggests that sex steroids are having an organisational effect upon finger lengths.

Secondly, certain aspects of morphological development lie under the control of Homeobox (*Hoxa*) genes with the *Hoxa* and *Hoxa* variants controlling development of the testes/ovaries, and the fingers and toes (Kondo *et al.*, 1997). Mutations affecting the *Hoxa* genes in particular result in a condition called 'hand–foot–genital syndrome' in which individuals show deformities in their fingers, toes and urinogenital system (Mortlock and Innis, 1997). There is a large and well-established sex difference in androgen exposure before birth (with males being exposed to higher levels) and if these genetic/morphological factors are linked by sex steroid exposure, then we would expect to see sex differences in certain physical characteristics.

Thirdly, humans who have been exposed to atypical prenatal hormonal environments display patterns of finger length ratio in accord with the hormonal environment experienced. For example, Brown *et al.* (2002b) and Ökten *et al.* (2002) have compared finger length ratios in males and females suffering from congenital adrenal hyperplasia (CAH), a condition in which the developing foetus is overexposed to androgens (see chapter 6). Both studies have reported more masculine-like digit ratios in males and females suffering from this condition. However, this is not clear cut as another study by Buck *et al.* (2003) reported no difference between 2D:4D in CAH girls and normal female controls.

Fourth, Lutchmaya *et al.* (2004) assessed foetal testosterone and estrogen via amniocentesis and found that 2D:4D measured at two years of age was associated with a high testosterone:estradiol ratio.

Finally, Manning *et al.* (2003) noted that variation in the alleles of the X-linked androgen receptor gene determines sensitivity to testosterone. In particular, androgen receptor alleles with low numbers of CAG triplets produce a heightened response to testosterone, while the opposite is true for alleles with high numbers of CAG triplets. In a sample of fifty males, Manning *et al.* (2003) showed that right hand 2D:4D was positively associated with the number of CAG repeats – the higher (more feminine) finger ratio being associated with androgen-insensitivity. However, as Manning admits, evidence linking 2D:4D with the amount of exposure, or degree of sensitivity to prenatal sex steroids remains circumstantial, as evidence is based upon relationships between characteristics that are themselves probably dependent upon sex steroids, e.g. physical characteristics (Fink *et al.*, 2003; 2005; Manning *et al.*, 1999) and autism (Manning *et al.*, 2001). It is thus impossible to be sure that 2D:4D is directly linked with prenatal hormone exposure – correlation does not mean causality. Nevertheless, the simple act of measuring someone's fingers might be the current best guess that we have concerning prenatal hormone exposure (McIntyre,

2006), even if it may only cast light on a fairly narrow window of early development (Putz *et al.*, 2004).

In a standard testing session the experimenter would measure the lengths of the second and fourth fingers (palm side facing upwards) from the tip of the finger to the most proximal crease at the base of each finger (not always easy to find!) using digital calipers capable of recording to 0.01 mm. Each finger would normally be measured twice and an average length for each finger calculated; fingers are pliable and not as easy to measure as one would expect, and single measures can lead to inaccuracies. Potential intraobserver and interobserver measurement errors can be assessed by establishing repeatabilities between the measurements, or by calculating various precision estimates (see Weinberg *et al.*, 2005) and absolute-agreement intraclass correlation coefficients used for assessing repeatability of the measurements (Voracek *et al.*, 2007). Where time is short, or participants are young and extremely fidgety, scans or photocopies can be taken of the hand. While there is a strong association between finger length measures obtained directly from the hand and from photocopies, ratios calculated from photocopies are lower than those obtained direct, owing to an increase in apparent finger lengths, perhaps because of spreading of the fat pads on the photocopier glass (Manning *et al.*, 2005). It is therefore advised not to mix recording methods within the same study, but using photocopies does appear to lead to stronger results. Evidence linking 2D:4D with various hormonal/behavioural characteristics will be considered where necessary in subsequent chapters.

## A re-evaluation of organisational versus activational effects

The distinction between organisational and activational effects of hormones has been used extensively to discuss the effects of hormones on brain and behaviour (especially the role of sex steroids in sexual differentiation – see chapter 5). Since its introduction, the organisational/activational hypothesis has proved an extremely valuable heuristic tool with which to conceptualise hormone–brain–behaviour interactions, and its success as a theory is due, in no small part, to the wealth of supporting evidence. Not surprisingly though, researchers have pointed out that such a simple classification is likely to form not quite the complete story. In a review of the evidence, Arnold and Breedlove (1985) argued that the wide variety of effects produced by hormones in the CNS cannot be simply placed into two discrete categories.

For example, in various studies involving birds and rodents, they note that steroid hormones can produce major morphological changes in the adult brain outside of critical or sensitive periods before or just after birth. Some changes are long lasting, and others appear to be permanent; this clearly undermines the notion of simple organisational versus activational effects. The authors do admit though that their argument is based upon extreme variations of hormonal action caused by deliberate experimentation (castration in males, androgen treatment in females) that falls outside of physiological events normally occurring in nature. This problem aside, we perhaps need to recognise that the original distinction between organisational and activational effects may no longer be appropriate. These authors suggest replacing it with a distinction between 'permanent' and 'impermanent' effects (Arnold and Breedlove, 1985: 490).

More recently, Forget and Cohen (1994) point out that the influence of testosterone is not limited to the perinatal period, but in fact has a lifelong influence upon various aspects of brain structure and function. Sisk and Zehr (2005) have also addressed the organisational/activational debate by considering the role of hormones in puberty and adolescence in humans. Puberty is defined as a period during which an individual achieves sexual maturity (i.e. is capable of reproduction) while adolescence is the time between childhood and adulthood which covers not only sexual maturation, but also emotional, social and cognitive maturity. During this time the endocrine system is extremely active, a process kick-started by the gradual increase in the frequency and strength of GnRH released from the hypothalamus which stimulates the secretion of the anterior pituitary gonadotropins LH and FSH; these then stimulate the gonads to produce their key steroids testosterone and the estrogens (Styne, 1997). This rapidly rising level of the sex steroids leads to diverse morphological changes in secondary sexual characteristics – physical growth, muscular development, fat deposition, etc.

Much attention has been paid to the obvious physical changes during puberty, but scientists are now beginning to understand that this often traumatic period is also accompanied by equally dramatic changes in the CNS. Animal studies have now shown that the adolescent brain is thoroughly reorganised by the same mechanisms (neurogenesis, apoptosis, axon sprouting, myelination, synaptogenesis and elimination) that sculpt neural circuitry during prenatal and perinatal development. For example, Meyer et al. (1978) demonstrated that dendritic branching in the hippocampus of male mice is normally increased at the beginning of puberty and then declines in the later stages of puberty. This morphological alteration is clearly governed by gonadal hormones as removal of the gonads prior to puberty abolishes these changes. In rats, primary visual cortex shows a sex bias in that this region in males is significantly larger than that of females; this is due to the fact that the female visual cortex experiences enhanced cell death during adolescence. This morphological sex difference is also governed by pubertal steroids, as ovariectomy before puberty eliminates this cell death, and such females do not differ to males in terms of adult cell number and volume in this region (Nunez et al., 2002).

In terms of normal adult behaviours, Schulz et al. (2004) compared sexual behaviours in male Syrian hamsters who had experienced adolescent brain development with normal gonadal hormone involvement, or without (individuals were castrated before or after puberty). Following castration, testosterone was replaced and the males were placed with sexually receptive females. Those males that had experienced adolescence without gonadal steroids showed abnormal sexual performance and behaviour compared with those that had experienced a gonadally normal adolescence. The authors argued that this represents a steroid-dependent organisation of reproductive behaviour circuits – as testosterone was replaced this cannot simply reflect activational deficiencies. In humans, similar structural changes appear to be taking place during adolescence, as several studies have shown that there are gross alterations in brain morphology during this period. In the hippocampus, for example, an increase in myelination leads to an increase in white matter volume, though it must be pointed out that such changes are not just limited to adolescence (Benes *et al.*, 1994). Girls normally reach puberty around one year earlier than boys, and this is reflected in a sex difference in peak grey matter thickness, with girls reaching this peak around a year earlier (Giedd, 2004).

While it is unethical to deliberately alter gonadal hormone secretions during development in humans, nature has provided its own series of case studies with which researchers can address the possible effects of pubertal steroids on brain morphology and thence behaviour. Delayed puberty is the result of the decreased ability of the hypothalamus to secrete GnRH, or of the failure of the pituitary gland to secrete sufficient levels of FSH or LH. Either problem (caused by a range of syndromes) leads to a condition called hypogonadotropic hypogonadism (Styne, 1997). Precocious puberty on the other hand is caused by the premature activation of the hypothalamic–pituitary axis (again due to a range of medical conditions).

Very few studies have assessed such individuals. One example was provided by Hier and Crowley (1982) who investigated spatial cognition in groups of males who had either developed hypogonadotropic hypogonadism after experiencing a normal puberty, or who had not experienced normal puberty because of failure of the hypothalamic–pituitary axis. The group who had not been exposed to the usual range of pubertal steroids showed impaired spatial cognition; those who had been exposed to gonadal steroids at puberty (and a control group of normal males) showed no such impairments in performance. Interestingly, the subsequent replacement of appropriate hormones in adulthood did not ameliorate such deficits in those who had not experienced a normal puberty. Sisk and Zehr (2005) thus proposed that gonadal hormones act to organise certain neural circuits and behaviours at puberty, and so puberty may in fact be a second key stage at which hormones permanently alter brain development. They pose the still unanswered question as to whether adolescence is a particularly sensitive period for steroid-dependent organisation (as is the prenatal brain). If so, then one might predict that individual differences in puberty onset might be mirrored by similar differences in behaviour.

## Comparing humans and animals

While this book is principally concerned with the possible effects of hormones on human behaviours, a necessary and important part of the evidence to be summarised will involve evidence from animal studies. The reason for this is fairly obvious in that certain experimental techniques are simply not possible in humans because of ethical considerations. One might be justified in debating the ethics involved in animal studies as well, but it is not within the scope of this book to do so; I will simply describe and evaluate the outcomes of such studies and how they have contributed to our understanding of hormone–behaviour interactions.

The 'comparative approach' was developed from the work of the naturalist George John Romanes in the late nineteenth century, who argued that animals possessed the necessary reasoning intelligence to solve certain problems. His theories remained speculation until Edward Lee Thorndike conducted empirical studies on how cats learned to escape from 'puzzle boxes', and formulated his 'law of effect' in 1898 (a key hypothesis in the understanding of animal learning as it stated that responses to stimuli that produce a satisfying effect are more likely to occur again in the same situation). The basic tenet of the comparative approach is that the behaviours of different species (including humans) can be addressed in a variety of ways, and the findings can be interpreted in terms of their differing ecological or phylogenetic backgrounds. Many efforts have focussed on comparative intelligence but others have addressed hormone–behaviour interactions, with a host of behaviours having thus far been addressed (e.g. communication, aggression, parenting, cognition, sensory and perceptual processing, reproductive and social behaviours).

Comparative endocrinological research has a long history, with certain species being favoured over others, rodents being by far the most 'popular' species investigated, but in addition numerous studies have focussed on primates, fish, birds, insects, amphibians, and reptiles (for reviews see Bass and Zakon, 2005; Crews and Moore, 2005; Fahrbach and Mesce, 2005; Wilczynski *et al.*, 2005; Wingfield, 2005). According to Rosen, 'much of the endeavor of animal research is to elucidate fundamental mechanisms that are applicable to humans and the human condition' (Rosen, 2006: 1). Rosen then admits that a key problem is that many of the methodological procedures and research paradigms used to assess physiology–behaviour relationships in animals are not comparable across species, or especially between say rats and humans. Humans are not large talking rodents, and rats are not small furry people! As we will see in future chapters, it may be impossible directly to translate research findings from behavioural endocrinological studies in certain species to humans because the functioning of the respective hormonal systems may be very different. However, it should be the case that broad comparisons can be made. For example, while McEwen (1981) notes that the location of estrogen- and androgen-sensitive cells in the CNS reveals a basic common plan between diverse vertebrate species, there are characteristic species differences.

An additional issue to consider is that comparative studies are typically conducted in two different settings. Within laboratory settings important variables like temperature, nutrition, social interactions, etc. can be rigorously controlled. Alternatively, studies are also conducted 'in the field', where free-living animals are studied in their home environment where they are naturally exposed to a wide range of ecologically relevant conditions and social stimuli. We can safely assume that their endocrine responses to such stimuli will thus be entirely normal and natural. This has led to a significant problem in that while laboratory studies are able carefully to control potentially confounding variables, the lack of ecological validity means that the expression of neuroendocrine/behavioural traits is likely to be incomplete (Fusani et al., 2005).

A good example is that of the dusky-footed woodrat. Studies addressing hormonal influences on territorial aggression have established that, in many species, animals defending what they perceive to be their territory fight with greater intensity and their hormone profiles (principally testosterone) show quantitative differences from animals not defending a territory – levels of testosterone being higher (see chapter 10). Monaghan and Glickman (1992) expected much the same in the woodrat, but when they compared the territorial behaviour of castrated and intact woodrats, both fought with the same ferocity, suggesting that differences in circulating testosterone were independent of these aggressive behaviours. However, the initial study was conducted in an 'open-field' laboratory setting (i.e. devoid of any natural features) and when they changed the setting by offering the inhabitants a 'house' of twigs to fight over, the non-castrated animals fought much harder and were more likely to prevail than their castrated counterparts.

Fusani et al. (2005) further point out that captivity itself can also have powerful effects on an animal's behaviour and indeed their physiology; for example, animals that are normally raised in large and complex social groups may show abnormal behaviours in adulthood if they have been reared in isolation, or in smaller groups during their development. Harlow's work on attachment behaviours in monkeys, for example, demonstrated the importance of tactile contact with an adult during infancy for the appropriate development of physical, social and emotional development (Harlow, 1958). Captivity is known to influence hormone levels and the physiological response to hormones. For example Wingfield et al. (1990) showed that captive birds had lower levels of circulating testosterone than those who were living wild. Canoine and Gwinner (2002a, b) found that the identical pharmacological treatment led to different aggressive responses in captive as opposed to wild European stonechats. During 120 hours of observation of groups of the domestic guinea pig and its wild ancestor, Künzl and Sachser

(1999) noted key behavioural and endocrinological differences. Domesticated males displayed less aggressive behaviours and increased social tolerance. In addition, basal activity of their sympathetic-adrenomedullary systems, and reactivity of their pituitary-adrenocortical system was also reduced. The authors suggested that their stress-response systems were downgraded, and were clearly adapted to their man-made housing conditions. It is obvious then that considerable care must be taken in evaluating results from laboratory-housed animals, especially when also discussing research based upon animals living in the wild.

## Testing hormone–behaviour relationships

Despite the issues outlined in the preceding section, it should be possible to devise fairly straightforward means by which to establish possible relationships between hormones and behaviour. While reviewing hormonal correlates of parental behaviours in doves, Silver (1978) set out a series of potential experimental conditions in which such relationships could be established. Needless to say, the utilisation of a single method on its own may be less effective than using several methods in combination; typically, though, owing to limitations in resources and time, most studies adopt a single paradigm. With different studies (within and between laboratories) conducting all three types of paradigm, the data from such converging operations should provide some fairly powerful evidence and lead to a unanimous conclusion:

### Removal

The first kind of experiment takes as its premise that any behaviour assumed to be dependent upon a particular hormone should disappear or decline when the source of the hormone is removed, or the actions of the hormone are blocked. The obvious example here is removal of the steroid-producing gonads in males (referred to as castration, orchiectomy or orchidectomy in humans; gelding in animals) or females (ovariectomy, oophorectomy in humans; speying in animals), generally before puberty. For example, Harding *et al.* (1983) castrated male zebra finches and monitored their sexual behaviours when they were placed with receptive females. The castrated males showed a significant reduction in their courtship behaviours and never attempted to mount receptive females. The clear implication here is that the missing gonadal sex steroids were directly responsible for the behavioural impairments. Note that this does not tell us the precise nature of the impairments – whether they are due to sensory, integrative or output mechanisms (or a mixture of one or more) – and this remains a key problem for many endocrinological studies: the behaviour has been impaired by hormone removal, but how?

## Replacement

The second kind of experiment leads on from the first and assumes that should a behaviour disappear or decline after the removal or blocking of a hormone, then logic dictates that the behaviour should return to its previously observed levels following the reintroduction of the hormone. In the 1950s Harris and colleagues had demonstrated that ovariectomised female cats would begin to show normal mating behaviours following the direct implantation of estrogen into the anterior hypothalamus (Beach, 1981). Taking the example previously provided by Harding *et al.* (1983), these experimenters did not just assess the effects of castration upon sexual behaviour in male finches, but also replaced the missing hormones using different groups. In fact, six different groups were castrated and then experienced different types of hormone replacement, covering not just testosterone but also androstenedione, androsterone, dihy-drotestosterone, estradiol and estradiol + dihydrotestosterone. These groups were compared with two control groups – gonadally intact males, and males who had been castrated but only received injections of cholesterol (which has no hormonal action). Using this careful replacement paradigm the authors were able to show that only those birds receiving testosterone, androstenedione or estradiol + dihydrotestosterone following castration subsequently showed normal sexual behaviours, with the androstenedione treatment being the most effective.

Care has to be exercised in the timing of the hormone replacement. If for example a hormone is reintroduced directly after the removal, then levels of the hormone may not have had chance to decline. It is usual that hormone replacement is delayed for several weeks/months in order to allow baseline levels to drop. A complicating factor is that when hormone levels are altered there are compensatory mechanisms involving up- and down-regulation of receptor numbers (see chapter 2). If receptors are for example down-regulated following a removal, then it may require higher than usual replacement amounts of the hormone in order to restore levels back to baseline; the opposite of course may occur with up-regulation (Brown, 1994).

## Correlation

These previous methods are routinely conducted on various animal species. However, such techniques are often not possible with human volunteers because of ethical or methodological considerations. However, as we shall see in subsequent chapters, nature has provided a range of human natural 'experiments' in which such techniques have been performed. For the most part behavioural endocrinologists have to be content with the logic that if hormones and behaviours are linked in some way then one should assume that relationships between the two should be evident and measurable. Circulating hormone concentrations and a particular behaviour should thus be covariant, i.e. the behaviour should only be observed when hormone concentrations are relatively high and never or rarely observed when the hormone concentrations are low. For example, the growth of the crop sac in birds (a structure which produces crop milk) is strongly dependent upon the release of prolactin, as this hormone stimulates the growth of the epithelial cells in the crop sac: the more prolactin, the thicker the growth of epithelial cells. Cheng and Burke (1983) measured serum prolactin levels and crop sac weight in male and female ring doves during the course of a normal breeding cycle. During early incubation and hatching there was no correlation, but during the midincubation period and while the chicks were growing, a significant positive correlation was observed. These relationships showed some predictable differences between males and females, and were clearly associated with the different behavioural/physical demands of the breeding cycle.

Such relationships can of course be problematic, as hormones are released in very small amounts, or are released in a pulsatile fashion such that single samples, or samples taken at the 'wrong' time, may give an inaccurate picture. In addition, while one might assume that such relationships may be linear in fashion (either positive or negative) it may well be the case that they are in fact curvilinear. For example, the first study that I ever conducted on hormone–behaviour relationships was concerned with possible links between circulating levels of testosterone and verbal and spatial performance. While we found no relationships at all between testosterone and performance on two verbal tasks, we observed a significant linear relationship on one spatial test and a significant curvilinear relationship on a different spatial test (Neave *et al.*, 1999). This suggests that higher levels of circulating testosterone were conducive to performance on one spatial test, but medium levels were related to better performance on another test, with low and high levels being associated with poorer performance. We will come across similar findings in subsequent chapters and address possible theoretical/methodological issues then, but suffice to say that this technique is straightforward to conduct in human volunteers and is thus very commonly used. A final caveat, of course, is that just because two variables are significantly correlated does not mean that they are causally related, e.g. just because levels of circulating testosterone may be positively correlated with aggressive behaviours, it cannot be inferred that changes in testosterone have caused aggression to increase. Further experiments utilising technique one or two might be required in order fully to address this putative relationship.

# 4 **Neurological effects of hormones**

In the first chapter I explained how cells within the CNS communicate with one another. At first glance it seems that neural signalling and endocrine signalling are quite different from one another. According to Rosenzweig *et al.*(2002) there are four key differences:

1 While neural communication is typically between fixed channels to precise destinations, hormonal signalling is rather more diffuse, as most hormones do not act immediately on localised areas but coordinate long-term changes in diverse regions of the body.
2 Whereas neural messages are very rapid (occurring over milliseconds), hormonal communication is slower and is measured in seconds and minutes.
3 Most neural messages are digitised, i.e. they either act or they do not ('all or none rule'). Hormonal signalling is analogue, i.e. graded in strength: the more of a hormone that is released, the larger the effect.
4 Some neural communication is under voluntary control while hormone release is not.

However, despite these differences, there are several similarities between hormonal and neural communication systems:

1 Neurons and endocrine glands produce chemicals, which are stored for later release.
2 Neurons and endocrine glands are both stimulated to release their chemicals.
3 There are many different neurotransmitters and hormones, each with specific functions. Indeed some chemicals serve exactly the same function, e.g. norepinephrine and epinephrine are both neurotransmitters and hormones.
4 Neurotransmitters and hormones react with specific receptor molecules at the postsynaptic receptor or at the target cell respectively. Neurotransmitters and hormones can only produce activation in synapses/cells which have the appropriate receptors for a particular transmitter/hormone.
5 Hormones exert their influence in a similar manner to neurotransmitters at metabotropic receptors. Hormones attach to receptors on the cell

membrane, where they activate an enzyme that produces a secondary messenger (e.g. cyclic AMP).

## Models of hormone effects

If hormones are to have any influence on behaviour then they must be able to modulate the functioning of the nervous system, by influencing either sensory systems, CNS integrative systems, output systems, or all three (see previous chapter). Peptide and steroid hormones do indeed regulate the activity of their target cells (though by different mechanisms). Steroid and thyroid hormones are small and fat soluble (lipophilic) and so can easily pass through cell membranes (as long as they are not bound to carrier proteins) where they bind to intracellular receptors. These intracellular receptors have been divided into two classes on the basis of their respective amino acid sequences, class I consisting of receptors for androgens, progesterone, glucocorticoids and mineralocorticoids, class II consisting of receptors for estrogens, thyroid hormones, retinoic acid and vitamin D (Evans, 1988). Each receptor is a simple protein housing a hormone-binding region (only certain hormones can bind to certain receptors, in the same way that certain neurotransmitters can only bind to certain receptors on the postsynapse: see chapter 1) and a DNA-binding region. After binding, the hormones and their receptors then form what is called a 'hormone-receptor complex' (or H-R complex) which serves to regulate gene expression within the nucleus of the target cell. Traditional explanations of how steroid hormones work in cells have been described as 'two-stage models' in that they assume that steroids first bind to their receptors in the cytoplasm, and then the H-R complex enters the nucleus of the cell.

In 'nuclear' models, the binding occurs directly within the nucleus of the cell. According to Harrison and Lippman (1989), nuclear models may well relate to estrogen receptors, but two-stage models may relate more to glucocorticoid and other steroid receptors. The extent of gene expression is determined not only by the amount of hormone receptors within a particular target cell, but also by the level of the circulating hormone. Alterations of hormone molecules in circulation can have a big impact upon the receptors: if target cells are repeatedly exposed to high concentrations of a hormone then the number of receptors drops – this is called 'down-regulation'. If circulating hormone levels decrease, however, then this leads to an increase in the number of receptors, and not surprisingly this is called 'up-regulation' (Martin, 1985). If a hormone is totally eliminated from circulation, its receptors decline markedly, as the presence of some amounts of a hormone is vital for the synthesis of new receptors. So, the number of receptors is not fixed but is partly determined by the amount of circulating hormones. Receptor numbers also alter over the lifespan. In the rat, for example, estrogen, progestin and androgen receptors are present in low amounts prior to birth, but their numbers increase markedly in the first few weeks after birth. Estrogen receptors are the first to expand in number, and this expansion leads directly to a surge in progestin receptors around postnatal days 8–10; the increase in androgen receptors occurs around a week post-birth. The aging process is associated with an equally dramatic fall in receptor numbers (MacLusky and Naftolin, 1981; McEwen, 1976; Roth, 1979). Whether this is also the case for humans remains to be verified.

## Autoradiography

It is only within the last few decades that neuroendocrinologists have been able reliably to quantify the number of receptors for a particular hormone, and their sensitivity to that hormone using a technique called 'autoradiography', which is particularly useful for detecting steroid hormone target cells. Such methods have led to a major leap in our understanding of how hormones appear to work within the brain. If we can locate cells sensitive to particular hormones in specific brain regions, and we understand the role of those brain regions in certain behaviours, then we can begin to derive hypotheses about the possible roles of those hormones in certain behaviours. In such techniques, a hormone that has been radioactively labelled (tritium – the radioactive isotope of hydrogen is commonly used) is injected into an animal that is no longer capable of producing the hormone in question (they have been castrated or ovariectomised) and works its way to the specific hormone receptors in the brain. The brain is removed, fixed (to prevent decay) and sliced, and the slices are coated with photographic emulsion. The radiation emitted by the decaying isotopes creates black dots on the emulsion, and the slices can then be stained to identify clearly the stained cell bodies (McEwen, 1976).

Things are not quite so straightforward though, as it is now understood that two or more hormones are able to bind to the same receptor. For example, androgen receptors have the greatest affinity for testosterone and dihydrotestosterone, but also bind with other androgens; progesterone also binds to androgen receptors and thus acts to block these receptors to the effects of androgens (Sheridan, 1983; McEwen, 1981; Wagner, 2006). In the case of steroid hormones, it is possible that within the same cell both androgen and estrogen receptors may be present; in this instance the two different hormones may act in conjunction within the target cell, or cancel one another out. McEwen (1981) points out that within the medial preoptic area of the hypothalamus (mPOA) and anterior hypothalamic nuclei, estrogens and dihydrotestosterone act together to trigger sexual behaviours. In various regions of the limbic system, however, it has been noted that glucocorticoids prevent gonadal steroids from acting, and thus inhibit certain kinds of behaviours (Sar and Stumpf, 1975). Animal studies (principally of rodents) have demonstrated that the following key hormone receptors are located in specific brain regions.

### Estrogen receptors

There is considerable overlap between androgen and estrogen receptors, such that the key locations for estrogen receptors lie within the mPOA, the anterior and ventromedial hypothalamus, and the amygdala, where concentrations of estrogen range between 3,000 and 5,000 molecules of hormone when fully saturated. Estrogenic receptors are also found in the pituitary gland, where concentrations can reach 12,000 molecules of hormone (McEwen, 1976). The localisation of neurons sensitive to estradiol appears to be consistent in a wide variety of animal species, including amphibians, birds, fish and mammals. Pfaff *et al.* (1976) conducted autoradiographic analysis of the brains of ten ovariectomised female rhesus monkeys and also confirmed that estrogen-binding was occurring in the same regions; we can perhaps thus speculate that humans may show the same pattern (this remains an educated guess). We can also speculate on the role of such regions in certain behaviours. For example, in animals, receptors within the ventromedial hypothalamus appear to regulate certain female sexual behaviours, while those in the anterior hypothalamus and amygdala play a role in emotional regulation, parental behaviours, aggression, hunger and body temperature (Brown, 1994).

In the 1970s, Naftolin and colleagues (cited in Balthazart and Ball, 1998) were the first to hypothesise that testosterone might undergo some sort of conversion to an estrogen before it could exert its effects on certain physiological and behavioural processes. It has now been established that within estrogen receptors in certain regions of the brain, testosterone is indeed converted into an estrogen (see diagram 2.2) via an enzyme called aromatase (also called estrogen synthase). Thus, within the target cells, molecules of testosterone attach to aromatase and are then converted into estradiol, and in the same manner androstenedione is converted into estrone; this process is called 'aromatization' (Callard *et al.*, 1978; Selmanoff *et al.*, 1977). The key regions at which aromatisation occurs strongly overlap with the location of estrogen receptors – preoptic area, amygdala, hypothalamus, septum and hippocampus (Brown, 1994). Aromatase regulation appears to be influenced by catecholaminergic neurons (principally those containing dopamine and noradrenaline) that are themselves influenced by social and environmental factors – another remainder of complex hormone/neurotransmitter/environment interactions (Balthazart and Ball, 1998). We shall see the importance of aromatisation for sexual differentiation in chapter 5, but it is important to note that there are significant species differences in the role of this process in behavioural activation. Specific examples will be mentioned as and where necessary (Adkins-Regan, 1981).

## Progesterone receptors

In rats it has been established that progesterone receptors are located mainly within the medial and lateral preoptic areas, the ventromedial and basomedial hypothalamus, the arcuate/median eminence, the amygdala, and the pituitary gland, and these overlap considerably with estrogen receptors (McEwen, 1981; Wagner, 2006). Indeed, progesterone and estrogen receptors in the ventromedial hypothalamus act in conjunction to trigger certain female sexual behaviours; progesterone receptors in the substantia nigra act alone to inhibit female sexual behaviour (McEwen *et al.*, 1979). Progesterone also appears to play a critical role in male sexual behaviours (see chapter 8), though its effects are complex, as it may have 'biphasic' or 'triphasic' effects depending upon dose and existing levels of testosterone (Wagner, 2006). Alternatively, progesterone has direct effects in the brain via rapid effects on GABA receptors and thus also acts as a neurosteroid.

## Androgen receptors

In the rat these receptors are densely located within the septum, amygdala, hippocampus, bed nucleus of the stria terminalis, mPOA, lateral and anterior nuclei of the hypothalamus, and pituitary gland (Sar and Stumpf, 1975). These brain regions have been strongly associated with masculine sexual behaviours, emotion, motivation, spatial ability and certain sexually dimorphic behaviours; the implication of course being that androgens contribute significantly to such behaviours (see subsequent chapters). In rhesus monkeys, Michael *et al.* (1989) have demonstrated that testosterone acts solely at androgen receptors in the mammillary bodies, arcuate nucleus and lateral septum. Androgen receptors are also located within the thalamus, cerebral cortex, brain stem and spinal cord (Brown, 1994). As we have already seen, androgen receptors bind most strongly to the principal androgen testosterone, but also bind to dihydrotestosterone after it has been converted from testosterone via 5α-reductase. In the mPOA, anterior and lateral hypothalamus, pituitary gland, gonads, prostate gland and penis, testosterone thus acts on target cells only after it has been converted into dihydrotestosterone.

In certain regions of the brain, testosterone can only act after it has been converted into estradiol via the actions of aromatase (aromatisation). If radioactively labelled testosterone is administrated to castrated male monkeys, much of the radioactivity in nuclei within the hypothalamus, preoptic area and amygdala is in the form of estradiol (Bonsall *et al.*, 1983). Michael *et al.* (1987) castrated eight male rhesus monkeys and injected all with radioactively labelled estradiol; beforehand, half had received a control injection, while the other half had received testosterone propionate; levels of radioactive estradiol were subsequently measured in brain slices.

In the testosterone-treated individuals, estradiol was reduced in the hypothalamus, preoptic area and amygdala. The authors hypothesised that the estrogenic metabolites of testosterone were preventing the uptake of radioactive estradiol. In the lateral septum and arcuate nucleus, however, this did not occur, suggesting that they contained estrogen receptors that were not blocked by testosterone pre-treatment. In monkey brains there thus appear to be two populations of estrogen target neurons, one being directly influenced by testosterone, the other by testosterone aromatised to estradiol.

In humans it is assumed that androgen receptors show similar patterns and characteristics, but, not surprisingly, evidence is hard to come by. In one study Fernández-Guasti *et al.* (2000) observed a sex difference in the distribution of androgen receptors within the human hypothalamus, while the pattern was only slightly different in the anterior hypothalamus; a conspicuous sex differences was found in several posterior hypothalamic nuclei. In a similar experiment Kruijver *et al.* (2001) focussed on this same region in forty-seven autopsied brains from a range of heterosexual/homosexual/transsexual/castrated individuals. A clear sex difference in androgen receptor expression was once more noted, this difference being more related to differences in circulating levels of testosterone than to sexual orientation or gender history. However, as circulating testosterone had not been directly measured, such a conclusion remains equivocal. Normal male sexual differentiation is determined by interaction of testosterone and dihydrotestosterone with androgen receptors in androgen-responsive target tissues (Hiort and Zitzmann, 2004) and so if the tissues are insensitive to androgens through failure of the androgen receptors, then a female phenotype will result (see chapter 6).

## Adrenal hormone receptors

Adrenal hormones are steroids and so they bind to receptors in the cell nucleus to form a H-R complex, which binds to DNA and initiates mRNA and protein synthesis. There is also evidence that they demonstrate the classical two-stage receptor action (Brown, 1994). As we have seen in chapter 2, there are two types of adrenal hormones – glucocorticoids and mineralocorticoids – and there are two types of receptor. Common sense would thus dictate that each receptor would bind to each type of hormone. However, this does not quite seem to be the case. In the liver, type I receptors bind principally to the mineralocorticoid aldosterone, but in the brain they also bind to the glucocorticoid corticosterone. It has thus been suggested that there are perhaps two forms of type I receptor, or alternatively, that the same receptor shows different binding characteristics in different circumstances. Evans and Arriza (1989) demonstrated that the key factor was the presence or absence of an enzyme called 11β-hydroxysteroid dehydrogenase. This substance deactivates the corticosteroids but has no effect upon aldosterone, as it is not present in the hippocampus. The type I receptors located here bind to both mineralocorticoids and glucocorticoids; in other regions it is absent, and so the type I receptors only bind to aldosterone. McEwen *et al.* (1986) noted that type I receptors are principally located in the hippocampus, septum, dentate gyrus, brain stem and various regions of cortex; they may well regulate locomotor activity, the sleep–wake cycle, appetite, mood and certain aspects of cognition.

Type II receptors only bind to the glucocorticoids (cortisol and corticosterone) and they are located principally in the hippocampus, septum, amygdala, paraventricular nuclei of the hypothalamus, anterior pituitary, and various regions of the cortex. They have a much lower affinity for glucocorticoids and only appear to be activated by high levels of glucocorticoids that are secreted during the stress response (McEwen *et al.*, 1986). In such situations they provide negative feedback to turn off the hypothalamic-pituitary-adrenal (HPA) stress-induced activation. It has been suggested that the two types of receptors which respond to glucocorticoids in a different manner may well serve different physiological/behavioural functions, because glucocorticoid action is not universal. At low levels the glucocorticoids enhance locomotor activity, trigger food-seeking behaviours and stimulate appetite. McEwen (1988) thus referred to them as the 'get up and go' hormones. These activational effects are associated with the daily rhythm of adrenocortical secretion. At higher levels the response to stress induces a cascade of adrenocortical hormones and a process of 'adaptation' as rising glucocorticoid levels exert a negative feedback loop in the brain, which reduces further secretions. This depends upon the nature of the stress. Moderate stress does not seem to depress glucocorticoid receptor mechanisms and may even increase receptor levels; severe stress, however, leads to neurotoxic effects on glucocorticoid receptors, in the hippocampus at least (McEwen, 1988).

Receptor capacity for corticoids shows large changes during the lifespan. Within the rat hippocampus, for example, low numbers are seen at birth but these rise rapidly and attain adult levels around week 4. It has been suggested that the glucocorticoids may thus play a developmental role, perhaps by limiting cell number, or by regulating phenotype expression (McEwen *et al.*, 1986). In aged rats, receptors steadily decline in the hippocampus, this age-related decline in hippocampal cells being preventable by conducting an adrenalectomy (Landfield *et al.*, 1981). Interestingly, there are considerable individual differences in corticosterone binding, and these may be genetically determined or the consequence of environmental experiences during early life. Such differences may also relate to behavioural differences; for example, rats displaying the best learning and retention of an avoidance response had a higher corticosterone-binding capacity in the hippocampus (cited in McEwen *et al.*, 1986).

## Thyroid hormone receptors

Target cells for thyroid hormones are located throughout the brain but the highest density is seen in the cerebellum, certain regions of the cortex, hippocampus, amygdala, medial basal nuclei of the hypothalamus, and brain stem (e.g. Kaplan *et al.*, 1981; Leonard *et al.*, 1981). Extensive evidence from a variety of sources has indicated a close relationship between thyroid hormones and noradrenaline in somatic tissue; in the brain, autoradiographic studies have shown that $T_3$ is localised in brain nuclei which are known to receive adrenergic projections (Dratman *et al.*, 1982). More recently, Rozanov and Dratman (1996) confirmed that in the rat brain there was a dense concentration of $T_3$ in nuclei and projection sites of the principal adrenergic systems: in particular, the locus coeruleus, lateral septum, dentate gyrus within the hippocampus, thalamus, hypothalamus, and various regions of the neocortex. These close links have led these authors to speculate that $T_3$ may be acting as a neurotransmitter/neuromodulator within the adrenergic system.

These target cells are activated in a slightly different manner from the steroid hormone target cells. First, the thyroid hormone thyroxine ($T_4$) is extracted from the blood plasma and converted to its active form triiodothyronine ($T_3$) by an enzyme called 5'-deiodinase. The $T_3$ is then able to bind to its nuclear receptor (it has a greater affinity for the receptor than $T_4$) and thus triggers the activation of specific genes by the H-R complex already described (Nunez, 1984). There are in fact two types of thyroid hormone receptor, the so-called TR-α and TR-β, which are encoded by different genes, each of which comes in two varieties that have different characteristics. Both forms are expressed in the telencephalon and cerebellum, but whereas the TR-$α_1$ form is expressed in all regions of the hippocampus, the TR-$β_1$ is only expressed within the CA1 subfield of the hippocampus. There are also developmental changes in these variants, as TR-$α_1$ is abundant during the foetal and early postnatal stages and then shows a decline, whereas TR-$β_1$ increases steadily from birth until adulthood (Bernal and Nunez, 1995). In humans it seems to be the case that very early in gestational life, around the nine-week mark, $T_3$ receptor occupancy begins to occur, as the foetal thyroid gland does not begin secreting thyroid hormones until around week 18. This demonstrates that thyroid hormones derived from the mother are beginning to influence receptor activity in their offspring (Contempré *et al.*, 1993).

## Hormonal effects on neuronal activation

In chapter 2 I noted that hormones work by modulating messenger RNA and protein synthesis; these indirect genomic effects subsequently induce changes in the number of receptors, and neurotransmitter synthesis, storage and release. Such changes are not instantaneous. In other cases, though, hormones do have immediate effects on the brain. The steroid hormones, for example, have direct, non-genomic effects in the cortex (recall that we talked about the so-called neurosteroids) that have an almost immediate influence upon the neurons to influence membrane potential and hence neurotransmitter release. For example, a series of pioneering studies conducted in the late 1960s and early 1970s (cited in Pfaff and McEwen, 1983) used single-cell recording techniques[1] to monitor electrical activity in various brain regions. These studies showed that alterations in the electrical activity of neurons within the arcuate nucleus and the medial anterior nuclei of the hypothalamus were associated with hormonal fluctuations during the estrus cycle in rats. Similar studies were undertaken comparing animals who had been ovariectomised, or who remained gonadally intact, and showed that estrogen treatment in ovariec-tomised individuals resulted in an increase in resting discharge rates in neurons in certain hypothalamic nuclei. Such alterations were noted almost immediately, suggesting that the hormones were having a direct effect on nerve cells and were not acting via gene transcription (McEwen et al., 1981).

Similarly, if glucocorticoids are injected into rats, the electrical activity of neurons in the hippocampus and hypothalamus is inhibited, seemingly by shifting the resting potential of the neuron further away from the threshold of excitation, i.e. hyperpolarisation (Pfaff et al., 1971). These effects are complicated by the fact that the same hormone can have inhibitory effects on some neurons, but excitatory effects on other neurons. For example, Pfaff and McEwen (1983) have noted that estrogen has excitatory effects on neurons within the medial basal region of the hypothalamus, but has inhibitory effects on neurons within the bed nucleus of the stria terminalis and the medial pre-optic area. Interestingly though, such differences can be related to behaviour. Pfaff and McEwen (1983) pointed out that estrogen acts to increase the electrical activity of neurons in brain regions which trigger female reproductive behaviours, but decrease the activity of neurons in other regions which inhibit reproductive behaviours. As complex behaviours do not just entail the triggering of one behavioural action, but also entail the inhibition of other actions, this dual role of certain hormones thus seems entirely sensible. Like estrogen, progesterone appears to have dual effects, but in the male rat at least, testosterone infusions seem only to produce excitatory effects which have been linked to the triggering of sexual arousal and certain sexual behaviours (Orisini, 1981).

## Human studies

In humans the picture is obviously more complex, and it is methodologically much more difficult to ascertain precise relationships between hormonal fluctuations and cortical activity. One method has been to monitor the gross

[1] A microelectrode is carefully inserted into a neuron and subsequent electrical activity can be recorded.

electrical activity of the brain and compare that with changes in circulating hormone levels. The technique used is that of electroencephalography, a non-invasive method of determining millisecond-changes in cortical activation. The first electroencephalography studies were conducted in the early 1900s, but the technique was popularised and named by Hans Berger in the 1920s. As we have seen in chapter 1, neurons produce electrical activity in the form of postsynaptic potentials. By placing sensitive electrodes on the scalp (or in some rare cases on the surface of the cortex) in a standardised pattern, and connecting them to an amplifier, a recording of activity can be made; the output is called an electroencephalogram (EEG). While individual brain-wave patterns are obviously quite different, there are characteristic wave forms[2] determined by their specific frequency characteristics.

In one study conducted by Vogel *et al.* (1971), volunteers were given continuous infusions of ethanol and saline, with some of the group also receiving testosterone. After two hours and again at four hours, EEG recordings were made while the participants engaged in the difficult task of serial subtractions over a three-minute period (in this case they were given the number 981 and asked to subtract 17 from it repeatedly). The infusion of testosterone appeared to have a slowing effect upon the alpha waves, and this group showed less deterioration in performance (alpha waves are associated with a relaxed, but alert state of mind). In females, Solís-Ortiz *et al.* (1994) recorded EEG activity over twelve sessions (one every two days) in nine women who were experiencing a regular menstrual cycle. A complex set of findings emerged in relation to differential menstrual cycle effects on the various frequencies, but the authors summed it up by suggesting that the central/parietal regions showed higher activation during menses, while the frontal regions of cortex showed lower activation during the premenstrual phase. These alterations in cortical activity during the different phases could thus be considered a factor in the supposed characteristic cognitive and mood changes associated with the different phases (i.e. deterioration during the premenstrual phase and an improvement during menses).

## Hormones and the hippocampus

Some studies have focussed on the effects of circulating steroid hormones within the hippocampus, the structure strongly associated with certain kinds of learning and memory. Within this complex structure various regions have been associated with different aspects of learning and memory, the pyramidal cells within the CA1 subfield being particularly important. It was assumed that organisational effects early in development carved out certain neural circuits which were then simply modified in later life by the activational effects of certain hormones. In the 1960s, however, researchers observed that neurons

---

[2] Alpha, beta, delta, gamma and theta.

within the hippocampus of adult female rats appeared to be very sensitive to fluctuating levels of gonadal steroids. These fluctuations led to dramatic physiological alterations which were assumed to go beyond simple modifications of pre-organised circuits (cited in Gould *et al.*, 1990a). It is now realised that adult neuronal circuits may be more 'plastic' than previously supposed; this seems to be particularly the case with the dendrites (the information-receiving regions of the neuron).

A key feature of dendrites are small extensions extruding from the surface, referred to as 'dendritic spines', which have been observed to change shape, extend or disappear – dependent upon appropriate postnatal stimulation (or lack of). These outgrowths have been linked with learning and memory processing as they are capable of producing action potentials (called 'dendritic spikes') which in turn leads to the strengthening of the synapse, which is referred to as 'Long-Term Potentiation' (LTP). Magee and Johnston (1997) demonstrated that if a synaptic activation and a dendritic spike occurred simultaneously, then calcium 'hotspots' were created, and the size of the EPSP was increased. When they infused a substance called tetrodotoxin (which acts to block the ability of the spines to produce a spike), then long-term potentiation did not occur following stimulation. But what of the role of hormones?

Gould *et al.* (1990b) first ovariectomised eighteen adult female rats; several days later one batch of six received an injection of estradiol; the second batch received estradiol and then two days later an additional injection of progesterone (this mimics the normal proestrus phase of the cycle); the final batch received injections of a neutral substance. After death, brain slices of the hippocampus were investigated. In those animals that had been ovariectomised but then did not receive replacement gonadal steroids, a profound decrease in dendritic spine density in the CA1 region was observed. In those animals who had received estradiol replacement, the decrease did not occur; the addition of progesterone seemed to have an augmenting effect, preventing the decrease in a shorter time scale.

Wooley and McEwen (1992) took daily vaginal smears from normal female rats for two weeks. In those with a regular five-day estrus cycle hippocampal brain slices were taken at various stages of the cycle. A selective and rapid increase in synaptic density in the pyramidal cells was observed during the proestrus phase when levels of estradiol are rising sharply in readiness for ovulation. However, this did not appear to be due to an increase in dendritic branching. Another key factor is that within the hippocampus the major neurotransmitter is glutamate, and it has been shown that the activation of glutamate receptors, especially the ionotropic NMDA receptor, mediates the synaptic changes associated with learning and memory (e.g. Morris *et al.*, 1986).

Is it possible then that estradiol treatment alters the sensitivity of neurons to glutamate activation via the NMDA receptor. Weiland (1992) ovariectomised thirty female rats. In subsequent days, twenty of the sample received slow-releasing capsules of estradiol, and ten of these animals also received a subsequent injection of progesterone. The densities of NMDA agonist and antagonist sites were determined, in those animals treated with estradiol alone, and with estradiol plus progesterone the density of NMDA agonist binding sites in the CA1 field was significantly increased. Such an increase would enhance hippocampal sensitivity to glutamate activation; thereby estradiol and progesterone are capable of mediating the behavioural effects of these neurons. The AMPA receptors are also implicated in learning and memory, but it is difficult to assess their specific contribution, as blocking these receptors leads to a general shutdown of neuronal communication. It is likely that such receptors are involved in neuronal excitation related to learning (Riedel et al., 2003).

Thyroid hormones have also been shown to influence dendritic spine density in the hippocampal pyramidal cells. For example, neonatal hyper- and hypothyroidism lead to significant alterations in the structural development of the pyramidal cells in rats (e.g. Rami et al., 1986). One way in which the thyroid hormones may produce such changes is via an amino acid protein kinase called neurogranin (or RC3). This protein is present in dendritic spines and appears to play a role in the influx and mobilisation of calcium in the spines, and hence may be a factor in long-term potentiation. Hypothyroidism during the neonatal period leads to a reduction in levels of neurogranin in the cortex, striatum and hippocampus, but levels can be restored with injections of $T_4$ (Iñiguez et al., 1993). To compare the structural effects of hyperthyroidism on hippocampal cells, Gould et al. (1990a) injected seven adult female rats with $T_3$ for five consecutive days, and seven other females with a neutral substance. In the hyperthyroid animals, the density of dendritic spines in pyramidal cells of the CA1 field was significantly reduced in comparison to the control group. This suggests that, in rats at least, certain cells within the brain maintain their sensitivity to thyroid hormones into adulthood. As hyperthyroid states in adult humans also lead to profound behavioural/cognitive changes that can be readily treated by reducing thyroid hormone levels (Foley, 1990), we can thus perhaps assume that an excess of these hormones is having similar neurological effects (see later section).

Finally, the effects of adrenocorticotropic hormone (ACTH) and corticosterone administration in the pyramidal cells and dentate gyrus of the dorsal region of the hippocampus have been assessed using single-cell recording in freely moving female rats. The rats were either intact, or had been hypophysectomised. Infusions of corticosterone led to a decrease in hippocampal cellular activity, while injections of ACTH led to an increase in cellular activity, the effects of ACTH being faster but shorter-lived than the slower, but longer-lasting effects of corticosterone. These hormones thus have independent effects on hippocampal activity. As the effects of ACTH were seen in both intact and lesioned animals, the authors suggested that its effects are not mediated by the inhibition of pituitary ACTH release

(Pfaff *et al.*, 1971). These same glucocorticoids may also be important in brain aging in structures like the hippocampus. Landfield *et al.* (1981) pointed out that adrenalectomy has been associated with a reduction in brain aging, as this drastic action leads to an elevation of ACTH which, as we have just seen, acts as a neural stimulant. In their study middle-aged rats were either adrenalectomised and chronically maintained with appropriate hormones, or left intact but supplemented with one of two neural stimulants. A batch of undamaged young and old rats served as controls. They found that the drug treatment groups showed neurological and cognitive characteristics more like those of the young animals than the old animals. Indeed the young animals and drug-treated group performed significantly better on a maze-learning task.

## Hormonal effects on neurotransmitters

Strong comparisons have been drawn between the localisation of steroid hormone receptors and the anatomical distribution of various neurotransmitter pathways. Grant and Stumpf (1975), for example, pointed out the close overlap between estrogen receptors and adrenergic, dopaminergic and serotonergic pathways. Similarly, glucocorticoid receptors show the same relationship with these three systems. Not surprisingly then, the steroids and glucocorticoids have powerful effects on noradrenergic, dopaminergic and serotonergic neurons, as these hormones alter the electrical activity of target neurons and trigger or inhibit neurotransmitter release.

For example, estradiol treatment decreases the activity of glutamic acid decarboxylase (GAD) in the ventromedial nuclei of the hypothalamus in ovariectomised rats. This enzyme is a direct precursor of the inhibitory neurotransmitter GABA, and so estradiol may directly interfere with GABA efficacy (Wallis and Luttge, 1981; cited in Pfaff and McEwen, 1983). Csakvari *et al.* (2007) have now shown that cyclical hormonal fluctuations during the estrous cycle in female rats parallel alterations in the number of GABAergic synapses in the arcuate nucleus of the hypothalamus. These synapses show a significant decrease around estrous compared to other days of the cycle, and this decrease in GABAergic synapses is accompanied by an increase in dendritic spine synapses. Thus, there is a rapid and selective turnover of synapses within this nucleus that is directly related to hormonal fluctuations.

The thyroid hormones have particularly strong relationships with the catecholamines adrenaline (epinephrine) and noradrenaline (norepinephrine) as thyroid hormones increase the capacity of the cells to respond to the catecholamines (Silva, 2000). In addition, thyroid hormones affect cytokine release (cytokines are a diverse set of compounds acting like neurotransmitters within the immune system) and their release may result in the excessive release of dopamine and noradrenaline (Rasmussen, 2000).

Adrenocortical hormones affect the metabolism of serotonin, especially in the hypothalamus, hippocampus and midbrain structures; in general the glucocorticoid hormones facilitate the development of the serotonergic system (McEwen *et al.*, 1986). These hormones have a similar effect on the catecholamines. For example, in humans, levels of dopamine in the blood are increased following an injection of dexemethasone, a powerful synthetic glucocorticoid (Rothchild *et al.*, 1984) and researchers have speculated that these glucocorticoid-dependent alterations in dopamine may underlie various behavioural/neuropsychiatric conditions.

Alterations in neurotransmitter release can thus result in motivational, sensory, cognitive and emotional changes within the individual. This relationship is reciprocal, as neurotransmitters can influence hormone release. For example, acetylcholine stimulates oxytocin and vasopressin release from the posterior pituitary; noradrenaline and adrenaline prevent the release of these hormones; and dopamine stimulates vasopressin release (Brown, 1994). Various neurotransmitters influence hormone release from the adrenal glands, pineal gland and thyroid glands.

## Thyroid hormones and brain development

In their review of the role of thyroid hormones in neurodevelopment, Bernal and Nunez (1995) make the point that thyroid hormones are a key physiological regulator of brain development in mammals. They suggest that 'normal' levels are required during embryonic life to ensure that certain development events are coordinated via specific effects on cell differentiation, cell migration and gene expression. While major anatomical changes are not evident, the cytoarchitecture of the neocortex and cerebellum can be permanently disrupted by thyroid hormone deficiency. In particular, reductions in circulating thyroid hormones, or impairments in the cellular response to normal levels of these hormones during foetal development (hypothyroidism), lead to impairments in cell migration, outgrowths of neuronal processes, growth of the synapses (called 'synaptogenesis'), and formation of the protective myelin sheath; other processes such as the proliferation of glial cells at the expense of neurons (called 'gliosis') and neuronal cell death show an increase. Thus, a state of hypothyroidism can lead to profound physical and intellectual retardation in humans. While the early symptoms may be subtle (with growth deceleration being perhaps the only sign), if the condition is not treated within a few weeks after birth then permanent mental and physical retardation will result (Foley, 1990). Fortunately early screening programmes and standard medication in the form of oral thyroxine have all but eradicated this condition in developed countries.

In adults it was not thought that hypothyroidism would have that great an effect on the brain, as adult brain metabolism was assumed to be unresponsive to thyroid hormones. As pointed out by Smith and Ain (1995), this was perhaps due to the fact that early studies of patients with hypothyroidism had demonstrated impairments in cerebral blood flow, but no alterations in cerebral oxygen use or glucose uptake. In their study, they recruited ten hypothyroid patients and assessed brain metabolism when they were unmedicated, and again when they were receiving thyroxine replacement therapy. Overall brain metabolism was significantly reduced in the hypothyroid state, and this was reversed whilst receiving medication.

The alternative state of hyperthyroidism (called 'thyrotoxicosis') also has negative effects on the brain, as an increase in thyroid hormones leads to an overstimulation of various metabolic processes such as oxygen consumption, energy expenditure, and basal metabolic rate. Such changes have knock-on effects on brain function as cell mitochondria, NA+ and K+ gradients across the cell membrane, and lipid metabolism, are all affected. In addition, an excess of thyroid hormones influences pituitary-gonadal function, with serum testosterone and estradiol being raised (Franklyn, 2000). As we have already noted, an excess of thyroid hormones leads to classic clinical symptoms in response to the increased activity of the noradrenergic neurotransmitter system, specifically by influencing the metabotropic β-adrenergic receptors by increasing the availability of cyclic-AMP, or by enhancing its effects (Silva, 2000).

Despite the evidence that a gross excess or deficiency of thyroid hormones leads to neurological impairments, studies have been unable convincingly to demonstrate gross abnormalities in the brain, perhaps because imaging techniques were not sufficiently sensitive. Oatridge *et al.* (2002) performed highly detailed magnetic resonance imaging (MRI) on eight patients diagnosed with hyperthyroidism and three patients diagnosed with hypothyroidism, before and after appropriate treatment. Following treatment, brain size and ventricular system volume changed significantly; in the hyperthyroid group brain size decreased and ventricle volume increased as their condition reverted to a normal (euthyroid) state. The converse was seen in the hypothyroid group. Despite the small sample size, this study showed a clear correlation between changes in brain size and thyroid hormone levels. The authors speculated that the brain size alterations may have come about as a result of the unbalancing of water/sodium in the cells.

## Synthesising evidence for hormone–neuro interactions

Thus far I have discussed the nature and location of hormone receptors, and the effects of various hormones on brain development and neurotransmitter action. Evidence is now overwhelming that hormones have a profound influence on the structure and function of the brain, and scientists of course have focussed on such hormone–neuro–behavioural relationships.

As we shall see in subsequent chapters, attempts at linking hormonal activity with neural architecture/function and thence specific behaviours have been more or less successful in certain instances. The key problems seems to be that the evidence has been of a piecemeal nature and is often conflicting, and there are probably variables at work that we do not yet fully understand or even yet consider. In many instances what is lacking is a kind of grand theory that can unify all of the different strands of evidence and provide testable hypotheses. Some attempts have been made to synthesise the various strands to provide all-encompassing theories that attempt convincingly to link a hormone with a set of neural/physiological/behavioural outcomes, and in doing so provide a series of testable hypotheses. In subsequent chapters I shall provide examples of such theories and provide some critical evaluations of them.

# 5 **Typical sexual determination/ differentiation**

The initial question that nervous parents ask when they attend their first routine scan during pregnancy is usually 'is it a boy or a girl?' We attribute major significance to the sex of our offspring, and throughout their lives these males and females will forever be labelled accordingly, and provided with numerous 'rules' from various societal, legal and religious sources, that will govern their interactions with one another. It is not surprising then that one of the key questions that has enthralled behavioural endocrinologists and social scientists, in almost equal amounts, concerns that of sexual determination/differentiation – how genes initially determine sex, and then how a variety of factors (principally hormonal) cause the sexes to differentiate in terms of their morphology, physiology and, most controversially perhaps, behaviour and psychology. From a psychological perspective, the study of such sexual differentiation in relation to cognition, personality, mood, etc. has formed major research topics that even now are dogged by controversy, hyperbole and downright sensationalism.

Feelings always run high when the topic of sex differences rears its head. I write this shortly after the resignation of Harvard president Lawrence Summers, for, amongst other things, suggesting that females were biologically less predisposed than males to succeed in mathematics/science. In fact it is only fairly recently that one could even use the term 'sex' in the context of such differences, the word 'gender' being the more 'politically correct' term (many psychologists in fact confuse the two and don't appear to understand the difference between them!). The debate concerns whether observed sex differences in behaviour (some are large and consistent, at other times they are small and less robust) are the result of biological or social forces. Of course in all likelihood both probably make significant and interrelated contributions (Breedlove, 1994). I shall avoid lengthy debate on the political whys and wherefores of this debate and simply try to focus on the evidence, in this and the next two chapters looking at sexual determination/differentiation in typical populations and atypical populations, and then focussing upon neurological differentiation.

## Historical background

The ancient Greeks, not surprisingly, had pondered over the issue of how males and females come to be the way they are. Empedocles had put forward the idea of the existence of male and female seeds that somehow blend together in the womb. Hippocrates was responsible for a pangenetic theory of sexual differentiation, arguing that male and female seeds are present in all parts of the body, the brain and marrow being the original source of the seeds, but the testes were assumed as being their storage and release sites. Aristotle was better versed in anatomy, botany, zoology and physiology, and based his theories on first-hand observations. He was one of the first to offer what we would now call an epigenetic theory, i.e. the concept that physical/sexual differentiations gradually emerge during foetal development.

A crude form of endocrinological manipulation was of course castration, a barbaric practice routinely carried out on slaves, on defeated enemies and in the priesthood. Numerous scholars described the effects of castration in men and boys and noted that the effects were dependent upon the age at which the procedure had been conducted. A late removal of the testes (post-puberty) may lead to lack of sexual function and desire, loss of fertility, and changes in physical appearance; an early removal (pre-puberty) means that secondary sexual characteristics never appear at all. For example Galen, often regarded as the founding father of experimental physiology, noted in his *Peri Spermatos* that castrated human males lost their libido and power of procreation, but also showed changes in fat deposition, hair growth and vocal characteristics. Galen further stressed that castration affected not only the functioning of the genital organs, but certain other sexually determined characteristics as well – the lion's mane, cock's comb, boar's tusk, etc. (Medvei, 1993). In the 1800s Johann Autenrieth also described the effects of castration, noting that once the testes were removed then the beard disappeared, but if castration took place prior to beard development, then it did not grow at all. He also noted similar effects in females who had had their wombs removed – the monthly period disappeared (or did not start) and the breasts failed to secrete milk (Medvei, 1993).

From the end of the 1500s castration was routinely carried out (despite being illegal) under the auspices of the Roman Catholic church to preserve the unbroken male voice and provide castrati singers for its choirs.[1] While the practice declined within the church, such was the popularity of this mutilation that the voices of the castrati then came to dominate opera throughout much of Western Europe up until the end of the 1900s. The most famous of the castrati was Farinelli,[2] the last 'great' castrati Giovanni Veluti gave his final public rendition in 1829 in London, but it was not until 1922 that the

---

[1] Women were barred from singing in church.
[2] Nickname given to Carlo Broschi (1705–82).

last resident castrato in the Vatican (Alessandro Moreschi) passed away, his voice actually being preserved on a gramophone recording (Jenkins, 1998). Interestingly, the practice of castration for religious reasons remained relatively popular among certain groups, the Skoptsy religious sect in Russia, for example, having thousands of willing recruits in the latter part of the 1800s and the early 1900s (Tulpe and Torchinov, 2000).

The testes were thus assumed to be the driving force behind male sexual differentiation, and by the 1700s theories were beginning to resemble more modern-day conceptualisations. In 1786 John Hunter (whom we met in a previous chapter) added the study of freemartins to his already impressive endocrinological discoveries. A freemartin is a cow possessing normal external female genitalia but whose internal genitalia are abnormal, with fallopian tubes and uterus being poorly developed, and with male-typical structures and connections being in place. The animal thus appears to be partly masculinised and remains sterile. Hunter recognised that the condition only seemed to arise when the cow had shared a womb with a male twin (who developed normally) and this was confirmed by Tandler and Keller in 1911 as they noted that the twins shared a common placenta (and hence a common blood supply).

## Sexual determination/differentiation up to puberty

In recent years great advances have been made in biochemistry and molecular genetics that have enabled researchers to investigate more fully the interactions between genes, endocrine glands, and the hypothalamus and pituitary, which together trigger and maintain sexual determination and differentiation. 'Sex' refers to the biological qualities that distinguish between males and females. In humans, as in other species, it is taken for granted that there are two sexes that are normally conceptualised as being at the opposite ends of a continuum. However, this supposedly clear dichotomy is actually more complex than it first appears as these qualities can be expressed by a person's chromosomal, gonadal, morphological and hormonal characteristics (Migeon and Wisniewski, 1998). Individuals can in fact be differentiated in several ways:

- **Chromosomal sex**: Males usually have one X and one Y chromosome in their body cells while females usually have two Xs (exceptions to this will be discussed later). This is true for mammals but not however for fish, amphibians and birds, in which the females have a shorter chromosome, while the males have two longer chromosomes.
- **Gonadal sex**: Males usually have testes, seminal vesicles, prostate gland and associated tubing, while females usually have ovaries, uterus and oviducts.
- **Hormonal sex**: In most vertebrate species females produce a high estrogen to androgen ratio while the opposite is true of males.

- **Morphological sex**: Males are typically larger than females and possess a penis and scrotum. In non-human species there may also be differences in colouration and secondary sexual characteristics (e.g. horns, antlers).
- **Sexual orientation**: Most males are sexually attracted to females and vice versa.
- **Gender identity**: Most males have the deep inner conviction that they are male, and most women that they are female.

I will address all of these differentiations to varying degrees in this chapter and the next.

### From chromosomes to gonads

The starting point for sexual differentiation is purely genetic and involves the chromosomes. Recall that the normal human cell contains twenty-two autosomal pairs of chromosomes alongside a pair of sex chromosomes (one X and one Y, or two Xs). The female ovum always contains an X chromosome, but the sperm from the male can contain either an X or a Y. In the behavioural endocrinological literature, individuals are often thus described in terms of their chromosomal make-up – thus normal males are referred to as '46, XY', while normal females are referred to as '46, XX' (Angelopoulou *et al.*, 2006). This looks a little odd at first, but it can be informative when comparing between individuals who possess a different number of chromosomes or a different complement of Xs and Ys. This simple difference can thus provide an explanation for much of an individual's morphological (and arguably psychological) characteristics.

There is no difference in male and female morphology during the first six weeks after conception; each individual possesses undifferentiated anatomical structures (gonadal ridges, internal ducts, germ cells and the external genitals) which are referred to as 'bipotential' as they can subsequently assume either the masculine or the feminine form. A key structure is the 'mesenephros' (a protokidney) on which a ridge of tissue called the 'germinal ridge' begins as 'indifferent' – i.e. it is morphologically 'plastic' and can develop into a testis or an ovary. What sex you will become is then determined by the TDF (testis determining factor), a protein encoded by the SRY gene (sex determining region on the Y chromosome, provided by the father). If the SRY gene is expressed, then the germinal ridge will develop into a testis, but if it is not expressed then an ovary will form. As only males possess a Y chromosome, the basic blueprint is therefore female. Male development thus involves differentiation from this standard female pattern (Gustafson and Donahoe, 1994), and all individuals therefore begin life as 'female', a fact which may cause macho males some degree of consternation.

Partial expression of this gene results in incomplete gonadal differentiation, and thus perhaps an individual who displays physical characteristics intermediate between those of a male or a female, or perhaps characteristics of both sexes. In the past such individuals were called 'hermaphrodites'.[3] Nowadays the term 'intersex' is most commonly used to describe individuals who show varying degrees of discordance between the sex of their gonads, external genitalia and internal ducts (Migeon and Wisniewski, 1998). Goodfellow and Lovell-Badge (1993) demonstrated that male mice that do not have the SRY gene develop ovaries instead of testes; if the SRY gene is inserted into developing female mice then they develop testes instead of ovaries. Other genes that are structurally related to the SRY genes (SOX genes) also seem to be involved in testicular development, while the DAX 1 gene is expressed during ovarian development, but remains inert during testicular development (Hiort and Zitzmann, 2004). Another important substance is SF-1 (steroidogenic factor 1), a product of the FTZ1-F1 gene which seems to play an important role in the formation of steroid-secreting glands, as it is required for the synthesis of testosterone. It is expressed in male and female urogenital ridges, and in the Sertoli cells; mice lacking SF1 fail to develop gonads, adrenals and a hypothalamus (Ozisik *et al.*, 2003).

## From gonads to genitals

In humans, under the direction of the SRY and other genes, the gonad begins to differentiate as a testis between weeks 6 and 7 of gestation. TDF stimulates the Leydig cells to prevent the formation of the female genital tract from the Müllerian[4] ducts by a substance called Müllerian-inhibiting hormone (MIH), also referred to as Müllerian-inhibiting substance (MIS). Levels of this substance remain at high levels in the bloodstream in males for several years postnatally, and it is only at puberty that levels drop to a low baseline state; in contrast MIH is not detectable in newborn females, but is found in low doses from puberty onwards (Gustafson and Donahoe, 1994). The Leydig cells then synthesise and secrete testosterone and its metabolites (principally dihydrotestosterone), which enter the bloodstream and guide the development of the entire body in the male direction. Androgen concentrations rapidly rise and reach a peak between weeks 15 and 18 of gestation, and the key action of this hormone is to 'switch on' the Wolffian[5] duct which develops into male internal genitalia (epididymis, seminal vesicles, vas deferens and prostate gland). In the absence of the SRY gene, sexual differentiation does not occur; the Müllerian ducts form the fallopian tubes, uterus and upper portions of the vagina, and the Wolffian duct degenerates.

Up to around week 8 of foetal development there is no observable difference between the sexes in their external genitalia. Up to that point these bipotential structures can develop into genitalia of either sex. The sexually

[3] Derived from Hermaphroditus, the son of Hermes and Aphrodite in Greek mythology, who was fused with a nymph.
[4] Named after Johannes Müller (1801–58).
[5] Named after Caspar Friedrich Wolff (1734–94).

undifferentiated foetus possesses a urogenital sinus, surrounded by urogenital ridges, flanked by the genital folds forming an outgrowth called the genital tubercle. Testosterone produced by the Leydig cells is converted into the powerful dihydrotestosterone (DHT) via the actions of the enzyme 5α-reductase, and this causes the urethral groove to fuse, the genital tubercle to develop into a penis, and the labioscrotal swellings to form the scrotum. Androgens also inhibit the differentiation of the vagina. If the individual is not exposed to these androgens then the clitoris develops from the genital tubercle and the labia develop from the genital folds (Conte and Grumbach, 1997; Gustafson and Donahoe, 1994).

## From genitals to sexual development

Thus, from a bipotential individual, the actions of certain genes and then specific androgens serve to masculinise (and at the same time defeminise) the male foetus; in the absence of these genes (and thus androgens) the bipotential individual will continue in its normal developmental path and will display characteristic female internal and external genitalia (feminisation and demasculinisation). The female ovaries appear to secrete low levels of estrogens, which it was assumed only played a small role in sexual differentiation (see later section for further discussion of this point). This is based upon studies showing that removal of the ovaries did not have a major effect upon the developing female (Breedlove, 1994). Thus during the first twelve weeks of gestation, alterations in exposure to androgens (too little in males or too much in females), or impairments in the androgen receptor in the presence of normal levels of androgens, will lead to major alterations in sexual development in both sexes (see next chapter).

Note that this explanation only applies to mammals. In reptiles the SRY is not testis determining; instead, differentiation of the gonads is controlled by the temperature at which the eggs are incubated. In alligators and some lizards the foetus is bipotential and if the eggs are incubated at a high temperature then a male will develop, at a low temperature then a female will develop. In many species of turtle, however, these temperature effects are reversed, males being produced in low temperatures and females under high temperatures (Crews, 1994). In birds, males possess a pair of ZZ chromosomes while females possess a W and Z combination. The default setting appears to be male as the absence of gonadal steroids will lead to male development, while such steroids are required for the female to develop (Balthazart and Ball, 1995).

## Example: sexual differentiation in animals

As summarised by Arnold and Schlinger (1993), sexual differentiation is caused by the secretion of steroid hormones by the gonads early in development. In particular, the testes secrete testosterone in high amounts;

in the body and brain testosterone is metabolised to other forms (i.e. dihydrotestosterone), and these bind to steroid receptors which influence gene expression; in turn this influences the formation and maintenance of neural circuits underlying masculine/feminine behaviours. If the masculinising effects of testosterone do not occur (for whatever reason) then feminisation occurs instead. This well-established hypothesis is based upon a series of pioneering studies where hormonal states were experimentally manipulated in animals. The crucial importance of the presence or absence of testicular androgens for normal sexual development in mammals was initially shown by Hamilton and Gardner (1937), who gave androgens to female rats during pregnancy, and noted that their daughters were born with masculinised genitals. Jost (1970) reviewed a series of pioneering studies on rabbit foetuses he had conducted in the 1940s and 1950s. If the developing male rabbit was castrated before the genital tracts began to differentiate, then, in the absence of gonadal steroids, the Wolffian ducts failed to develop, while the Müllerian ducts continued to develop (as in females); the external genitalia also became feminised as these males lacked a scrotum, but developed a vagina and clitoris. If female rabbits were treated with androgens in the womb then the opposite effects occurred – the Wolffian duct developed and the genitals became masculinised; however the Müllerian ducts did not degenerate (as is normally seen in males). Jost thus speculated that androgens lead to masculinisation of the Wolffian duct and external genitals, but another substance (now known to be MIH) must be influencing the Müllerian ducts.

Phoenix *et al.* (1959) published a classic study on the effects of prenatal and early postnatal androgen treatment on both physiology and behaviour in guinea pigs. In many species, females and males show typical mating postures, with females standing immobile with arched backs (lordosis) and males exhibiting mounting behaviours. It was already established that castration of males early in development prevented mounting behaviour in adulthood, while testosterone administration to some of these castrated males restored mounting behaviour. It could be thus assumed that testosterone causes such behaviours, but testosterone administration to adult females does not produce mounting behaviours. Similarly estrogen administration to castrated males did not produce female-typical sexual behaviours – such behaviours are thus established early in development, with males becoming masculinised/defeminised and females becoming feminised/demasculinised.

Phoenix and colleagues administered testosterone to female guinea pigs during pregnancy, with some being given very high doses. At birth, the female offspring of high-dose mothers possessed male-typical external genitalia, while the offspring of mothers exposed to lower doses had normal female genitalia. In adulthood, all females and a group of males had their gonads removed, received androgen injections, and were paired with opposite-sex individuals. Androgens given to females early in life reduced lordosis in adult-hood, and led to displays of male-typical mounting behaviour. No effects were seen on male offspring. We will further evaluate the effects of hormones on sexual behaviours in chapter 8.

## Mechanisms of hormone action

A puzzling finding in many early animal studies was that estrogen (considered as having feminising/demasculinising influences) seemed to mimic the effects of androgens and actually have masculinising effects. For example, injections of estrogen before ten days of age in rats had a stronger masculinizing effect on physiology and behaviour than did injections of androgens (Booth, 1977). Sexual behaviour was abolished in male rats castrated neonatally, but these behaviours could be reinstated by injections of a synthetic estrogen such as diethylstilbestrol, or estradiol itself (e.g. Doughty *et al.*, 1975). In fact, testosterone exerts its masculinising effects by the fact that it is converted into estradiol via the enzyme aromatase, a process called 'aromatisation'. Testosterone can thus bind to both androgen and estrogen receptors (only in the presence of aromatase for the latter). Dihydrotestosterone is non-aromatisable and thus only acts via the androgen receptor. Not surprisingly then, aromatase is found in high concentrations in brain regions that also have high concentrations of estrogen receptors (MacLusky and Naftolin, 1981).

More significant in terms of evidence for its role in sexual differentiation is the finding that drugs that inhibit aromatase also interfere with the masculin-isation process; in addition, drugs which block the effects of estrogens (e.g. tamoxifen) block behavioural masculinisation and defeminisation in the rat (studies cited in Arnold and Schlinger, 1993). This strongly suggests that estro-gens and not androgens are the real cause of masculinisation. This then raises the tricky question of why females are not also masculinised by estradiol? The answer is a glycoprotein called alpha-fetoprotein (AFP) which is only pro-duced by the female foetus during the same stages of early development when testicular androgens are exerting their masculinising effects. This protein binds with molecules of estradiol and blocks most of it from entering the sen-sitive cells, but this protein has no effect upon testosterone (MacLusky and Naftolin, 1981). In the human female foetus AFP is produced by the liver, with peak levels being attained around the end of the third trimester, and then levels decline. It is excreted into the amniotic fluid and can thus cross the placenta into the mother's bloodstream. Levels in the mother mimic those of the foetus but are much lower and reach a peak around week 32. Levels of AFP are routinely determined by a test, as high levels can signify a foetal abnormality.

## The case of the spotted hyena

In the examples described above, it appears to be the case that sexual differentiation (both physical and behavioural) is entirely under the command of the foetal testes. One interesting case is the spotted hyena,[6] a pack-living animal native to the savannah and desert regions of Africa, regarded for many years by hunters as being hermaphrodite. This assumption was due to the fact that people would take one look at the pack and assume that all were male, and indeed notice that these 'males' also appeared to have sex with one another, and one of them would subsequently give birth! How did such misperceptions come about? The answer was provided by Watson (1877), who presented a detailed account of the reproductive organs of a female spotted hyena that had perished at London Zoo. He noted that the female did not possess a vagina but instead displayed an elongated penis-like organ, surrounded by a prepuce and having a glans perforated by a single urogenital canal; in addition, surrounding the anus were two small spheres giving the appearance of a scrotum. The penis-like structure is actually an erectile clitoris which projects forwards and downwards, measuring some 6½ inches (approx. 14 cm). Keen observers of these animals have noted, however, that it is possible to tell the sexes apart as the male penis is longer and thinner then the female clitoris, and has a more angular glans (the female 'glans' is more rounded). The female urinates, mates and gives birth through this pseudo-penis, the latter two actions providing a significant physical challenge to the male: as Watson coyly stated 'the mode of coupling of these animals also is worthy of observation, as, from what has been stated, it will be seen that the arrangement of the parts is not such as to facilitate this act' (Watson, 1877: 378). The internal reproductive organs, however, approximate those of a typical female mammal.

Glickman et al. (2005) have recently provided some updated information concerning sexual differentiation of physiology and behaviour in this animal (alongside information concerning elephants and tammar wallabies). During mating the clitoris is retracted, thus providing the male easier access. This retraction is under the voluntary control of the female and thus she belongs to one the few species in which it is impossible for a male to copulate forcibly with a female (the same being true for elephants). It was thus assumed (in line with evidence provided by Jost, Phoenix, etc.) that androgens acted strongly to masculinise the external genitals to make them assume a more masculine shape, and at the same time defeminise the female external genitals (causing the vagina to disappear). Some support for this was provided by Lindeque et al. (1986), who captured sixty specimens from different clans in Natal. Single blood samples were collected from fifty-two of the sample, and in the remainder serial samples were obtained every fifteen minutes. Concentrations

---

[6] Often called the 'laughing hyena'.

of both hormones were significantly higher in pregnant females compared to non-pregnant females, though no significant differences were revealed between concentrations of testosterone and androstenedione in adult males and females.

However, Cunha *et al.* (2005) established that the masculinised clitoris begins to take its characteristic shape well before the ovaries begin to differentiate and start secreting androstenedione. Another major problem for any 'androgen hypothesis' was that when anti-androgens (these prevent androgens from working) were administered to pregnant females on a daily basis starting from day 12 of gestation, no effects were seen on the development of the phallus and scrotal region. In fact, both male and female offspring developed a large phallus and fused scrotal region (typical of females). However, following such treatment the male offspring did display pronounced feminisation, in that the penis much more closely resembled the female clitoris than the usual male penis. In addition, they showed female-typical morphology in their CNS and hypothalamic-pituitary axis (Drea *et al.*, 1998). Glickman *et al.* (2005) suggested that the difference between the penis and the clitoris is thus androgen-dependent, contrary to initial predictions that females were being exposed to higher amounts of androgens during development than males. Both males and females receive androstenedione from their mother via the placenta, but during key stages of development this dose is supplemented by testicular androgens in the males, thus turning the clitoris into a penis.

In terms of social behaviour, spotted hyenas live in a matrilineal society in which females take the active social role, and whereby the offspring assume the rank of their mother at a kill. Females are larger than the males and more aggressive, and the males are totally subservient to them during social interactions (Frank, 1986). Again, it has been tempting to link such social behaviours with the effects of androgens, but the picture is clearly more complex than that, as young males can dominate adult immigrant males and lower-ranking adult females. Glickman *et al.* (2005) point out that the role of ovarian hormones on physiology and behaviour in this species remains to be fully determined.

So, it is an easy trap to fall into to assume that androgens primarily serve to masculinise and also defeminise the body (and brain), while if androgens are absent then the body and brain will continue being feminised. While there is in fact strong evidence for this supposition, McEwen (1981) pointed out the difficulties in this broad assumption by noting that there is considerable diversity within mammals, and even between different strains within the same species in terms of masculinising/defeminising effects of steroids. The hormonal mechanisms underlying such effects are also likely to show species differences; for example, defeminisation in rats appears to be mediated by the process of aromatisation at the estrogen receptors, but in rhesus monkeys masculinisation is via the androgen receptors. Indeed, defeminisation may not even occur in all mammals: as Arnold and Schlinger (1993) noted, the 'zebra finch is not just a flying rat'. One must therefore be cautious in explaining sexual differentiation. It is clear that we are still a long way from understanding this complex process.

## Genes, gonads or local action?

Established wisdom thus spoke of a two-process theory of sexual differentiation, the first process being genetic, the second hormonal (triggered by the first). Arnold (1996) pointed out that the gonads themselves are not differentiated by the actions of steroid hormones. If steroids are administered to either sex at various stages of development then there is little effect on the developing gonads. He thus concluded that 'sexual differentiation of the gonads is genetic, whereas sexual differentiation of the brain is hormonal' (1996: 496), though of course one could easily argue that since the primary factor is genetic, then all the subsequent mechanisms are genetic, as they are under the control of the genes. In birds, there are several lines of evidence to suggest that sexual differentiation is dependent not upon gonadal steroids but rather on the genes.

For example, the plumage of adult house sparrows is sexually dimorphic: males have black throat feathers while females have brown throat feathers. Mueller (1977) grafted patches of skin from young males to young females and vice versa before the dimorphism had developed, and noted that the feathers in the grafted section always develop into the colour of the donor but not of the recipient. If circulating hormones were responsible for altering feather colour then one would expect the feathers to display characteristics of the recipient. Plumage colour thus appears to be purely under genetic control, but it is difficult to be certain as hormonal secretions in the egg or shortly after hatching could of course play an important role. Many similar plumage-swapping studies have been conducted in the zebra finch, another species with sexually dimorphic plumage. Such studies (reviewed in Arnold, 1996) have involved various treatments with androgens, estrogens, anti-androgens and anti-estrogens, aromatase inhibitors, and combinations of each, to try and tease apart the relative contributions made by various steroids. In each case the plumage colour in the recipient remained that of its genetic sex. Certain neural regions were altered by steroid action, however.

More recently, an additional mechanism has been proposed specifically to account for brain sexual differentiation in songbirds. Schlinger *et al.* (2001) pointed out that some sexually dimorphic brain development can occur autonomously, independent of circulating hormones in the zebra finch. In studies cited in their review they describe a sexually dimorphic connection within the neural song system that may only develop in males due to the fact that estradiol is being synthesised in greater amounts directly within their brains. Powerful evidence for this stems from the finding that genetic females induced to develop with fully functioning testes, secreting normal amounts of androgens, fail to develop a masculinised song system. This, then, is a neurosteroid mechanism (chapter 2). It is still of course possible that genetic or hormonal events during very early development could later prime certain brain regions to be more responsive to local signals in the form of neurosteroids. So, at present we seem little nearer to unravelling the complex interplay between genes, gonads and neurosteroids. It suffices to say that the three mechanisms are undoubtedly important and most certainly related in a complex manner.

## The role of ovarian steroids

Thus far I have focussed on the significant role of testicular androgens in sexual differentiation, their role appearing to be to divert the developing male foetus away from the standard female blueprint and towards a male phenotype. The evidence in support of this hypothesis has mainly come from the effects of castration in males (demasculinising), and overexposure to testicular androgens in early development in females (masculinising). In addition, studies assessing the effects of ovariectomy in females typically showed that following such procedures female sexual differentiation proceeds as normal. The possible role of the ovarian steroids has thus tended to be overlooked, and some authors have even noted that 'the ovaries and their secretary products do not have a role in the differentiation process' (Svare and Kinsley, 1987).

However, Döhler et al. (1984a–c) pointed out that such conclusions were not that surprising, but are in fact based upon false assumptions: the ovaries are not in fact the main source of foetal estrogens; rather the foetal and maternal adrenal glands also secrete high amounts of estrogens over the course of gestation. Removing the ovaries does not thus completely remove circulating estrogens. An additional factor to consider is AFP. Recall that molecules of estrogen bind to AFP. While this means that the estrogen is unable to act at a biological level, it also means that these estrogens are able to circulate for much longer, and these 'bound' estrogens may be 'on call', and could be made biologically available if required. Indeed, these authors point out that AFP has been found within brain tissue. As it is not synthesised within the brain then it must have got there by some other means – i.e. transported there along with the estrogen it was bound to. Döhler et al. (1984a–c) described a series of studies involving the use of the potent estrogen antagonist tamoxifen.[7] The rationale for such studies was that if female differentiation genuinely occurs in the absence of estrogens then treatment of

---

[7] A popular and effective treatment for breast cancer.

females with tamoxifen should lead to defeminisation, and also perhaps masculinisation. Subsequent sexual behaviours did indeed appear to be defeminised but not masculinised. Under estrogen-free conditions, then, normal female sexual differentiation is impaired.

More recently, Fitch and Denenberg (1998) also assessed evidence that estrogen plays a role in sexual differentiation. They note that AFP (in rats) seems to 'switch off' around postnatal day 7 and is followed by a rise in estrogen, thus providing a possible window of opportunity for ovarian estrogens to exert differentiating effects, which may not become evident until after puberty. Some researchers have noted, for example, that certain components of female sexual behaviour are enhanced following estrogen priming in animals who have been ovariectomised after puberty, compared to a group of females ovariectomised neonatally (e.g. Gerall *et al.*, 1973). Interestingly, a group of male rats gonadectomised neonatally, and who then received ovarian transplants or treatment with estrogen at puberty, displayed characteristic female sexual behaviours. In support of this, some studies have compared differences in brain morphology between groups of rats treated with different hormonal regimes. For example, in a series of studies Bloch and Gorski (1988) have pointed out that the anteroventral preoptic nucleus in the hypothalamus (AVPv) is normally much larger in females than in males. If males are castrated postnatally and then treated with combined low doses of estrogen plus progesterone then this structure becomes comparable in size to that of a normal female; males who were simply castrated did not show these morphological changes.

We have already seen that spine density in the hippocampus of the female rat is regulated by the hormonal changes during the estrous cycle (chapter 4). In a similar manner it has been reported that dendritic spine density in the ventromedial hypothalamus also varies across the cycle; ovariectomy in adulthood reduces this density, while estrogen and progesterone replacement therapy increase spine density (Frankfurt *et al.*, 1990). While Fitch and Denenberg (1998) admit that such evidence is more fitting for an activational hypothesis of steroid function, they point out that such evidence strongly indicates that ovarian steroids are capable of modifying neural structures. Of greater relevance is the finding that estrogen and progesterone during the early postnatal phase (when organisational effects are still underway) exert different developmental effects on cortical thickness in female rat brains – estrogen leads to a thinner cortex while progesterone serves to thicken it (Pappas *et al.*, 1979).

Fitch and Denenberg (1998) concluded that feminisation is a process which occurs in tandem with masculinisation. They speculate that the two processes may have common hormonal underpinnings (gonadal steroids) but these are qualitatively different and operate during different stages of development. It is assumed that, for normal sexual differentiation to take place, males must be exposed to testosterone and its metabolites during foetal life and the early postnatal period (in rodents this crucial stage seems to be from foetal day 17 to postnatal day 10). For feminisation to occur in females they also need exposure to estrogens and progesterone during a later period, which may even extend into puberty and beyond. In the open peer commentary following their review, Halpern (1998) reminds us to consider the facts that gonadal hormones do not act independently, but interact with one another, and, perhaps more significantly, also interact with the environment. There are thus possibly multiple answers concerning sexual differentiation, and the adoption of univariate answers is thus perhaps overly simple.

## Models of hormone action

The preceding sections have laid out a variety of possible hormonal actions that are related to sexual differentiation. The classic view has been that testicular hormones serve both to masculinise and to defeminise the body, brain and behaviour, while lack of exposure to these hormones is necessary for feminisation and demasculinisation (Goy and McEwen, 1980; Naftolin, 1981). However, as we have seen, ovarian secretions may also play some role in this process, so the explanation thus offered is far from complete. In their extensive review Collaer and Hines (1995) provide several theoretical models which could explain the observed influences of gonadal hormones on human behavioural sex differences.

The first model is called the 'Passive Feminisation Model' and reflects the classic view already described in that it assumes that testicular hormones masculinise and defeminise, while the ovarian steroids contribute little to sexual differentiation. In the absence of testicular steroids the individual will become feminised and demasculinised. Their second model, called the 'Gradient Model', is a modification of the first model in that testicular hormones are still assumed to masculinise and defeminise but that ovarian estrogens also cause some degree of masculinisation and defeminisation. Their third model is called the 'Active Feminisation Model' and this is derived from suggestions that ovarian hormones (most probably estrogens) serve to feminise and demasculinise. Testicular hormones are still assumed to masculinise and defeminise. At the end of their review (which focusses on human behavioural sex differences) they conclude that the evidence is still not sufficient to determine which of the models is likely to be correct and that all to some degree fit the data they present (some of these data will be reviewed in this and the next chapter). Of course it could be that all of the models are correct to some degree as it is possible that sexual differentiation may involve not a single underlying mechanism, but rather several different mechanisms operating for physical, neural and behavioural characteristics.

## Human psychosexual differentiation

In the preceding sections I have addressed the hormonal influences on physical sexual differentiation in some detail, but of key interest to psychologists are the processes which underlie psychosexual differentiation – namely the development of gender identity, gender role and sexuality. In humans 'gender identity' can be described as the gender with which an individual identifies him/herself. This is the personal manifestation of 'gender role', the behaviours, attitudes and personality traits which, within a given society, are ascribed to, or expected from, individuals of one sex or another (Cohen-Kettenis and Pfäfflin, 2003). For an individual to have a gender role, then, they must first be capable of differentiating between the genders. Studies using the habituation paradigm have attempted to see if very young infants can indeed tell the difference between the sexes. In one example, Fagot and Leinbach (1993) showed nine-month-old babies a series of faces from one gender group. The babies soon lost interest in this task, but when a face from a different gender appeared in front of them then their level of interest was reawakened, and they looked (fixated) at the new stimulus for longer. This showed that these infants were capable of discriminating between the sexes.

Children soon learn to identify their own gender, and understand that this is a stable feature of their life, and that gender is a permanent factor not dependent upon one's physical appearance or choice of activities. Children rapidly learn gender stereotypes, with such knowledge developing around the age of three and increasing rapidly thereafter. Once such gender stereotypes are established, they can influence the way new information is processed. Children rapidly come to the understanding that gender is not a neutral term, but rather brings with it an array of affective meanings and values that can be placed on the sexes. Social learning theorists have provided a great deal of information on how children learn about gender by observing the actions of peers and family, and by the portrayal of the sexes in the media. Despite the undoubted effects of external influences on perceptions of one's own and other people's gender, it would be surprising, given what we have already discovered about the effects of hormones on physical differentiation, if the same substances did not play some role in the social manifestations of biological sex.

It would be ideal, of course, to be able to have a measure of foetal hormone exposure as well as circulating hormone levels post-birth, in order to be able to tease out possible influences of organisational versus activational effects on subsequent gender behaviour. Udry *et al.* (1995) were fortunate enough to obtain frozen serum samples obtained from pregnant women who were taking part in a large-scale study of child health and development. The authors interviewed the female offspring when they were aged in their late twenties to early thirties to assess gender behaviour, and also obtained measures of circulating androgens. Adult testosterone and androstenedione were significantly inversely correlated with gender score (made up of nineteen independent measures) – a high feminine score was associated with low circulating androgens. In addition, maternal androgen exposure in the second trimester of pregnancy (as assessed by levels of SHBG) was significantly related to more masculinised gender behaviours. The authors concluded that adult gender behaviour was related to the maternal hormonal environment but also to circulating androgen levels in the individual.

In a similar study Hines *et al.* (2002a) took maternal levels of testosterone and SHBG from around week 16 of gestation and compared these values with gender role behaviours in 342 male and 337 female children aged around three and a half. They predicted that higher levels of prenatal testosterone (or lower levels of SHBG) would be associated with more masculine-typical gender role behaviours, especially in the female offspring. Gender role was assessed by the PSAI (Pre-School Activities Inventory), a questionnaire in which carers indicate the child's involvement in certain sex-typical behaviours (e.g. playing with sex-typical toys). On the basis of their scores the children were classified as either 'extremely', 'moderately' or 'low' masculine/feminine, and these six groups were then compared in terms of prenatal hormone exposure. For the girls, a significant relationship between maternal testosterone and behaviour was found, with the more masculine girls being exposed to higher levels of testosterone *in utero*. There was no relationship between maternal testosterone and boys' gender role behaviours.

As other background variables (e.g. maternal education, presence of older brothers, parental adherence to traditional sex roles, etc.) did not appear to play a significant role, the authors concluded that testosterone exposure during pregnancy has a key influence on the expression of masculine gender behaviours in girls. One could ask why such relationships did not hold for boys – as they demonstrated differences in their degree of gender role behaviours, then why was this also not related to prenatal testosterone? The authors addressed this issue by pointing out two possible explanations for the more consistent relationship between variability in prenatal hormone exposure and postnatal gender behaviour in girls but not boys. First, studies have consistently demonstrated that the male foetus is exposed to much higher levels of testosterone (from their own testes and from their mother) than the female foetus. Normal maternal variability in testosterone may therefore be of less significance in comparison to the high levels of testosterone experienced by most males. For females, however, they are exposed to much lower levels, and any fluctuations in maternal testosterone might therefore have significant masculinising effects. Secondly, studies (e.g. Fagot, 1978) have demonstrated that boys are more strongly encouraged to conform to gender-typical stereotypes, and thus girls may be more likely to display hormone-related gender atypical behaviours because such predispositions are less likely to be countered by other social influences.

In a study apparently involving the same participants, however, Hines *et al.* (2002b) provided contradictory evidence to their paper previously discussed. Here their focus was on maternal perceptions of stress in relation to gender role behaviours in their offspring, the rationale being that prenatal stress leads to hormonal changes that influence gender development. This hypothesis (to be discussed in more detail in the next chapter) was derived from rodent studies showing that if female rats are stressed during pregnancy their male offspring show reduced masculine-typical, but increased feminine-typical behaviours (e.g. Ward, 1972). Mothers completed a stress questionnaire at eighteen weeks of gestation, and eight weeks postnatal, and this stress score showed a small relationship to gender role behaviour in the female children, with higher stress being related to higher masculine gender scores. No relationship was seen in males. In both sexes, however, key variables such as maternal education, presence of older brothers and sisters, parental adherence to traditional sex roles, etc. made significant contributions to the child's sex role behaviours. Obviously, more work is required to assess the relative contributions of hormonal versus environmental factors to gender role identity in children.

The final examples concern possible relationships between organisational levels of sex steroids (as assessed by 2D:4D ratio) and scores on a measure of self-perceived gender: the Bem Sex Role Inventory (BSRI) is a commonly used questionnaire assessing gender identity, which requires the person to indicate how well each characteristic fits his or her own self-perception (there are twenty male, twenty female and twenty neutral items). Csathó *et al.* (2003) examined 2D:4D and performance on the BSRI in forty-six adult females. On the basis of their scores the women were characterised as either 'masculine' or 'feminine', and these groups were compared on 2D:4D ratio. The more masculine sex type was associated with a more masculinised (lower) finger length ratio; the more feminine sex type was associated with the feminised (higher) ratio. In a much larger sample, Rammsayer and Troche (2007) assessed the same variables in 423 male and 312 female university students. While there was no relationship between 2D:4D and female gender-role orientation, in the male sample those with a higher (more feminine) ratio scored higher on the 'feminine' items.

It must be pointed out, though, that a problem for all studies using such self-report measures of gender role is that other researchers have pointed out that they may not actually be measuring what they are supposed to be measuring (e.g. Lubinski *et al.*, 1983). Much better, of course, is to focus on behaviours that are more amenable to objective analysis. An example here is that of gender-linked play and toy behaviours. There is a large and robust sex difference in terms of toy preferences, with girls preferring toys such as dolls while boys prefer toys such as vehicles and balls (Alexander and Hines, 1994). Such preferences emerge early in childhood and are undoubtedly influenced by gender socialisation. However, such preferences have also been noted in monkeys (studies cited in Alexander, 2006) and are presumably not created by gender-related socialisation processes. Alexander (2006) gained retrospective reports from thirty-five adult males and twenty-nine females of their gender-linked childhood activities using the PSAI. They measured 2D:4D and assessed preferences for toys using the novel technique of eye-tracking – pairs of gender-linked toys (e.g. a ball and a doll) appeared on a computer screen and the number of visual fixations to them were recorded. The assumption is that greater preference for one over the other is dependent upon the number of fixations each receives. As predicted, males showed a clear preference for masculine toys, and females for feminine toys, and interestingly those individuals with lower, more masculinised 2D:4D ratios (irrespective of gender) showed a greater preference for masculine toys. Obviously, similar studies conducted in children may shed further light on prenatal influences on gender-linked toy preferences.

## Sexual differentiation at puberty

After an interval of relative hormonal inactivity throughout child-hood, the hypothalamus shows a marked increase in activity in the period up to and including puberty, which leads to a dramatic surge in pituitary gonadotropins and thence sex steroids, which bring about the characteristic morphological changes associated with puberty. In particular, pulses of gonadotropin-releasing hormone (GnRH) trigger the anterior pituitary gland to secrete luteinising hormone (LH) and follicle-stimulating hormone (FSH). In males LH stimulates the Leydig cells in the testes to secrete testosterone, and FSH stimulates the Sertoli cells to produce inhibin, which feeds back to inhibit FSH. In females, LH triggers ovulation at menarche and FSH stimulates the granulosa cells in the ovaries to produce estrogen (promoting breast development) and the follicles to produce inhibin. In prepubertal children GnRH secretion increases during the early stages of sleep, with peaks of LH and FSH occurring several hours later. As puberty progresses there is little diurnal variation, and levels of LH and FSH remain constantly high. Gonadal hormone secretion follow the same pattern (Styne, 1997).

In addition the adrenal cortex secretes dehydroepiandrosterone (DHEA), its sulfate (DHEAS) and androstenedione in increasing levels as puberty approaches. This commences at around the age of six to seven in girls and seven to eight in boys, but what triggers this process remains as yet unknown. This is called 'adrenarche', and some of the physical effects include increased sweat production, oily skin, pubic hair growth, acne and body odour; as these coincide with pubertal increase in sex steroids it is still not certain which hormone relates to which process. In both sexes, males and females also show a growth spurt which is under complex endocrine control, including the thyroid gland, growth hormone, and IGF-1 (insulin-like growth factor) produced by the liver in response to direct and indirect stimulation by the sex steroids. An objective assessment of puberty is provided by the 'Tanner stages'[8] – a five-stage definition covering physical measurements of developments (e.g. pubic hair) on external primary and secondary sexual characteristics. Three specific examples of the role of pubertal hormones on physical sexual differentiation are provided below.

## Body shape

Changes in body composition are also apparent, as prepubertal girls and boys have an equally lean body mass, but postpuberty males demonstrate more lean mass, skeletal mass and muscle mass, while females have twice as much body fat (Styne, 1997). This leads to characteristic morphological changes in male and female bodies which make them readily identifiable as typically male or female (android versus gynoid body shapes respectively). Females show a marked change in their waist-to-hip ratio (WHR), a standard morphometric measure assessed by measuring the waist at its narrowest point, the hip at the level of the buttocks, and dividing the former by the latter. The typical female WHR becomes significantly lower than that of the male, ranging between 0.67–0.80; while the typical male range is 0.85–0.95 (Singh, 1993). The WHR is unique to human females and may be an adaptation signalling fertility. Body fat distribution as assessed by WHR is correlated with pubertal endocrinological activity, as well as the probability of successful conception in females receiving artificial insemination (DeRidder et al., 1990; Zaastra et al., 1993).

   In contrast, males deposit adipose and muscle tissue on their upper body and thus demonstrate an inverted-triangle shape, with broad chest and shoulders and a narrow waist, the measurement of which can be assessed by taking the waist-to-chest ratio (WCR), the waist circumference divided by the chest circumference. Direct links between body fat distribution and hormones have been shown in studies assessing the effects of exogenous hormone administration to various patient groups. For example, Vague et al. (1984) showed that male to female transsexuals given estrogen supplementation as part of their treatment develop a gynoid fat distribution, while female to male transsexuals given testosterone develop an android body shape. Elderly males prescribed testosterone supplementation demonstrated increases in their WHR and lean body mass (e.g. Vermeulen et al., 1999).

   Testosterone alters body composition by promoting lean mass over fat mass, the assumption being that this occurs at puberty solely in response to activational mechanisms. There has been speculation as to the possible role of hormones at the organisational (i.e. prenatal) phase on subsequent body mass at puberty. McIntyre et al. (2003) employed the 2D:4D ratio to explore

---

[8] Named after the paediatrician James Tanner.

possible prenatal androgen effects on abdominal adiposity in middle-aged men. Prenatal androgen exposure was related to waist circumference in middle-aged men, with higher prenatal levels being associated with an increase in the proportion of abdominal fat. However the sample consisted of gay men (whose finger length ratios may differ from heterosexual males – see next chapter), and more worrying was the fact that participants conducted the anthropometric assessments on themselves. Fink *et al.* (2003) also assessed relationships between 2D:4D and morphology in heterosexual males and female in their twenties, with the aim of determining to what extent adult sexually dimorphic physical traits determined at puberty relate to traits determined *in utero*. In males, only body mass index (BMI) was related to left-hand 2D:4D (higher ratio = higher BMI); in females a lower (more masculine) ratio in both hands was associated with a higher WCR, chest circumference and hip circumference – thus androgenisation before birth may lead to a more masculinised body shape during puberty in females.

## Bone metabolism

A key sexual dimorphism at puberty is that of body size, as males on average are taller then females. Another key dimorphism relates to face shape (telling male and female faces apart is much easier after puberty) as testosterone is thought to affect a number of facial features, in particular the lateral growth of the cheekbones, jawbone and chin, the forward growth of the eyebrow ridges, and the lengthening of the lower face, leading to a more robust face shape. The absence of androgens, or the presence of estrogens, is thought to lead to a more gracile face shape with high eyebrows, smaller and more rounded jaw line and fuller lips (Enlow, 1996). Both dimorphisms are thought to derive from differences in bone growth which is mediated by cells called osteoblasts (derived from the Greek words for 'bone' and 'embryonic'). The complementary process of bone resorption is mediated by osteoclasts (derived from the Greek words for 'bone' and 'broken'). Their relationship is complementary such that bone renewal and turnover are held fairly constant.

Receptors for androgens and estrogens are found in both types of cell, with androgens increasing the proliferation and differentiation of osteoblasts (Kasperk *et al.*, 1997). Some effects of testosterone on bone tissue may also be facilitated in an indirect manner by growth hormone and IGF-1; both of these substances act to increase bone mass and density. As aromatase and 5α-reductase are found in bone tissue, it is likely that testosterone may have its effects after being converted to an estrogen, or to dihydrotestosterone (Kung, 2003). Estrogens increase osteoblast formation, differentiation and proliferation, but decrease osteoclast formation. This is the key reason why menopausal females are prone to osteoporosis (a condition leading to a reduction in bone mineral density and hence to an increased likelihood of bone fracture). Elderly males also lose considerable bone mass, but as their bones are typically longer and thicker to begin with this is less of a problem for them. During puberty boys acquire around 25% greater peak bone mass compared to girls, and this is due to greater bone size, as testosterone particularly promotes growth in the long bones of the arms and legs (Seeman, 1997).

The effects of hormones on bone development have been assessed in experimental animals, with the most straightforward technique involving the castration of male animals (usually rodents). In younger male rats orchidectomy leads to a reduction of calcium in the long bones and an increase in osteoclasts, leading to a significant loss of bone tissue. Such effects can be prevented by the administration of aromatisable or non-aromatisable androgens (studies cited in Zitzmann and Nieschlag, 2004). As stated previously, estrogen is also important, as knock-out mice models in which individuals have been bred to lack one or both types of estrogen receptor have demonstrated a decrease in bone growth in animals lacking the ER$\alpha$ receptor.

In human males whose testes do not produce sufficient levels of androgens (they are referred to as hypogonadal) several studies have shown that testosterone administration enhances markers of bone growth. When treatment was stopped, then levels of these markers also dropped (e.g. Wang *et al.*, 2001). As in the mice studies, human males who have mutations in the ER$\alpha$ receptor or aromatase genes fail to develop normal bone density despite having circulating testosterone levels in the normal or high range (e.g. Grumbach, 2000). Falahati-Nini *et al.* (2000) conducted an ingenious study in order to assess the relative contributions of estrogen and testosterone on bone turnover. They took a sample of otherwise healthy elderly males and rendered them temporarily hypogonadal by a GnRH agonist, while at the same time blocking the conversion of androgens to estrogens by administering an aromatase inhibitor. The volunteers then received replacement doses of testosterone and then estrogen. While testosterone had a modest effect on bone resorption, estrogen showed a much stronger effect; both hormones had a similar effect on bone formation.

In boys without obvious gonadal dysfunction, delayed growth and puberty are the commonest reasons for them to be referred to endocrine clinics, and androgenic steroids are routinely administered until endogenous puberty advances sufficiently. In one study, Mayo *et al.* (2004) conducted a randomised crossover, assessing the effects of newly devised testosterone skin patches worn overnight (oral and injected supplementations are usually unpopular) on eight boys referred for pubertal delay. Hormone profiles were continually taken over the two eight-week treatment periods and various anthropometric measures recorded. Significant changes in circulating testosterone were observed, as were sustained improvements in growth and bone formation. A potential problem is that androgen supplementation may lead to excessive growth in the bones of the face and jaw. In rats, for example, Noda *et al.* (1994) had established that injections of an anabolic steroid to young female rats accelerated craniofacial growth, significantly increasing the total skull length. In a study of boys with delayed puberty, Verdonck *et al.* (1999) monitored craniofacial growth following testosterone supplementation therapy over a six-month period. Compared to a control group of age-matched boys going through normal puberty, the supplementation group showed accelerated facial bone growth. However, as the treatment group had demonstrated significantly shorter facial bone development prior to treatment, the effect of this treatment was simply to bring them up to normal facial growth standards. After one year of assessments the delayed-puberty boys displayed completely normal craniofacial measurements.

As reported previously, some studies have assessed possible links between the prenatal hormonal environment (by markers such as 2D:4D) and subsequent bodily characteristics at puberty. Fink *et al.* (2005) hypothesised that individuals with a low (masculinised) 2D:4D ratio might display facial characteristics judged to be more 'robust' and masculine than those with the higher (more feminised) ratios. In their study, 2D:4D and frontal facial photographs were taken in fifty males and fifty-six females. Facial shape was analysed by placing sixty-four predetermined feature points on each face. These landmarks were subsequently analysed by a geometric morphometric toolkit, with the result that shape regression of the landmarks upon 2D:4D could be calculated. They found that for both male and female faces some facial characteristics regarded as 'typically' male corresponded to lower finger length ratios while typical female features corresponded to higher finger ratios.

## The voice

A final sexual dimorphism which becomes transparent during puberty (often embarrassingly so) is to do with the characteristics of the voice, the 'breaking' of the voice being a key indicator of pubertal change in males. The principal structure is that of the larynx, an organ in the neck consisting of a framework of cartilage with surrounding soft tissue, which plays a crucial role in breathing and speech production. The anterior (or forward-facing) portion of the larynx can often be seen in the neck as it protrudes to form the laryngeal prominence (or Adam's apple). In the centre of the larynx are the vocal folds (otherwise known as the vocal cords), a V-shaped muscle which opens the airways during breathing, and the air vibrating over the vocal folds produces sounds which are then modified by the vocal tract to produce our characteristic speech sounds. There are two acoustic components to the human voice: fundamental frequency (pitch) determined by the vibration of the vocal folds, and formant frequencies, which are determined by the size and shape of the vocal tract, and by movement of the articulators (tongue, lips, etc.). The average adult male voice has a much lower fundamental frequency than that of an adult female owing to the actions of testosterone permanently lengthening and thickening the vocal folds: they reach around 23 mm in adult males and 17 mm in adult females, compared to 5 mm in prepubertal children (Abitbol *et al.*, 1999). There is also a simultaneous but independent descent of the larynx, resulting in a lowering of mean formant frequency (Fitch and Giedd, 1999).

Up to puberty, male and female voices are very similar in terms of fundamental and formant frequencies, but as puberty approaches then the voice in both sexes begins to change. Vuorenkoski *et al.* (1978) found that between the ages of eight and ten (before puberty had started) fundamental frequency fell from 259 Hz to 247 Hz in boys but not in girls (253 Hz), lowest fundamental frequency fell from 234 Hz to 203 Hz in boys, and in girls from 230 Hz to 218 Hz, and a sex difference became apparent. During puberty, male voices dropped further to around 100 Hz and female voices also fell to around 213 Hz. In a longitudinal study Hollien *et al.* (1994) tracked vocal and physical changes in forty-eight boys over a five-year period, covering pre- and postpuberty. The preadolescent group (twelve years old) displayed a fundamental frequency typical of a child (around 233 Hz); by the age of thirteen and a half this frequency had dropped to a mean of 174 Hz, and in the postadolescent period (nearly fifteen years old) voice pitch had dropped to around 122 Hz, a level almost equivalent to that of most adult men (around 100 Hz).

Animal studies have shown that androgen stimulation has direct effects upon the larynx which leads to such changes. For example, Beckford *et al.* (1985) castrated forty-two rams at around two months of age. Upon recovery they were assigned to various treatment groups to assess different hormone regimens (including low doses of testosterone, high doses of testosterone, etc.). After treatment their larynges were studied, and in short, the higher the dose of testosterone the greater the laryngeal changes, especially in the thyroid cartilage. The same structure appears to undergo similar changes during puberty in humans. Kahane (1982) described preadolescent and adolescent laryngeal growth changes in twenty human cadavers aged nine to nineteen. The most striking developmental change was the development of the thyroid cartilage, which enlarged three times as much in males as in females over the course of puberty. The vocal folds also demonstrated significant growth in males, increasing by 63% from prepuberty to puberty (female growth was 34% over the same period). In 129 live individuals Fitch and Giedd (1999) assessed the development of the vocal tract using MRI. They found a significant difference between male and female vocal tract morphology, notably in the length of the vocal tract and in the relative proportions of the oral and pharyngeal cavities, which were not evident in children.

As regards associations between hormonal changes and vocal tract development, Harries *et al.* (1997) recorded both singing and speaking frequencies over a period of twelve months in a group of thirteen to fourteen-year-old boys passing through the established Tanner stages of puberty. Salivary testosterone was also measured, and abrupt vocal changes were observed between Tanner stages III and IV. While circulating testosterone levels did not appear to be related to these changes, testicular volume was – the larger the volume, the lower the voice pitch. Males with clinical impairments in gonadotropin secretion (e.g. idiopathic hypogonadotropic hypogonadism: IHH – see next chapter) do not achieve sexual maturation without exogenous androgen supplementation. Akcam *et al.* (2004) followed such a group of twenty-four IHH patients and compared their voices pre- and post-androgen treatment with normal males and females (who were not receiving any treatment). Pre-treatment the IHH males displayed a mean fundamental frequency of 229 Hz, a value intermediate between the normal males and females (150 Hz and 256 Hz respectively). Following three months of androgen therapy mean voice pitch had fallen to 173 Hz, though serum hormone levels did not directly correlate with voice pitch.

In females the absence of circulating androgens during puberty thus leads to a characteristic female voice and the introduction of such hormones at any point in a female's life will lead to a permanent (masculine) change to her voice. However, hormonal changes during the normal menstrual cycle can influence the female voice. Abitbol *et al.* (1999) point out that estrogens and progesterone lead to thickening of the laryngeal mucosa and dryness of the vocal folds just prior to menses, leading to what they refer to as a 'premenstrual vocal syndrome' characterised by vocal fatigue, decreased range and a huskier voice. Such changes may be more pronounced in women who suffer from premenstrual syndrome (Chae *et al.*, 2001). During the menopause, the production of estrogens and progesterone stops, but circulating androgens remain free to have some vocal effects (this can be dependent upon body morphology) – one being to thicken the vocal folds and produce a more masculine-sounding voice.

As vocal changes appear to be completed after puberty there is no reason to suppose that voice pitch will show any relationship to circulating androgen levels later in life. However, Dabbs and Mallinger (1999) measured salivary testosterone in sixty-one male and eighty-eight female college students. They found that higher levels of circulating testosterone were indeed related to lower voice pitch in the males, but not in the females. The authors provided two explanations, the first a physiological one relating to physical effects of testosterone on the vocal apparatus, the second a psychological one relating to the assumption that higher-testosterone males might deliberately adopt a lower voice pitch to reflect their social dominance status. As this study only took one sample of testosterone and did not appear to control for time of day then such results remain unconfirmed. More recently Bruckert *et al.* (2006) have also reported that salivary testosterone levels in young adults are significantly associated with voice pitch – higher testosterone = lower pitch – but as they used a cotton-based material to collect the samples (for problems with this method see chapter 2), only took one sample, and did not control for time of day, then again this relationship remains unproven.

# 6 Atypical sexual differentiation

As I have explained in the previous chapter, at a very basic level normal sexual differentiation seems to be a two-part process. For an embryo to develop into a female then it must become both feminised and demasculinised; normal male development on the other hand depends upon both masculinisation and defeminisation. There are many stages to this complex process and at each stage errors can occur. It is therefore likely that while most individuals will be strongly physically and behaviourally masculinised/defeminised or feminised/demasculinised, some may only partly develop these characteristics, either at a neurological, physical or behavioural level, or at all levels. Research questions concerning the role of the gonadal steroids in sexual differentiation in humans cannot of course be directly tested because of ethical considerations; however, certain developmental quirks have cast considerable light upon sexual differentiation in our species. Specifically, such conditions have enabled researchers to try to ascertain the possible effects of the pre- and perinatal hormonal environment upon subsequent psychosexual differentiation. There are a considerable number of such abnormalities and a thorough discussion of each is beyond the scope of this text. I will instead focus upon the main syndromes that have provided important information not only concerning physical sexual differentiation, but, of key interest to this text, also concerning psychological (gender) differentiation (chapter 11 will discuss cognitive characteristics observed in such syndromes).

## Congenital adrenal hyperplasia (CAH)

There are six different types of CAH (also referred to as adrenogenital syndrome) but all share the same genetic cause – an autosomal recessive disorder which leads to a deficiency in the adrenal enzyme P450, which mediates 21-hydroxylase activity. This creates a deficit in the ability of the individual to produce cortisol, which acts to inhibit the release of adrenocorticotropic hormone (ACTH), and thus to control steroid synthesis. This leads to the massive over-production of adrenal androgens, which have a masculinising effect upon the female foetus (the male foetus remains largely unaffected), with varying degrees of virilisation of the external genitals being common. Around 1 in 16,000 births shows a deficiency in 21-hydroxylase, making it a relatively common disorder, and thus enabling some large-scale studies to be conducted (Speiser and White, 2003). High foetal androgen levels prior to week 12 of gestation in females leads to a marked level of virilisation, with external genitalia resembling a penis and empty scrotum, while individuals exposed to androgens after week 12 of gestation may only show an enlargement of the clitoris (Cohen-Kettenis and Pfäfflin, 2003). In the most serious forms of the disorder, the 21-hydroxylase deficiency is accompanied by deficits in aldosterone, and thus the individual loses salt (called 'salt-wasting CAH'), leading to electrolyte and fluid losses, and a range of serious medical complications. If left untreated the virilisation (in males and females) continues after birth and there may be rapid bone growth, muscular development, acne, and premature development of pubic and axillary hair (Conte and Grumbach, 1997). Treatment is usually in the form of corticosteroid administration, and, in the salt-losing type, the additional administration of mineralocorticoids.

So, affected females are concordant for genetic sex (46,XX) and their internal ducts have developed according to the normal female blueprint (Müllerian development and Wolffian regression). However, they are discordant for hormonal sex (high levels of androgens) and external genital sex (masculinised). In most cases, if the condition is correctly diagnosed shortly after birth the individuals are almost always assigned a female gender because they have ovaries, a uterus and a vagina, and will feminise at puberty. In rare cases the virilisation is such that a correct diagnosis is not made within the first eighteen months and gender reassignment becomes more complicated (Dessens *et al.*, 2003).

As the diagnosis of this disorder typically takes place after birth, it is of course very difficult to ascertain precisely the extent of androgen exposure in the affected individuals, and thus to be able to correlate such levels with subsequent behaviours. One possible method is to use the previously described putative marker for prenatal hormone exposure – the second to fourth finger length ratio (2D:4D). Recall that a low ratio is assumed to reflect a masculinised hormonal environment, while a high ratio is assumed to reflect a more feminised environment (Manning, 2002). If androgen exposure is related to the degree of masculinisation then one would hypothesise that individuals with a lower ratio should display more physical, and perhaps behavioural, masculinisation.

Brown *et al.* (2002b) assessed 2D:4D from photocopies in sixteen male and thirteen female CAH patients, and seventy-two controls. Despite low numbers in the patient groups they found that female CAH patients were significantly more likely to possess a masculine-typical right-hand 2D:4D ratio than the control females; male CAH patients had a significantly lower left-hand ratio than control males. Interestingly, in six of the male CAH patients the authors also compared their finger ratios with a male relative who did not have CAH – the affected males had significantly lower ratios on both hands. This hypermasculinisation of digit ratio in the males was slightly unexpected, as previous accounts of this disorder have not suggested that males are hypermasculinised in other physical/behavioural traits.

This initially seems odd, as such males are being exposed to androgens from their gonads (as is normal) in addition to an extra excessive dose of adrenal androgens – one might therefore assume that they would display hypermasculinisation in a variety of traits. However Brown *et al.* (2002b) offer some explanations for this apparent discrepancy. First they point out that once androgen receptors are saturated, an additional influx of steroids is unable to have any further effect. Alternatively, it could be the case that the male foetus is able to regulate circulating androgens within a specific range such that the extra dose of adrenal androgens is countered by a decrease in gonadal androgen output, and homeostasis is thus maintained. Such speculations sound plausible but remain as yet only hypothetical.

In a similar study Ökten *et al.* (2002) assessed 2D:4D via photocopies and X-ray images in seventeen female and nine male CAH patients all aged under thirteen, and in 104 control children. As in the previous study, female patients displayed significantly lower (masculinised) ratios in comparison to healthy controls; male patients also displayed lower ratios. Curiously the X-rays revealed only slight differences between the length of the metacarpal and phalangeal bones of the second and fourth fingers in patients and controls. So, the presumed virilising effects of androgens on finger lengths were presumably not due to alterations in bone length, but rather due to influences on the epidermis and dermis of the digits, notably with thicker soft tissue being found on the top of the fourth finger. This could explain why Buck *et al.* (2003) failed to find significant differences in 2D:4D between sixty-six CAH female patients and sixty-nine female controls as they only took measurements from X-ray photographs. In addition, they only measured 2D:4D from the left hand and it has been argued that many 2D:4D associations are more strongly expressed in the right hand, for reasons not yet fully understood (Manning *et al.*, 2003).

## Gender identity and behaviour in CAH

Some early studies described CAH girls as being 'tomboyish' in behaviour and attitude. For example, Ehrhardt *et al.* (1968) noted that in comparison to control girls, female CAH patients showed greater interest in 'rough and tumble play', preferred playing with male-typical toys, and showed little interest in 'normal' female-type play activities. This preference for heightened physical activity drew comparisons with a study conducted by Young *et al.* (1965) in rhesus monkeys. If female monkeys were injected with androgens during pregnancy then their daughters displayed levels of rough and tumble play similar to that of male controls.

In a study of toy preferences, Berenbaum and Hines (1992) recruited twenty-six females and eleven males (aged three to eight) with CAH and used unaffected same-sex relatives as controls. The children were provided with a range of gender-typical toys (e.g. construction sets, dolls, etc.) and some gender-neutral toys (e.g. books) to play with in an informal setting. The investigators observed the children interacting with the toys for ten minutes, scored the amount of time the child played with each toy, and summed the time spent in play with toys in each of the three categories. The CAH girls spent significantly longer playing with the male-typical toys than did the control girls, in fact around the same time as the control boys; the male CAH and control boys did not differ. This then indicates some degree of masculinisation of toy preferences in the androgen-exposed females. However, other studies have provided conflicting evidence by finding that CAH girls were not more tomboyish and did not differ on a questionnaire assessing sex-typed play activities (e.g. McGuire *et al.*, 1975).

But are these behaviours the direct result of prenatal hormones or are they due to other factors? Recall that female CAH patients often present with masculinised external genitals, and the masculine appearance of the genitals could influence parental perceptions of the child, or the self-perceptions of femininity in the children themselves, and thus affect their sex-typical behaviours (Quadagno *et al.*, 1977). CAH girls are sometimes raised as boys for perhaps the first few years of their life; even after diagnosis is made, parents may continue to have doubts as to the appropriate gender of their offspring. Social psychologists have shown on many occasions that adults behave very differently towards children they perceive as being either male or female, and it is possible that this differential treatment may strongly influence a child's behaviours. In addition, CAH children (especially those with the salt-losing variety) are often seriously ill for the first few years of their life and spend considerable time in hospital. Increased stress and anxiety could thus manifest itself in alterations of gender-typical behaviours. Indeed, Slijper (1984) compared gender role behaviours in CAH girls and boys (non-salt-losers, and salt-losers), in other children who were chronically ill (diabetes), and in a sample of healthy controls. It was found that girls who were chronically sick (CAH and diabetic) scored significantly more on the 'boyish' scale of a gender test, with the salt-losing CAH girls scoring the most masculine.

Money *et al.* (1984) questioned thirty female CAH patients and twenty seven-female controls on their erotosexual status and found a much higher incidence of self-reported bisexuality in the patient group. Dessens *et al.* (2003) reviewed the literature on studies concerning gender identity and behaviour in 250 CAH patients, most of whom suffered from classic CAH and who had experienced mild to severe genital masculinisation. Out of this sample the majority were raised as females and 95% of them developed a strong female gender identity. However the remaining 5% did show serious problems with their gender identity – a prevalence much higher than comparative groups showing strong gender dysphoria (such as female to male transsexuals).

Meyer-Bahlburg *et al.* (2003) assessed gender identity using a range of measures in adult patients displaying various forms of CAH, and in control females. A retrospective measure of gender role behaviour in childhood was markedly masculinised in CAH patients with the salt-losing form; no differences were found between the other groups. All patient groups, however, had lower romantic involvement scores and significantly fewer reported having heterosexual coitus. Those that did experienced it later in life, and the salt-losing group also appeared to be shifted towards a bisexual/homosexual direction. The authors explained this as a masculinisation of gender role caused by prenatal androgen exposure, but in a series of in-depth qualitative interviews their patients provided telling evidence that extensive genital surgery and frequent genital examinations by male physicians may have resulted in greater embarrassment with the opposite sex, and thus could possibly have influenced their sexual behaviours.

## Androgen-insensitivity syndrome (AIS)

This syndrome is an X-linked recessive genetic disorder in which the androgen receptors are partially or completely unresponsive to the binding or utilisation of androgens, resulting in the failure of the male foetus to masculinise. As the default setting is female, such 46,XY individuals display normal female genitalia and show breast development at the appropriate time (in those with partial AIS, the external genitals may be more ambiguous), despite the fact that they have functional testes which produce normal levels of androgens. Anti-Müllerian hormone is produced normally, so the Müllerian ducts regress, but the Wolffian ducts remain undeveloped and so the internal reproductive system does not develop along typical female lines (McPhaul and Griffin, 1999). At birth (depending upon the degree of genital feminisation) AIS children are labelled as 'female' and raised accordingly, an action made easier by the fact that their behaviour and appearance is completely feminine (Cohen-Kettenis and Pfäfflin, 2003). It is not normally until months or even years after birth that certain physical abnormalities give away the 'true' sex of the individual – for example, what appears to be a hernia is found to be testicular material, and subsequent examinations and genetic tests reveal the true story. In some children the correct diagnosis is not made until the teenage years when pubic and axillary hair fail to appear, and menstruation does not occur. It is common to perform gonadectomies on diagnosis, and to alter the vagina surgically to allow later sexual intercourse; at puberty AIS individuals receive hormone therapy to promote and maintain breast development.

## Gender identity and behaviour in AIS

In this syndrome the picture is fairly clear as these individuals are not responsive to androgens and so develop along female lines. They are also raised as girls from birth and are thus 'female' both physically and psychologically. Melo *et al.* (2003) described the clinical and psychological features of twenty-five Brazilian AIS patients studied over the long term. In this sample, twenty were suffering from the complete clinical syndrome and all were raised as girls, maintaining their feminine gender role into adulthood. The remaining five cases were suffering from partial AIS but were also raised as girls despite some degree of genital virilisation; they also maintained their female status.

Cohen-Kettenis and Pfäfflin (2003) summarised several studies comparing gender role development in individuals with complete AIS (CAIS) and normal females. These studies report that CAIS individuals have a completely female gender identity, are heterosexual in behaviour, are described by others as having a female gender identity, and do not differ from other women in marriage and relationship patterns. However, these authors site the case of Betty, a CAIS patient referred to their clinic who had a clear preference for boys' toys and activities, and displayed masculine gender role behaviours. When seen several years later 'she' stated that she wished she were a boy, wanted to have a penis, and planned to become a truck driver when she grew up. Other individuals where androgen insensitivity is not complete (partial AIS) often display confused gender identities. Perhaps because of their ambiguous genitalia they are classified as the 'wrong' sex and are surgically altered (sometimes wrongly) according to the whim of the clinician. One would have thought it would perhaps be sensible actually to ask individuals, at the point at which gender identity becomes established, what sex they thought they were, before surgically reassigning them! In fact Betty may perhaps have been wrongly classified from the outset, and despite having unambiguous external genitals may have been only partially affected psychologically.

## Klinefelter syndrome (46, XXY)

Individuals with this syndrome[1] are male but have an extra X chromosome, and are thus usually referred to as 'XXY males'. The addition of the extra chromosome leads to primary hypogonadism and thus sterility; they have small testes and penis, and may develop breasts at puberty (gynecomastia). Sufferers tend to have long legs and poor muscular

---

[1] Named after Harry Klinefelter, a medical researcher who first described the condition in the 1940s.

development, show a lack of facial and body hair, and demonstrate intellectual and behavioural problems; in particular deficits in verbal IQ are noted (e.g. Rovet *et al.*, 1996). Testosterone production is minimal and thus circulating levels of bound and free testosterone are low, while levels of plasma estradiol are high. Testosterone treatment at puberty is thus commonly conducted in order to enhance secondary sexual characteristics (Conte and Grumbach, 1997).

### Gender identity and behaviour in 46,XXY

Despite being exposed to very low levels of androgens during embryogenesis and up to puberty (and often high levels of estradiol after puberty) XXY males generally demonstrate male-typical behaviours and interests, though they have been described as being 'less masculine' than other males. Nielson and Pelsen (1987) conducted a twenty-year follow-up of thirty-four males with Klinefelter syndrome and found that 59% of them had married, or were in a long-standing heterosexual relationship.

## Idiopathic hypogonadotropic hypogonadism (IHH)

This syndrome is caused by the insufficient release of gonadotropin-releasing hormone from the hypothalamus, and is sometimes referred to as 'Kallmann's syndrome'[2] when it is accompanied by the developmental absence of the olfactory bulbs, causing a lack of the sense of smell (anosmia). It can affect both males and females but is more common in males. These males are genetically normal, but do not receive sufficient testosterone prenatally. Their external genitals can be very small (micropenis) and their testes do not produce sperm, so at puberty secondary male sex characteristics fail to appear. Treatment consists of androgen and gonadotropin replacement therapy.

### Gender identity and behaviour in IHH

Males with Kallmann's syndrome display male-typical genitalia at birth and are raised accordingly. Few studies have actually been conducted that assess psychosexual orientation. One employing a single case study reported that the individual was heterosexual and displayed a male-typical gender identity (van Seters and Slob, 1988). However another study (which did not employ a control group) reported that IHH males showed a reduced interest in sex (Bobrow *et al.*, 1971).

---

[2] Named after geneticist Franz Kallmann, who described the syndrome in the 1940s.

## Turner's syndrome (TS)

This syndrome is named after endocrinologist Henry Turner who first described the condition, though did not recognise the genetic cause (Turner, 1938). It is also referred to as '45,X gonadal dysgenesis' and, as this term suggests, individuals only possess one chromosome, an X, which in around 70–80% of cases derives from the mother. Individuals also demonstrate absent or poorly functioning ovaries. Individuals are assigned and raised as females, but as ovarian function is grossly impaired these females do not enter puberty spontaneously; they remain infertile, and thus the key hallmark of Turner's syndrome is sexual infantilism. Other characteristic physical features include cardiovascular problems, short stature, a short webbed neck, a shield-like chest, and a distinctive facial appearance, with small jaw (micrognathia), epicanthal folds, prominent low-set ears and drooping eyelids (ptosis) all being commonly reported (Conte and Grumbach, 1997). Emotional and behavioural problems are routinely reported, as well as lower IQ, with specific visuospatial, social and attentional cognitive impairments being observed (see chapter 11). Interestingly, those individuals who posses the paternally derived X chromosome have been shown to be better adjusted, and display superior verbal and attentional skills, than those receiving the X chromosome from their mother (Skuse et al., 1997). Treatment normally begins around the age of twelve and typically consists of estrogen supplementation to induce puberty and prevent osteoporosis, and growth hormone therapy to address short stature.

### Gender identity and behaviour in TS

Reports appear to be unanimous in ascribing a female gender identity to Turner's syndrome individuals as they consistently demonstrate stereotypical feminine interests and appearance combined with a low sex drive. However, Pavlidis et al. (1995) noted that such studies had consisted of relatively few participants, generally drawn from a clinical sample. In their study they assessed self-perceived gender role, body image, self-concept and sexual functioning in eighty adult Turner females ranging in age from nineteen to fifty-six. The Turner females were significantly slower to achieve adult sexual milestones, regarded themselves as being significantly more conservative in their sexual attitudes, and were more likely never to have had sexual intercourse in comparison to a normative sample. The key factors appeared to be their self-perceived health status and poor body image; interestingly a small subsample of the group (nine females) were not currently taking ovarian hormones and they scored significantly lower on body image.

## Enzyme deficiencies (pseudohermaphroditism)

These syndromes are characterised by the failure of critical enzymes such that normal gonadal steroid production is impaired. Testosterone is converted to the much more powerful dihydrotestosterone (DHT) by the actions of the enzyme 5α-reductase, but in 5α-reductase deficiency this conversion cannot take place (Russell and Wilson, 1994). As DHT is critically involved in the formation of the external genitals, male sufferers display ambiguous genitals ranging from micropenis to an apparent vagina. Bizarrely, at puberty some degree of virilisation occurs and the testes enlarge and descend, the phallus lengthens, the voice deepens and muscle mass increases. In another condition, known as 17β-hydroxysteroid dehydrogenase deficiency, the lack of this crucial enzyme in the synthesis of testosterone (and thus DHT) in the Leydig cells means that genetic XY males demonstrate female-typical external genitalia; again, at puberty virilisation occurs and testosterone levels approximate that of normal males. In both disorders the children are normally assigned to the female sex and raised as girls.

### Gender identity and behaviour in enzyme deficiency syndromes

The enzyme deficiency syndromes provide a unique window into gender role and psychosexual development because here we have the highly unusual case of a genetic male beginning labelled throughout life as 'female' and reared as such, but then at puberty showing significant physical masculinisation. If androgens are truly involved in gender role development then we would perhaps predict that such individuals would 'switch' gender. In fact initial reports made much of the fact that such individuals had adopted a feminine gender role for much of their early life but because of the sudden surge in androgens at puberty did reverse their gender identity and 'change' sex (e.g. Imperato-McGinley *et al.*, 1974). More recently Mendonca (2003) reported that half of a sample of twenty-six 5α-reductase individuals did 'change' sex after puberty. There was however no relationship between the extent of virilisation and likelihood of gender change, and it is possible that testosterone may have masculinised the brain to some degree before birth.

Similarly, in a review of studies assessing gender outcome in enzyme deficiency syndromes, Cohen-Kettenis (2005) noted gender role changes in 56–63% of 5α-reductase cases and 39–64% in 17β-hydroxysteroid dehydrogenase individuals, with most of the gender role changes taking place during late adolescence. Such studies have led researchers to speculate that sex of rearing is less important than androgen exposure, but others have pointed out that such a strong conclusion may not be justified, as rearing may have been ambiguous and changes in sexual identity may result from changes to the genitals, or from the considerable social advantages in being male in the societies where the mutations are relatively common (Herdt and Davidson, 1988).

Cohen-Kettenis (2005) concluded 'it seems that a masculine appearance in childhood, in association with masculine behaviour (perhaps both partially caused by a prenatal exposure to androgens), make gender role change likely after pubertal changes reinforce an already existing gender discomfort'.

## The case of John/Joan

What would be very interesting, of course, is to get hold of set of male monozygotic (identical) twins, castrate one of them shortly after birth, modify his external genitals, and raise him as a girl to see what would happen to his gender identity and psychosexual development. Ethically of course this would not be allowed to happen, but through an instance of medical incompetence this unfortunate but fascinating 'experiment' has occurred. While there have been several instances of genetic males being reared as females because of the accidental destruction of the penis (most often during botched circumcision operations), the 'John/Joan' case remains the most influential because the hapless individual happened to have a normal male twin brother who was to act as an unwitting control. When I was studying for my undergraduate Psychology degree in the early 1980s the established dogma (based almost entirely on this case) was that while biological sex was indeed determined by one's chromosomes, the social manifestation of this (gender identity, gender role and possibly sexual orientation) were determined entirely by powerful social forces acting upon the infant, who was assumed to be like a 'blank slate' upon which such forces would scrawl out their instructions. Thus, male infants could be socialised to be feminine and vice versa, because their biological sex was of much less importance than their socialisation. Indeed, as late as 1997 Herdt stated 'the sex of rearing outweighs the biological sex in the development of gender identity and social identity', a statement undoubtedly influenced by this notorious case but which only a year later would appear downright misleading (Herdt, 1997).

So, how did such dogma arise and last for so long? In 1975, charismatic psychologist and influential expert on intersex individuals, John William Money, reported a series of cases in which forty-five genetic males had been assigned and reared as females, the majority of these cases being intersex conditions in which the infants had been born with ambiguous genitalia. Two cases, however, were not intersex; they were normal males whose penises had been accidentally destroyed – in the case of 'John' this occurred at seven months of age (in 1966), but what made his case so interesting was the existence of his twin brother. The case came to Money's attention when the infant was some seventeen months old and it was decided to reassign 'John' to 'Joan': his name was changed, a female hairstyle was adopted, clothing was amended accordingly, and four months afterwards the first stages of genital reconstruction were commenced. For the first nine years of John/Joan's life, annual visits were made to Money and colleagues at Johns Hopkins University, and these indicated that Joan was developing as a well-adjusted (though somewhat tomboyish) girl. Money in fact concluded, 'her behaviour is so normally that of an active little girl, and so clearly different by contrast from the boyish ways of her twin brother, that it offers nothing to stimulate one's conjectures' (Money, 1975: 71).

The research team lost track of Joan when she was in her early teens, but for almost the next thirty years the 'success' of this case was widely acknowledged in research papers and textbooks, and at conferences. The case fitted well with the current concept of 'psychosexual neutrality', the idea that at birth our sex is not fixed, but is rather fluid and amenable to manipulation by the many social forces surrounding us. The implication was enormous – a genetic male, who had received normal androgen exposure in the womb and during the first few months of life, had been successfully reared as a female; nurture could thus outweigh nature, and humans were thus not bound by their biological roots. In fairness to Money, he did not personally deny the role of biological forces in shaping gender and sexuality, but rather considered that sex of assignment was more important (Money, 1981). His considerable error (which was to haunt him for the rest of his scientific career) was tacitly to allow the rest of the world to assume that all was fine with Joan when in fact long-term follow-up studies had not been conducted, and even in the early days considerable doubts as to the success of the gender reassignment were being raised.

In fact, other scientists had tracked down 'Joan', who was found to have reverted to a masculine existence from the age of fourteen (changing 'her' name to David), receiving a mastectomy and testosterone therapy, followed by phallic constructive surgery at age sixteen. When interviewed in his thirties, David was living as a heterosexual male with his wife and adopted children. He was completely unaware of the 'success' of his gender reassignment, as he had experienced a miserable childhood unable to comprehend how as a 'boy' he was made to dress, act and behave as a girl (Diamond and Sigmundson, 1997). The case was publicised by journalist John Colapinto, firstly in *Rolling Stone* magazine and then in a popular book (Colapinto, 2000), and the story achieved international notoriety as the incredible story of the twins Bruce (who later became 'Brenda') and Brian Reimer became known. The story has a tragic ending as unaffected twin Brian committed suicide in 2002, and David, unable to cope, took his own life in 2004.

## Summary of psychosexual differentiation in atypical groups

In the previous chapter I provided strong evidence of the physically masculinising effects of sex steroids, especially androgens; however, the evidence concerning the masculinisation of psychosexual development was less conclusive. In the atypical hormone exposure groups described above an equally complex picture emerges. In the most extreme group, genetic males who remain unresponsive to androgens (AIS) are physically and psychologically feminine, a fact which lends some support to the 'Passive Feminisation Model' (Collaer and Hines, 1995) and which also demonstrates that the nature of the chromosomes or gonads does not dictate gender role (Gooren, 2006). In cases of partial androgen resistance, the majority develop a gender role in accord with their sex of rearing, but more female-assigned partial AIS patients initiate gender change to male, than do their male-assigned equivalents, which may well indicate the prenatal effects of androgens (Meyer-Bahlburg, 2002).

Female CAH patients have been exposed to extremely high levels of androgens prenatally but in most cases are happy with their assigned female gender. A confounding point remains, of course, that CAH individuals have a serious medical condition requiring hospitalisation, drugs, and often radical surgical intervention. It is commonly the case that their external genitals are not normal, and this may well affect their self-image and self-esteem, and have a negative effect on their normal psychosexual development, particularly leading to deep embarrassment when meeting potential romantic partners (Gooren, 2006).

Males with Klinefelter syndrome or Kallmann's syndrome have a male phenotype and a male gender identity; female Turner's syndrome patients also demonstrate gender-typical behaviours, and as they are profoundly estrogen-deficient this may indicate only a minor role for estrogens in human psychosexual development (again supporting the 'Passive Defeminisation Model'). The complex cases of individuals with one of the enzyme deficiencies changing gender role at puberty are clouded by lack of information concerning their social/rearing environment and must thus be treated with caution.

Despite the varied problems with all of these lines of evidence, not the least the lack of information concerning the effects of prenatal hormone exposure on brain structure and function, and the lack of long-term follow-up studies, Wilson (1999) concluded that gender identity and gender role behaviour most probably develop in accord with the predominant prenatal hormonal environment, and this can withstand some degree of virilisation/feminisation of the external genitals. Wilson also points out that it is virtually impossible to determine the degree to which psychological/social/endocrinological factors contribute to psychosexual development in intersex conditions because the psychological/social forces almost always correspond with the anatomical and endocrine factors.

The John/Joan case has achieved much publicity and is a fascinating tale, but unfortunately may not be all that well suited to inform us about the role of androgens in gender development. Meyer-Bahlburg (1999) points out that the gender reassignment probably occurred too late to discount the possible effects of social experience – for seven months he was raised as a male along with his twin brother, with another fourteen months elapsing before a decision was made concerning gender-realignment and the surgery being conducted. This is on the very edge of the border for what is normally considered an appropriate time-window for sex reassignment in intersex children. In addition, a similar case of ablatio penis, where the male infant was reassigned to female aged seven months, appeared to be much more successful (though 'she' developed into a bisexual 'woman') with no apparent gender dysphoria (Bradley *et al.*, 1998).

## Other atypical 'conditions'

The previous examples have described individuals with a range of identifiable medical conditions which lead to some degree of phenotypic (and possibly neurological) alteration. There are several other 'conditions' where there appear to be no underlying hormonal, metabolic, physiological or physical abnormalities, yet the individuals display atypical gender role/sexual orientation.

### Transsexuality

A transsexual is someone who displays a gender identity that is not in accord with their internal and external genitalia and secondary sexual characteristics. Thus, a phenotypic male may state that they feel (and have always felt) themselves to be a 'female', trapped in a male body. As there are no signs of internal or external genital abnormalities, phenotypic feminisation or abnormalities in chromosomal patterns, and normal secondary sexual characteristics appear at puberty (deep voice, muscles, facial hair, etc.), it must be assumed that this 'feeling' has a brain substrate (Gooren, 1990). Transsexualism can thus be described as an extreme form of gender dysphoria – a discrepancy between gender identity/gender role on one hand, and physical characteristics on the other, though technically one may argue that transsexualism in fact constitutes physical body sex dysmorphia, as the individuals are happy with their gender identity, but unhappy with the surrounding physical architecture. The incidence of transsexuality is rare, but appears to be consistent across cultures, and classes within a culture, with figures of between 1 in 13,000–15,000 for male-to-female and 1 in 30,000–35,000 for female-to-male transsexuals being quoted (van Kesteren *et al.*, 1996).

There appear to be two subtypes of transsexual. One group displays what is called 'early-onset transsexualism' and these individuals demonstrate gender nonconformity from a very early age, stating that they are the 'wrong' sex, or are in the 'wrong' body. They are almost always sexually oriented towards males, and their sex-reassignment is often successful. Another group are 'late-onset transsexuals' who gradually develop a gender dysphoria, often following episodes of overt or covert transvestite behaviours. They are more likely to be sexually oriented towards women, and the outcome of sex reassignment is much less likely to be successful (Gooren, 2006).

If some kind of hormonal alteration during prenatal or early postnatal development is a causal factor in this condition, then as the male phenotype emerges from the basic female blueprint following considerable hormonal activity, we might predict that certain hormonal perturbations might affect developing males more so than developing females. One might predict, then, that male-to-female transsexualism might be much more common than female-to-male transsexualism, especially in those individuals described as 'early-onset'; this does indeed appear to be the case (see figures quoted above by van Kesteren *et al.*, 1996). There has thus been a long-standing search for female biological/hormonal traits in male-to-female transsexuals, and male biological/hormonal traits in female-to-male transsexuals, though it is perhaps unlikely that such a straightforward dichotomy will exist. Several researchers have proposed that some kind of aberration in the early organisational influence of sex steroids may play a key role in transsexualism. For example Dörner *et al.* (1991) reviewed several lines of evidence and concluded that the lower the levels of circulating androgens (due to genetic or environmental factors) then the greater the predisposition towards transsexualism in males, though the evidence cited seems predominantly to come from studies of homosexual males! This tendency to lump together homosexuality and transsexuality leads to great confusion and is probably an incorrect assumption, as transsexualism should not be confused with sexual orientation; and like non-transsexuals, transsexuals may be heterosexual, homosexual or bisexual (Gooren, 2006; Levy *et al.*, 2003).

Bosinski *et al.* (1997) conducted physical and endocrinological examinations on twelve female-to-male transsexuals and fifteen women not experiencing gender dysphoria. In the transsexual group 83% showed clear evidence of hyperandrogenic action, with levels of testosterone, androstenedione and DHEAS being elevated. The majority of the clinical sample also presented with polycystic ovaries, a common endocrine disorder referred to as 'polycystic ovary syndrome' (PCOS).[3] This condition affects around 10% of normal women and the key clinical feature is that the ovaries produce excessive amounts of androgens, leading to menstrual/fertility problems, hirsutism and adiposity. There is thus a temptation to suppose some link between transsexuality and PCOS, but Bosinski and colleagues urge caution, pointing out that psychosexual assessments of women with PCOS do not report problems of gender identity (e.g. Raboch *et al.*, 1985) and, as PCOS is very common, one would then assume that female-to-male transsexualism would be much more common than it in fact is. Employing larger samples, Meyer *et al.* (1981; 1986) have investigated physical and hormonal characteristics in male-to-female and female-to-male transsexuals. In the earlier study, thirty-eight non-castrated male-to-female transsexuals and fourteen non-castrated female-to-male transsexuals demonstrated no physical or hormonal abnormalities prior

---

[3] Known clinically as Stein-Leventhal syndrome, after it was first described by them in 1935.

to receiving standard hormone therapies. The later study, utilising sixty male-to-female and thirty female-to-male participants, found that only two individuals (both in the female-to-male group) had a congenital defect in hormone production or abnormal genital development.

Using the technique of dermatoglyphic analysis (see chapter 3), Slabbekoorn *et al.* (2000) assessed total ridge counts and finger ridge a symmetries in a large sample of 184 male-to-female transsexuals and 110 female-to-male transsexuals. They predicted that the dermatoglyphic characteristics of the transsexual groups would show similarities with opposite-sex control groups (i.e. male-to-female transsexuals would display dermatoglyphic characteristics similar to those of normal women). Contrary to their expectations, the fingerprints of the transsexual groups showed marked similarities to their genetic sex controls. As they also failed to find significant differences in dermatoglyphic characteristics in the control males and females, this technique might thus not be sensitive enough to support a prenatal hormone exposure hypothesis. Schneider *et al.* (2006) have instead relied upon the other putative 'marker' of prenatal hormone exposure (2D:4D), and measured this ratio in sixty-three male-to-female transsexuals, forty-three female-to-male transsexuals, and male and female non-transsexual control groups. After controlling for handedness (by excluding all the non-right-handed participants), they reported that the ratio was significantly different between normal males and male-to-female transsexuals, the latter group showing a higher ratio that was no different from that seen in the normal female group. This then hints at a potential causal role for prenatal testosterone exposure.

More recently, Henningsson *et al.* (2005) have focussed attention not on absolute levels of circulating sex hormones but rather on the genes coding for the receptors sensitive to them (androgen, estrogen β and aromatase receptors). In their study twenty-nine male-to-female transsexuals provided a blood sample from which DNA was extracted, and various polymorphisms of the three receptor genes under consideration were examined. The estrogen β receptor (ERβ) repeat differed between controls and transsexuals, the mean length being significantly longer in the transsexual group. In addition there was a significant interaction between the androgen and aromatase receptor polymorphisms. Thus, the authors suggested that the presence of a long ERβ repeat, or a long AR repeat, could predispose towards transsexualism (it is unclear in the paper which could be the more important, or precisely how such polymorphisms could lead to transsexualism).

## Homosexuality

The degree of sexual attraction to the same sex or to the opposite sex is called 'sexual orientation' and this shows within-sex variation. The majority of individuals are heterosexual, but around 2–5% of the male population and 1–2% of the female population are exclusively homosexual (approximately 10% of males show bisexual behaviours), irrespective of culture and environment (studies cited in Rahman and Wilson, 2003a). In males, the distribution of sexual orientation appears to be bimodal (heterosexual versus homosexual), but amongst females it is more variable in the form of different degrees of bisexuality. This is consistent with the notion of female 'erotic plasticity', in that the female sex drive appears to be more influenced by situational and cultural factors (Baumeister, 2000). This indicates that male and female sexual orientation may have divergent but perhaps overlapping causal pathways. Numerous theories have arisen as to the possible causes of homosexuality. It is beyond the scope of this text to review them all; instead I will focus on the more relevant biological/hormonal explanations.

It should first be noted that homosexuality is not an exclusively human trait. In his extensive text Bagemihl (1999) provides a wealth of observational evidence which attests to the existence of 'homosexual-like' behaviours in a wide variety of species. Many animals thus display aberrant sexual preferences, and if such phenomena correspond to human homosexual behaviours (some authors argue they do not), then this provides strong support for a biological 'cause'. The idea that homosexuality is a learned process has now largely been discounted because of two lines of evidence. First, sexual orientation congregates within families, and while environmental influences cannot totally be excluded, this suggests that homosexuality may be partly heritable. Bailey and Pillard (1991) interviewed 115 homosexual men and their twin brothers (identical:MZ and non-identical:DZ), and a further forty-six homosexual males with their adopted brothers. They reported that 52% of the MZ co-twins, 22% of the DZ co-twins and 11% of adopted brothers were either homosexual or bisexual.

In a later study Bailey et al. (1993) carried out a comparable study in female homosexuals and reported similar results, i.e. 48% of MZ co-twins, 16% of DZ co-twins and 6% of adopted sisters were either homosexual or bisexual. Some studies have suggested that X-linked genes may influence male sexual orientation, as gay men have more homosexual uncles and cousins amongst their maternal relatives (Hamer et al., 1993), but this has not always been found (Bailey et al., 1999). Studies utilising molecular genetic techniques have revealed evidence of a genetic marker for homosexuality on chromosome Xq28 in males (Hu et al., 1995) but a more recent study has failed to confirm this (Rice et al., 1999). While the direct genetic basis of sexual orientation remains elusive, evidence that homosexuality is somehow influenced by genetic mechanisms is strong.

Secondly, there appears to be a strong relationship between childhood gender nonconformity and adult sexual orientation, in boys at least. Zuger (1984) carried out a long-term follow-up of fifty-five boys showing signs of gender nonconformity. They were first seen between the ages of three and fourteen, when they displayed symptoms of effeminate behaviour. The children were seen again approximately twenty-seven years later and were questioned on their sexual preferences: 73% of the sample described themselves as homosexual, 6% as heterosexual and 21% as bisexual. In a similar study Green (1985) compared two groups of boys on measures of gender identity in childhood and adolescence. One group consisted of sixty-six clinically referred boys whose behaviour showed clear signs of gender identity disorder, and fifty-six boys who were demographically matched. During childhood, extensive data were gathered on their sex-typed behaviours, relationship with other children and relationships with parents. In adolescence, a sexual orientation score was determined, and 68% of boys in the referred group demonstrated significant homosexual/bisexual orientation, whereas none of the boys in the control group did.

## Hormonal contributions to homosexuality

Initial thoughts concerning a biological/hormonal explanation of homosexuality were provided by the legal adviser Karl Heinrich Ulrichs, who, from an early age, had shown clear gender nonconformity, and became a passionate advocate of equal rights for homosexuals. He argued that homosexuals[4] were distinctly different from heterosexuals, and coined the term 'Urning' to describe them[5]. In 1864 he proposed a theory to account for this difference, namely that the human embryo can develop in either the male or the female direction: in most individuals physical development and sexual orientation were concordant, but in homosexuals the body had developed along male lines while mental development was along female lines. The opposite process was thought to occur for female homosexuals.

Later on, Ulrichs realised that this simple explanation was incorrect, as he met many homosexual men who were not feminine in behaviour; some were extremely masculine apart from their sexual orientation. He thus revised his theory to describe a spectrum of male homosexuality ranging from female types (a male, feminine in appearance and behaviour, who is attracted to masculine men and perhaps prefers a passive sexual role) to male types (a male, masculine in appearance and behaviour, but attracted to other males and who prefers a more active sexual role) (LeVay, 1996). Henry Havelock Ellis, the noted doctor and sexual psychologist, also argued that homosexuality was inborn, as he had failed to find any differences in social experiences between homosexuals and heterosexuals, though he did not discuss a specific biological cause (Ellis, 1915). Around the same time, sexologist Magnus Hirschfeld addressed possible hormonal influences by speculating that if the balance between male and female hormones was upset in some way, then homosexuality could result (cited in LeVay, 1996).

---

[4] This term was first used by Karl Maria Kertbeny in 1869.
[5] This is based on one of Plato's works whereby a character refers to same-sex lovers as the offspring of Aphrodite, daughter of Uranus.

When the measurement of hormones became practical and reliable, experimenters were able to assess Hirschfeld's predictions by comparing levels of various hormones in heterosexual and homosexual volunteers. For example, Loraine *et al.* (1970) measured various hormones in the urine of three male and four female homosexuals, and heterosexual controls. Two out of the three homosexual males showed abnormally low levels of testosterone, while all of the homosexual women displayed higher levels of testosterone and luteinizing hormone. Similarly, Gartrell *et al.* (1977) found that blood plasma testosterone levels were 38% higher in a sample of twenty-one homosexual women compared to heterosexual controls. However, such studies were heavily criticised because of perceived problems with their design and interpretation. Meyer-Bahlburg (1979), for example, reviewed studies thus far conducted on female homosexuals, and pointed out that in many individuals hormone levels fell within normal limits when menstrual cycle phase was controlled for; time of day was usually not considered, and the existence of potential disease states leading to a hormone abnormality not fully addressed. In more carefully controlled studies, homosexual and heterosexual women were closely matched in terms of behavioural variables known to influence hormone levels (e.g. stress, mood, exercise) and analysis of a range of plasma hormones revealed no significant group differences (Dancey, 1990; Downey *et al.*, 1987). So, circulating levels of various hormones do not seem to differ between homosexuals and heterosexuals, and of course if homosexuality is caused by prenatal hormonal events then there is no reason to suppose that differences in circulating hormones should be apparent in later life. The focus then shifted to more neurologically based theories attempting to deal with prebirth hormonal influences.

## Initial explanations

Feldman and MacCulloch (1971) proposed a tentative theory, suggesting that the brains of 'primary' male homosexuals (those reporting exclusively homosexual preferences) had a sexually undifferentiated brain of the female pattern, hypothesised to arise from a lack of hypothalamic exposure to androgens during prenatal development. Several years later Dörner *et al.* (1975) revised this theory slightly by proposing that an absolute or relative deficiency in androgens during the phase at which the hypothalamus is being organised leads to a failure of the male brain to masculinise sufficiently. Dörner (1976) then formulated a 'dual mating centre' theory in which he argued that in the rat the medial preoptic nucleus of the hypothalamus regulated male sexual activity, while the ventromedial nucleus of the hypothalamus mediated female sexual activity. The morphological differentiation of these nuclei lies under the control of prenatal hormones: if levels of androgens are high then the male centre will develop strongly; if androgens are low then the female centre will predominate. If the female centre predominates in a male individual (because of an early lack of androgens) then that individual will become homosexual. But what may trigger this alteration in prenatal hormone levels?

In the 1970s and early 1980s, a possible answer came to fore as a result of a series of studies investigating the physiological consequences of stress in rats. In such studies, groups of pregnant female rats were exposed to high levels of stress in a 'restraint paradigm' in which the animal is confined to a small space and is exposed to intense sensory stimulation, such as light and/or noise. This is very stressful for rats, and not surprisingly the individuals displayed elevated levels of adrenaline, corticosteroids and adrenocorticotropic hormones in their blood. Interestingly, the stress experienced by the mother also had a knock-on effect for her unborn male offspring, as these stress hormones cross the placenta and block the action of androgens, thereby disrupting normal sexual development in male offspring only (Ward, 1972; 1984; Ward and Weisz, 1980). Timing of the stress was found to be important, as one study showed that if mothers were exposed to the stressor up to one week after giving birth, their offspring would still demonstrate reduced levels of testosterone and higher levels of stress hormones, presumably via the mother's milk; stress experienced early on in pregnancy had lesser effects on the foetus (Dörner, 1979).

In a series of experiments on male rats, Dörner and colleagues showed that altering levels of various hormones at the critical times could indeed alter the morphology of certain brain regions and create 'homosexual' individuals. More recently, these data have been confirmed by Meek et al. (2006) in mice. In their study, pregnant mice either were exposed to random bouts of stress (handling in noisy, brightly lit environments) three times per day for forty-five minutes during the last week of pregnancy, or remained stress-free. At three months of age, the offspring of these mothers were allowed access to sexually experienced male and female individuals and measures of partner preference and sexual behaviour were taken. The stressed males made significantly fewer visits to the female's compartment but significantly more visits to the male; they showed a longer mean time to mount the female and made fewer mounts; they also displayed lordosis to the other male, significantly more often than did their non-stressed counterparts. They did not, however, display other characteristic female-like mating behaviours such as dart-hopping or ear wiggling (see chapter 8). This study clearly showed that the offspring of stressed mothers showed certain female-typical sexual behaviours, though the authors admitted that prenatal stress may have perhaps merely delayed the onset of male-typical behaviour.

There are other criticisms that question the concordance between such studies and human homosexual behaviours. First, 'homosexual' male rodents behave more like female rodents (i.e. display lordosis); and it could be argued that human homosexual males behave like typical males apart from their sexual orientation (i.e. take an active role in sex), though of course this is not always the case with some individuals preferring the more passive role. Second, the rats did not show other alterations in sex drive and other sex-typical behaviours were not affected. Third, early manipulation of gonadal hormones in animals affects not only sexual activity but also the structure of the genitals. Human homosexuals do not show genital anomalies concomitant with increased or decreased androgen exposure.

These criticisms aside, the stress theory led to direct predictions concerning homosexuality in humans, i.e. it should be the case that the mothers of human male homosexuals would have experienced significantly higher levels of stress during certain phases of pregnancy than the mothers of heterosexual male offspring. Dörner *et al.* (1980) did indeed propose that maternal stress is a key factor in the aetiology of human male homosexuality, and in support he noted that among males born in Germany between 1934 and 1953 an unusually high proportion of homosexuals were born between 1941 and 1946, a period of immense social upheaval and stress during and immediately after the Second World War. In a later study, Dörner *et al.* (1983) also found that 75% of the mothers of homosexuals, compared to 10% of the mothers of heterosexuals, were able to recall stressful episodes during pregnancy.

Such post-hoc studies have been severely criticised on methodological grounds, and other studies have only been able to find partial support for the theory or have failed to find any relationship between prenatal stress and homosexuality. For example, Schmidt and Clement (1990) found no increase in homosexuality in German males conceived during the Second World War; another study found a small significant difference between thirty-nine homosexual and sixty-eight heterosexual males in reports of maternal stress during the second trimester, but other phases of pregnancy showed no clear relationships (Ellis *et al.*, 1988). In another study, involving 143 males and 72 females, Bailey *et al.* (1991) revealed no association between recollections of maternal stress and sexual orientation in males, but for the females in this sample prenatal stress was associated with a reduction in heterosexuality.

In a review article, Dörner *et al.* (1991) further speculated on the neuro-hormonal effects of maternal stress. One particular deficiency related to the production of 21-hydroxylase is hypothesised to act in combination with stress to cause an increase in maternal androstenedione. In the placenta androstenedione is aromatised to estrone and conjugated to estrone sulphate, a substance which in animals acts to inhibit testicular androgen production during foetal development, and thus leads to feminisation of specific brain regions, and of certain sexual behaviours. The authors note an increased tendency for homosexual males and/or their mothers to display heterozygous forms of 21-hydroxylase deficiency.

If male homosexuals do have a 'feminised' brain then perhaps there are other elements of their physiology that more resemble females than males. It is known, for example, that there is a specific sex difference in how the hypothalamic–pituitary–gonadal axis responds to steroids, especially the estrogens. In normal women, an injection of estrogen will lead to a characteristic rise in luteinising hormone within the pituitary gland; this positive feedback response is not normally seen in males. Dörner *et al.* (1975) demonstrated that the majority of exclusively homosexual men (13/21) did indeed show this LH response in response to an injection of estrogen, while only 2/25 non-exclusively homosexual/heterosexual males showed that response. Gladue *et al.* (1984) confirmed this response. They injected heterosexual and homosexual men and a control group of heterosexual women with estrogen and monitored their LH levels for several days. While the homosexual males displayed an LH surge in response to estrogen and the heterosexual males did not, the LH surge in the homosexual group did not fully match that of the female group. The authors pointed out that this may be due to relationships with testosterone. When injected with estrogen, testosterone levels drop rapidly (in all males) and then gradually return to baseline; testosterone levels returned to normal much more slowly in the homosexual males, indicating that brain–pituitary relationships associated with sexual orientation are quite complex (Gladue, 1994).

In support of this, an unpublished report by Gladue (cited in Gladue, 1994) demonstrated that homosexual females displayed a hyper-feminine LH response to estrogen, not a more masculinised response as perhaps would have been predicted. This (and other evidence) seems to show that female homosexuality is not a simple 'mirror image' of male homosexuality. However, other authors have failed to replicate this response in homosexual and transsexual volunteers (Gooren, 1986a), and Gooren (2006) has argued that the design of the studies purporting to demonstrate the LH response was insufficient to demonstrate that all requirements of an unequivocal estrogen-positive feedback were achieved. Moreover, male-to-female transsexuals receiving hormone replacement therapy in the form of estrogens to establish a female hormone milieu did demonstrate the estrogen-positive feedback. Current endocrine status rather than prenatal endocrine history thus appears to be the crucial factor (Gooren, 1986b).

## The 'big brother effect'

Over the years various researchers have considered diverse family/environmental factors in the search for the 'causes' of homosexuality. Some have turned out to be confounds and red herrings, but one of the most consistent correlates has been found to be the presence of older brothers. Since the mid-1990s, Blanchard and colleagues have published data from large numbers of homosexual participants in various studies from all over the world, and have demonstrated that each older brother significantly increases the odds of homosexuality in their younger male siblings (Blanchard and Bogaert, 1996). So how strong is this effect? In other words, of all gay men, how many have acquired their sexual preference through the effect of their older brothers? Blanchard (2001) provides the answer in that almost a quarter of gay men with only one older brother owe their sexual orientation to his presence. Paternal or maternal age, birth intervals or the presence of older sisters appear to play no significant role, and so this phenomenon has been termed the 'fraternal birth-order effect' or 'FBOE' (Blanchard, 2001).

So how does this seemingly robust effect come about? Blanchard and Bogaert (1996) speculated that the key factor may be a maternal immune reaction, a response which is only provoked by male foetuses, and which increases with every male foetus carried. A likely candidate for this immune response could be the H-Y antigen present on all cell surfaces but which is only expressed by male foetuses. The antigen can enter the maternal bloodstream and its presence there triggers the release of antibodies by the mother's immune system. When triggered, these maternal antibodies cross the placenta into the brain of the foetus and could interfere with neurological sexual differentiation: the stronger the immune response the greater the chance of abnormal neurological sexual differentiation (Blanchard, 2001; Blanchard and Bogaert, 1996). As the maternal immune system has been hypothesised to be capable of 'remembering' previous male foetuses, then the strength of maternal immunisation may increase with every subsequent male foetus, and thus increase the probability of them being homosexual. While evidence for such an immune response in humans remains to be outlined, animal studies have shown that the maternal immune system can and does respond to H-Y antigens expressed by the male foetus (reviewed in Blanchard and Klassen, 1997).

An additional factor appears to be birth weight. Blanchard (2001) hypothesised that a mild maternal immune response may lead to a slight reduction in birth weight in a male foetus, while a much stronger response (caused by a history of pregnancy with male foetuses) could lead to a markedly reduced birth weight (along with a greater predisposition towards homosexuality). In support of this conjecture, Blanchard and Ellis (2001) derived information on birth weight and found that, as suspected, homosexual males with older brothers weighed significantly less at birth (around 170 g less) than did heterosexual males with older brothers. Subsequently, birth weight was assessed in 250 boys referred to a gender identity clinic and assumed to be 'pre-homosexual' and in 739 control boys and 261 girls. Feminine boys with two or more older brothers weighed 385 g less at birth than control boys with fewer than two older brothers. Feminine boys with fewer than two older brothers showed no weight difference at birth compared with the control boys (Blanchard et al., 2002).

This theory clearly cannot, of course, explain all incidences of homosexuality as there are many homosexual males who have no older brothers. The supposed explanation has also come under criticism as it remains unclear exactly how the proposed mechanism might actually work. More importantly however, as pointed out by Rahman and Wilson (2003a), H-Y antibodies are present in all brain tissue, and so the effects on sexual differentiation should be generalised, i.e. they should result in global neurological feminisation, when in fact homosexual males display a composite of male-typical and female-typical somatic and neurocognitive traits.

## Evidence from finger length ratios

The hypothesised marker of prenatal androgen exposure is of course the 2D:4D finger length ratio. An initial report investigating this ratio in homosexual and heterosexual participants was published by Robinson and Manning (2000); in several studies, they measured 2D:4D in homosexual and heterosexual males, and the homosexual sample displayed a masculinised (lower) ratio, indicating that homosexual males may have been overexposed (or were more sensitive) to prenatal testosterone. Interestingly the authors were able to split the homosexual sample into 'exclusive' and 'non-exclusive' (i.e. bisexual) homosexuals, and while the 'exclusive' group showed a lower ratio than controls, the 'non-exclusive' group displayed an even lower, more masculinised pattern. Fraternal birth order was not related to 2D:4D in that study, but in a report published in the same year Williams *et al.* (2000) only found a difference between heterosexual and homosexual males in 2D:4D when taking birth order into account; thus males with more older brothers had a lower 2D:4D ratio than males with fewer or no older brothers. These authors were also able to sample a female homosexual population and found that right-hand 2D:4D ratio was masculinised in homosexual females and did not differ from that seen in the heterosexual males.

This finding of a masculinised finger length ratio in homosexual females was replicated by McFadden and Shubel (2002), but they noted that 2D:4D in homosexual males was feminised – ratios of both these groups were intermediate between heterosexual males and females. Another study has also revealed that homosexual males show feminised finger length patterns (Lippa, 2003). More recently, one study has confirmed the finding of masculinised ratios in both homosexual males and females relative to controls (Rahman, 2005a), while another failed to find any difference between heterosexual and homosexual females (van Anders and Hampson, 2005). The data (especially for homosexual males) now appear slightly confusing, with several groups reporting a hypermasculinisation of the finger length ratio in homosexual males, but others indicating the exact opposite.

A possible explanation for these discrepant findings comes from the study of Brown *et al.* (2002a), who assessed finger length ratios in homosexual females, but took care to split the group into self-reported 'butch' (masculine) and 'femme' (feminine), though this separation was not exhaustive as it only relied upon an answer to a single statement. This issue aside, the 'butch' group displayed significantly more masculinised (lower) finger length ratios than their 'femme' counterparts. This could be a crucial point as thus far all studies assessing 2D:4D in homosexual males have simply categorised their samples into heterosexual or homosexual, and have ignored possible within-orientation variations. As a general point, recall that Ulrichs had proposed a spectrum of homosexuality ranging from female types to male types in recognition of the fact that homosexual men are not simply feminised versions of heterosexual men. In the sex differences literature it is now recognised that simply to classify participants into males and females may well ignore significant overlap between the groups in terms of behavioural/cognitive characteristics, and the idea that males and females are located at the opposite ends of a continuum now seems very oversimplistic. This confusion may be solved when studies routinely take robust measures of physical and behavioural masculinity/femininity (perhaps by using both self-perceptions and more objective measures).

## A developmental theory

Developmental instability (DI) is the term given to the way in which the organism copes (or not) with the variety of developmental stresses it experiences during prenatal and perinatal development. Such stresses can be caused perhaps by genetic factors, maternal disease, pathogens, exposure to environmental teratogens (poisons), medical interventions, etc. (Møller, 1998). These factors are hypothesised to shift the individual's ontogenetic trajectory from an 'ideal' phenotype of heterosexual orientation towards homosexuality; homosexuality may thus represent a kind of neurodevelopmental perturbation (Lalumière et al., 2000). The prediction is therefore clear in that homosexual individuals should be more likely to display minor physical anomalies reflecting an increase in developmental instability. One such hypothesised marker is handedness, in which 90% of individuals are consistently right-handed, which reflects left hemisphere dominance. In individuals known to have experienced developmental perturbations then the incidence of left-handedness rises significantly (studies cited in Coren, 1992).

In a review of the literature, Lalumière et al. (2000) noted elevated frequencies of left-handeness in homosexual males (34% were left-handed) and in homosexual females (94% were left-handed). Another marker of DI is that of fluctuating asymmetry (FA) defined as 'random deviation from perfect bilateral symmetry in a morphological trait for which differences between right and left sides have a mean of zero and are normally distributed' (Watson and Thornhill, 1994). Thus far, however, studies have not been very supportive of this model. For example, Rahman and Wilson (2003b) assessed FA by measuring the differences between the lengths of the second and fourth fingers in homosexual and heterosexual males and females, but reported no differences. Similarly, Mustanski et al. (2002) measured FA in dermatoglyphic characteristics of the fingers and also found no differences between sexual-orientation groups. A possible limitation with all such studies, however, is the focus on a very narrow range of FA measures, and perhaps studies utilising multiple markers may have more success (Rahman, 2005b).

## Neurohormonal theories

Thus far the dominant neurohormonal theory has been that of Ellis and
Ames (1987), who argued that sexual orientation is determined by the degree
to which the nervous system is exposed to testosterone and its metabolite
estradiol while sexual differentiation of the brain is occurring. During this
organisational phase, testosterone serves first to masculinise the genitals and
then to masculinise the brain. So human sexual orientation may be determined between the middle of the second month and the end of the fifth
month of gestation; overlapping this period and extending by two to three
more months is the phase during which sex-typical behaviour patterns are
organised. The model generates several predictions that subsequent research
has either supported or questioned. These are as follows:

1 Homosexuality should be more common in males. This is supported.
2 Homosexuals of both sexes should demonstrate cross-sex shifts in neu-
  robehavioural characteristics in line with their sexual partner preference.
  Thus, for example, homosexual males should demonstrate more female-
  typical neurological/cognitive characteristics. This is partly supported, as
  some studies demonstrate more feminine characteristics in homosexual
  men and more masculine characteristics in homosexual females. There is
  also considerable evidence that such groups show behaviour characteristic
  (or even hypercharacteristic) of their genetic sex.
3 Gender atypical behaviour should be evident from birth. This is supported.
4 Homosexuality should be non-randomly distributed along family lines. As
  we have seen there is strong evidence that homosexuality is heritable.
5 There need not be major differences between circulating hormonal levels
  in later life. This appears to be supported.
6 Attempts to alter sexual orientation after birth should fail. None has yet
  proved successful.

McFadden (2002) points out that this theory does not address why in some
instances homosexual males appear to be hypermasculinised but in others
appear to be hypomasculinised. A possible solution is that of 'localised'
effects in that different structures and neural circuits are responsible for
different traits compared within the sexes. These different structures and circuits can be differentially and perhaps independently affected by androgens
during development; they may either be differentially exposed to androgens,
or be differentially sensitive, perhaps at different times during development.
McFadden (2002) also points out that the effects of prenatal androgens may
not be monotonic, i.e. an increase in androgens has masculinising effects up
to a point, beyond which increases produce a reversal of effects. Rahman
(2005b) adopts a similar approach by arguing that homosexual males may
show a 'mosaic' pattern of features that are mainly cross-sex shifted (feminised) but they may also demonstrate hypermasculinised features owing to

differential effects of localised androgen action on specific neural tissues, perhaps acting at different times during development.

An additional factor to consider could be the process of aromatisation. In certain species of sheep some males show an exclusive same-sex preference even if provided with access to receptive females. It has been found that these males show reduced aromatase activity in regions of the hypothalamus known to mediate certain sexual behaviours and thus are not experiencing estrogen-mediated masculinisation (Roselli *et al.*, 2004; Morris *et al.*, 2004). In humans the same process could occur in that homosexual males (through several potential causes) may be androgen insensitive in certain key brain regions and this may explain the mosaic of traits – certain brain regions responsible for sexual orientation are not being masculinised, but other phenotypic traits (e.g. 2D:4D) are. The focus of current research is thus to explore the aromatase–estradiol pathway and possible variation in estrogen receptors.

# 7 Neural differentiation

The previous chapters have established the key role played by the gonadal steroid hormones in sexual differentiation of the body, and we have also seen evidence that certain behavioural indices (such as gender role, sexual orientation, etc.) may be related to differential hormonal exposure, these indices presumably reflecting differentiation of the central nervous system. This chapter will thus focus more closely on sexual differentiation of the brain, assessing evidence from brain regions involved in sexually dimorphic behaviours (in animals and humans), and those that are assumed to subserve certain aspects of cognition (in humans).

## The avian song centres

In many animal species, individuals show different patterns of behaviour, especially within contexts related to courtship and reproduction. Such sexually dimorphic behaviours are likely to be subserved by neurological differences, perhaps to a greater or lesser degree triggered by hormonal changes. A good example is that of bird song. Nottebohm (1970) described in detail the development of bird song, using as an example the wild chaffinch, a species in which adult males sing but adult females do not. The young male has to learn his songs from adult males in the nearby environment; these songs last around two seconds, and consist of two or three phrases, ending with a complex set of notes. This learning process takes place during the first year. A set of rambling vocalisations called 'subsong' increase in complexity, and develop into 'plastic song', very similar to the final polished version but lacking full complexity and well-defined phrasing. The final adult song is permanently acquired at around ten months of age: birds deafened before this stage produce grossly abnormal songs, while birds deafened after this stage produce normal songs, though these can regress in quality after time (studies cited in Nottebohm, 1970). If male chaffinches are reared in isolation then they never learn to 'sing' like their wild counterparts; instead they produce songs of normal duration and pitch but with no phrasing and lacking the complex ending. Once the song has developed during the first year of the bird's life, then it remains very stable and will not change in subsequent years.

Thus, if early in life, during a 'sensitive period', the male he is exposed to adult males singing, then he will later produce a polished version of the songs he has been exposed to. Importantly, the onset of his singing coincides with a seasonal rise in testosterone levels. If the male is not exposed to normal levels of testosterone at the right time (e.g. following castration) then he will not sing. It is thus interesting to speculate on the kinds of neurological changes which might be associated with the onset of singing when exposed to the appropriate hormonal environment. Of key interest is the fact that at the onset of the breeding season adult males display a rise in circulating testosterone that has a direct effect on the morphology of the brain. Nottebohm (1981) demonstrated that testis volume and serum androgen levels showed marked seasonal variation, and were closely related to the onset and termination of singing. Those regions of the brain underlying singing showed dramatic changes in size over the course of the year, expanding as testosterone levels rises when the breeding season begins (when singing starts), shrinking when the breeding season ends and testosterone levels drop (and singing declines). Nottebohm poetically noted 'the plastic substrate for vocal learning is renewed once yearly, a growing, then shedding of synapses, much the way trees grow leaves in the spring and shed them in the fall' (Nottebohm, 1981: 1370).

Like chaffinches, the adult male canary sings while the adult female does not, and Nottebohm and Arnold (1976) discovered a striking sexual dimorphism in certain regions of the canary brain that are strongly implicated in the vocal control of singing. All four areas were significantly larger in the male birds compared to the female birds. The authors were careful to control for possible sex differences in overall brain weight, and noted that two regions of the thalamus which are not involved in singing showed no such differences between males and females. Later studies established that these differences reflected an increase in nuclear volume, an increase in dendritic length, and also a greater number of synapses within these 'singing centres' (Nottebohm, 1981; DeVoogd and Nottebohm, 1981).

Adult female canaries can be stimulated to 'sing' following injections of testosterone propionate (though this does not occur in adult female zebra finches). However, the song shows considerably less variation than that of the normal adult male. Arnold (1980) compared the volumes of various brain regions in normal male and female zebra finches, and in castrated males, and in adult females receiving testosterone injections. No significant differences were established between intact and castrated males in the volume of the song production regions; paradoxically the castrated males showed greater volume in several different regions not limited to the 'singing centres'. There was a significant difference between the female groups however, with those receiving testosterone displaying greater volume in one 'singing' centre. As this nucleus still remained much smaller than that seen in a normal male, Arnold concluded that the sexual dimorphism in this nucleus was only partly explained by sex differences in circulating androgens.

## The rodent hypothalamus

In the 1960s Pfaff reported subtle morphological differences in the hypothalamus between castrated male rats and those who remained gonadally intact (Pfaff, 1966). Several years later Raisman and Field (1971) proposed that female rats showed a greater number of certain types of synapses in a specific region of the hypothalamus called the preoptic area (POA) than did males. However, such differences could only be seen using a microscope, and some doubts were raised as to the reliability of these findings. The important finding by Nottebohm and Arnold (1976), that the brains of songbirds contained sexually dimorphic regions that were so apparent that they could be identified by the naked eye, led to greater confidence in the search for rodent neural dimorphisms. Subsequently, Gorski et al. (1978) also focussed on the POA and once more noted that it was significantly larger in male rats, this enlargement apparently being due to the greater number of neurons within a specific region of the male POA (Jacobsen and Gorski, 1981). This nucleus has since been referred to as the 'sexually dimorphic nucleus of the POA' (SDN-POA). It shares dense connections with other regions of the brain that are targets for sex steroid hormones, and are also sexually dimorphic (De Vries and Simerly, 2002). It is probable that the SDN-POA is responsible for integrating sensory, somatic and humoral information to coordinate appropriate sexual behaviours in response to certain sexual cues.

The work by Pfaff some years previously had suggested that male sex hormones might be critical in the development of this structure. Jacobsen et al. (1981) confirmed this by castrating one-day-old male rats (at this stage male rat brains are still being 'organised' by androgens) and demonstrated that they showed a significantly reduced SDN-POA in adulthood. To further strengthen the possible involvement of testosterone in sculpting this neurological sexual dimorphism, neonatally castrated male rats and whole female rats both given exogenous testosterone showed a male-typical volume of this structure in adulthood (Jacobsen et al., 1981). This finding was confirmed by Döhler et al. (1984b), who found that if females were injected with testosterone throughout their pregnancy, and their pups continued to be injected up to postnatal day 10, then these female offspring displayed a completely masculinised SDN-POA. No added effects were noted for males. In a different species (the Mongolian gerbil) Commins and Yahr (1984) compared the characteristics of the SDN-POA in gonadally intact males and females, and in males and females gonadectomised, or gonadectomised and given testosterone. Gonadectomy decreased the volume of the SDN-POA in both sexes, but testosterone treatment prevented these changes.

Some studies have assessed possible developmental changes in the SDN-POA by injecting the autoradiographic tracer [$^3$H] thymidine to pregnant female rats on different days of gestation. Such studies have revealed that the SDN-POA actually shows a sex reversal during gestation: up to day 17 it is larger in females than males, but after day 17 (when male animals receive a surge of testosterone) it then becomes larger in males (Jacobsen and Gorski, 1981). Interestingly, perinatal exposure of female pups to the non-steroidal estrogen diethylstilbestrol (DES), which does not bind to alpha-fetoprotein (AFP), also leads to a sex reversal of the SDN-POA, thus suggesting that estrogen rather than testosterone might be crucial. Indeed, male rats with testicular feminising mutation show a marked reduction in androgen receptors, but have normal levels of estrogen receptors, and possess an SDN-POA equivalent in volume to that of normal males (Gorski et al., 1981). Postnatal administration of the anti-estrogen tamoxifen not surprisingly then leads to a reduction in the volume of the male SDN-POA (Döhler et al., 1984c); however, it also reduces female SDN-POA volume, so there is clearly more to be discovered about the precise hormonal mechanisms underlying sexual dimorphism of this structure.

A study assessing dimorphism of this nucleus in sheep suggests a possible role for sexual orientation and the role of aromatase. Roselli et al. (2004) note that around 8% of rams exhibit a clear sexual preference for male partners (even if provided with ample opportunities to mate with ewes). The SDN was compared in a group of these 'male-oriented' rams and a group of female-oriented rams, the volume of the SDN being found to be significantly larger in the female-oriented group. In addition, the volume of aromatase mRNA expression was significantly higher in the SDN of the female-oriented males than in male-oriented males and in ewes.

Gorski (1985) in fact suggested six (possibly interrelated) mechanisms that may determine neuronal volume in this structure (and perhaps in other brain regions as well).

1 Steroids may stimulate neurogenesis (neuronal development), or prolong the time during which neurogenesis occurs.
2 They may modulate the migration of newly formed neurons to the SDN-POA.
3 Steroids may prolong cell survival during migration, or prevent cell death.
4 They may influence the process by which neurons aggregate into the SDN-POA.
5 Steroids may prevent histogenic cell death after migration has taken place.
6 They may influence the specification of neurons in terms of functional and/or neurochemical identification.

Such mechanisms may operate alone or in tandem with each other, and some mechanism may be more important in the development of some structures but not of others.

McCarthy and Konkle (2005) speculated that steroid hormones may not affect the development of the cells in these nuclei that are destined to become sexually dimorphic; rather, these hormones may determine whether pre-existing cells will survive or die. In support, newborn males and females seem to have the same amount of neurons in the SDN-POA, the adult difference being due to cells dying off in the female nucleus in the first few weeks of life. Whatever the precise mechanisms, in rodents at least we can safely say that exposure to gonadal hormones leads to certain structural sexual dimorphisms in the CNS.

## Differentiation of the human brain

The topic of human brain differentiation has a long and controversial history, especially when suggestions are aired as to the possible causes of any observed differences. At the beginning of the 1900s it was first suggested that hormones might be involved in sexual differentiation of the genitals and reproductive organs (cited in Swaab and Hofman, 1984) and by the 1930s the focus had switched to the brain, with Pfeiffer (1936) arguing that the pituitary gland was sexually dimorphic, and that such differences resulted from differential hormone production from the gonads. As we have already seen, Phoenix *et al.* (1959) led the way in showing that manipulation of the prenatal hormonal environment led to physical and behavioural sex differences in adulthood in guinea pigs. The key problem for scientists when analysing possible human neurological sex differences was casting off the unsavoury reputation that had come about through early investigations. The existence of morphological differences between males and females was littered with sexist and racist bias, and poor methodology.

For example, Hushke in the 1850s (cited in Swaab and Hofman, 1984) demonstrated that the frontal lobe in female brains was 1% smaller than that of male brains. He noticed some other minor differences in shape and size of various structures, and from such tiny differences boldly concluded that women were somehow inferior. Other researchers pointed out that such minor differences probably owed more to the bias of the researcher than to some objective identifiable difference, but these remained isolated voices as many scientists sought to 'prove' the intellectual inferiority of women and certain racial groups. Great attention was paid to measuring skull circumference and to assessing cranial capacity, all typically showing the 'expected' outcome that white Caucasian males had bigger brains, and were thus arguably more intelligent (Gould, 1981).

In the 1800s the noted comparative anatomist and famous discoverer of the speech production centres in the left hemisphere of the brain, Paul Pierre Broca, himself stated 'the brain is much larger in mature adults than in the elderly, in men than in women, in eminent men than in men of mediocre talent, in superior races than in inferior races' (cited in Gould, 1981: 83). With little trace of irony, esteemed sociologist and founding father of social psychology Gustave le Bon noted: 'In the most intelligent races, as among the Parisians, there are a large number of women whose brains are closer in size to those of gorillas than to the most developed male brains' (cited in Gould, 1981: 105). With statements like these coming from such eminent scholars, it is little wonder that even today suspicion surrounds researchers treading the same path, the danger being of course that such researchers are utilising methods perhaps equally flawed, and with preconceptions equally (if unconsciously) biased. With this caveat established, I will review certain key morphological differences ascribed to the human brain, and discuss possible hormonal mechanisms derived from pertinent animal and human studies.

## Brain size/weight

More than a hundred years ago several researchers reported statistically significant differences between the sexes in brain size and weight (cited in Kretschmann *et al.*, 1979). Dekaban and Sadowsky (1978) confirmed such differences, and noted that they existed early in life. However, reported values for such effects varied markedly, and it is likely that numerous factors play a role. It is, for example, generally the case that male infants are both heavier and taller than female infants; it is thus likely that sex differences in neonatal brain weight reflect these differences in stature. Indeed, when allometric scaling is applied to such data then female infants are found to have similar brain weights to males of a comparable weight and size.

However, sexual dimorphism in relative brain size appears at around two years of age, when the brain has reached around 85% of its adult value, and this cannot be fully explained by differences in height or weight (Swaab and Hofman, 1984). Amongst normal adults there is a difference of around 120–160 grams between male and female brains, though whether this difference is due to the amount or the size of individual neurons or glia remains to be established (Breedlove, 1994). Rabinowicz *et al.* (1999) provided some evidence in the form of a morphometric study of neuronal density in thirty bilateral brain regions in six males and five females. This participant group is small, and the age range wide (twelve to twenty-four) and so one can only draw tentative conclusions; nevertheless, the researchers observed significantly higher neural density in the male brains: males displayed around 299,000 neurons per $1\,mm^2$ of cortex while the females had around 265,000 per $1\,mm^2$. As more nerve cells imply a corresponding increase in axon number, then this would explain the greater brain weight. An increase in brain size/weight of course does not necessarily imply greater intelligence: brain function is not simply to do with size but with other factors such as processing speed, connectivity, etc. De Courten-Myers (1999) pointed out that female brains contain more cortical neuropil – the patchwork of unmyelinated neuronal processes (both axonal and dendritic) within the grey matter. This suggests that female brains possess more dendritic branching, leading to more connections between the neurons, and hence perhaps greater processing capacity.

To my knowledge (and hopefully someone reading this will correct this ignorance), research has not yet identified links between hormones and human brain weight, though a likely candidate could be the thyroid hormones, the lack of which during foetal development are clearly associated with neurological abnormalities such as a reduction in synaptogenesis and myelin production which would clearly affect brain weight (see chapter 4).

## The hypothalamus

In light of the significant sex differences in various rodent hypothalamic nuclei, researchers have, not surprisingly, focussed their attention on the equivalent structures within the human brain. One region of interest has been the bed nucleus of the stria terminalis (BNST), a structure that exhibits a clear sex difference in rodents by being much larger in males (Hines *et al.*, 1992). This structure shares connections with the amygdala and nucleus accumbens, contains both androgen and estrogen receptors, and in may species has been identified as a key area where aromatisation is known to take place (Commins and Yahr, 1985; Sheridan, 1979). Allen and Gorski (1990) reported that part of this region was two to three times larger in adult human males than in females, though this difference does not appear to be present before the age of ten (Breedlove, 1994).

Interestingly, Zhou *et al.* (1995) compared the size and volume of the BNST in heterosexual, homosexual and male-to-female transsexual individuals. Heterosexual males displayed a significantly larger volume compared with heterosexual women, but did not differ from that seen in homosexual males. The male-to-female transsexuals, however, displayed a BNST volume 52% that of the heterosexual males, smaller (but not significantly so) than the female volume. Such differences were independent of levels of circulating sex steroids. Zhou and colleagues suggested that the dimorphism in the BNST is probably established during early development by the organising effect of sex hormones, a suggestion supported by the fact that neonatal castration in male rats and androgenisation of female rats leads to reversals of this sex dimorphism (del Abril *et al.*, 1987). As transsexuals are administered cross-sex hormones as part of the reassignment process, this group provides a unique window in which to see if the provision of certain hormones can alter brain morphology. Thus far studies have not been able to investigate this. However, Pol *et al.* (2006) took high-resolution brain scans of female-to-male transsexuals and male-to-female transsexuals, before and after hormone therapy. The provision of estrogens and antiandrogens to males led to a decrease in brain volume, while androgen treatment in females led to an increase in brain volume. These changes appeared to be due particularly to alterations in total brain volume, but specifically to alterations in the hypothalamic nuclei.

The POA of the hypothalamus has received much attention in rodents (see previous section) and not surprisingly researchers have looked for a similar dimorphism in the human brain. Swaab and Fliers (1985) did indeed find a sexually dimorphic structure within the human hypothalamus that was more than twice as large in males than in females. In terms of its cyto-architecture and locality it appeared homologous to that observed in the rat. The human POA has in fact been divided into four regions, referred to as the interstitial nuclei of the anterior hypothalamus (INAH) and commonly abbreviated to INAH 1-4, with INAH-1 being considered equivalent to the rodent SDN-POA. Allen *et al.* (1989) reported no clear sex differences in INAH-1 but their sample was biased in terms of age. Swaab *et al.* (1992) pointed out that differentiation of this structure only seems to occur after around the age of four (the nucleus degenerates in females after this point) and this is perhaps why Allen and colleagues failed to find a difference.

As this structure differentiates long after the major gonadal hormonal changes during development, and well before the next series of hormonal events at puberty, it seems likely that this structure is not directly affected by the gonadal hormones, though it could of course be organised by these hormones early on and then later activated by other hormonal events that we do not yet understand. The animal literature clearly points to some involvement of the gonadal steroids, but of course manipulation studies are ethically difficult to conduct in humans, and as yet cases of 'quirks of nature' involving prenatal hormonal abnormalities have not yet been examined in this field of study. Interestingly, LeVay (1991) reported that in homosexual men the INAH-3 does not differ in size from that of females, and is clearly different from that of heterosexual males. However, as all of these males died of AIDS (which is known to reduce brain weight and testosterone levels) the cause of this difference remains unknown. Other studies have also failed to confirm this finding (Byne *et al.*, 2001). Thus far, the link between hormones and the development of this structure remains unconfirmed; however, using immunocytochemical techniques Fernández-Guasti *et al.* (2000) have demonstrated that the male INAH contains greater numbers of androgen and estrogen ($\alpha$ and $\beta$) receptors than the INAH in females, which clearly points to some role of the gonadal steroids.

## Cerebral asymmetry

In 1836, French doctor Marc Dax reported his observations concerning some of his patients who displayed severe disruption in their ability to produce and comprehend speech following damage to their left hemisphere.[1] His announcement was greeted with total apathy and he died a year later unaware of the impact that his observations would have on future generations of

---

[1] Such deficits are called 'aphasia', from the Greek word meaning 'without speech'.

neurologists and psychologists (Springer and Deutsch, 1993). In fact Dax had unwittingly paved the way for a considerable body of research concerned with hemispheric specialisation – the understanding that the two halves of the brain are not mirror images of one another, but in fact are responsible for different types of processing. The evidence from such as Dax and Paul Broca led neurologist John Hughlings Jackson to propose the idea of a 'leading' hemisphere, and he noted that in most individuals the left hemisphere is the dominant one. Over the years systematic neuropsychological testing, utilising a range of diverse neurological groups and normal controls, has indeed shown that the left hemisphere is primarily involved in the processing of language/communicative information, while the right hemisphere is more important for the processing of spatial (non-verbal) information (Springer and Deutsch, 1993).

At a simple level, each hemisphere is responsible for controlling the opposite side of the body: the left hemisphere controls the right side and vice versa. It has since been noted that hemispheric specialisation is not a constant factor, but instead varies between individuals, especially in relation to handedness and sex. Numerous studies involving diverse methodologies have now demonstrated that, for the processing of certain types of information, males tend to be more strongly lateralised (i.e. one hemisphere bears the brunt of the responsibility for the processing) whereas females tend to show more equity in cortical effort between the hemispheres. For example, Shaywitz et al. (1995) conducted functional MRI scans of two areas known to be important for language processing – extrastriate cortex and the inferior frontal gyrus. Right-handed males and females performed a series of language tasks, during which brain activation in males was found to be lateralised to the left inferior frontal gyrus; in females the pattern of activation engaged more diffuse areas in both hemispheres.

Another common (and cheaper) technique for assessing cerebral lateralisation is known as the 'dichotic listening' task. When two different words are presented simultaneously to both ears, those words presented to the right ear tend to be more accurately reported than those presented to the left ear. This right-ear advantage is assumed to reflect the specialised role of the left hemisphere for language/speech processing. In contrast, melodic patterns (processed by the right hemisphere) are better identified with the left ear. Males are slower and make more mistakes in responding to auditory information presented to their left ear, while women show similar performance with both ears. Interestingly, women exposed to testosterone in the womb display a male-typical lateralisation compared to their unexposed sisters (Hines, 1991). A recent meta-analytic review by Voyer (1997) considered the evidence for sex differences in cerebral lateralisation in auditory, visual and tactile modalities, and confirmed that males were more lateralised in all three modalities, regardless of whether verbal or non-verbal tasks were used.

## Hormones and cerebral asymmetry

As sex appears to have a considerable influence on the degree of cortical asymmetry and, as we have seen in previous chapters, sexual differentiation is determined by prenatal hormone exposure, then logically we should expect to find links between certain hormones and cerebral lateralisation. In rats, males display a cerebral cortex thicker than that of female rats (Stewart and Kolb, 1988). There is some asymmetry apparent in that males appear to show greater cortical thickness in the right hemisphere compared to the left, but the reverse pattern seems to be true for females (Diamond et al., 1975). However, in an analysis of discrete cellular regions of rat cortex, Reid and Juraska (1992) confirmed sex differences in cortical thickness in numerous areas, but could not confirm the existence of consistent cortical asymmetries. The role of hormones in such dimorphism appears fairly strong; for example, female rats ovariectomised at birth display the more male-typical pattern of right > left cortical thickness in adulthood, while male rats castrated at birth show the more female-typical pattern (Diamond et al., 1981; 1979). It is tempting to conclude that testosterone or estrogens are responsible for such morphological characteristics. However Lewis and Diamond (1995) failed to find androgen receptors in prenatal rat brains, and the presence of alpha-fetoprotein in rat neocortex suggests that estrogen may be unable to act at a morphological level (Soloff et al., 1972). Therefore the likely candidate could be the conversion of testosterone to estradiol via aromatisation, the presence of aromatase being confirmed in various brain regions (Roselli et al., 1997).

Like handedness in humans, rats display a bias in the way their tail lies: males typically show a right-facing tail bias, while females typically show a left-facing tail bias. Rosen et al. (1984) injected pregnant female rats with either testosterone propionate (aromatises to estradiol), dihydrotestosterone propionate (cannot be aromatised), or a control substance. While the dihydrotestosterone propionate and control substance had no effect on tail posture in female pups, injections of testosterone propionate led to a significant shift towards a male bias in the exposed females, indicating that testosterone may exert its effects after being converted to an estrogen.

Wisniewski (1998) has reviewed the evidence concerning the organisational and activational effects of hormones on cerebral asymmetry in humans. With regard to organisational effects, one line of evidence concerns relationships between testosterone levels and functional lateralisation. Grimshaw et al. (1995a) took samples of testosterone from amniotic fluid during foetal development, and when the children were ten their behavioural asymmetries were assessed via handedness questionnaires and two dichotic tasks (a left-hemisphere verbal task, and a right-hemisphere emotional task). In boys, prenatal testosterone was positively related to their performance on the right-hemisphere task. In the sample as a whole, the authors found a positive correlation between prenatal testosterone and levels of right-handedness, with testosterone being associated with an increase in cerebral lateralisation.

Another line of evidence concerns exposure to the synthetic estrogen diethylstilbestrol[2] (DES) during foetal development. As it acts like an estrogen, DES has masculinising/defeminising effects, and in support of this Hines and Shipley (1984) noted, for example, that DES-exposed females exhibited dichotic processing more akin to that of males than females, in comparison to their unexposed sisters. In males, those exposed to DES during development showed a more feminised pattern of cortical lateralisation compared to their unexposed brothers (Reinisch and Sanders, 1992). Such data appear rather contradictory in that females exposed to this synthetic estrogen show an increase in lateralisation, whereas exposed males show a decrease. Wisniewski (1998) points out that methodological differences between how laterality was assessed in the two studies, and the time and duration of gestational exposure between the male and female samples, may account for this contradiction. However, perhaps the data are not so contradictory, as animal studies have in fact demonstrated that the same sex steroid treatment can have a masculinising effect in females, but a feminising effect in males (e.g. Diamond *et al.*, 1973).

A third line of evidence concerns lateralisation in individuals with certain clinical conditions in which prenatal hormonal exposure has been abnormal (see chapter 6). CAH women have been exposed to high levels of androgens pre- and postnatally and it would thus be expected that they might show masculinised cerebral lateralisation. However, Helleday *et al.* (1994) assessed lateralisation via a handedness questionnaire, a finger tapping test and a dichotic verbal test in twenty-two CAH women and age-matched controls. Contrary to their expectation, the CAH females did not display a more masculinised pattern of lateralisation, but Wisniewski (1998) notes that the authors had tested a small sample, and used tasks that were not that appropriate to the research question. Evidence from girls with Turner's syndrome is slightly clearer. Recall that such individuals have been exposed to very low levels of estrogens; thus one might again assume that they would display more masculinised patterns of cerebral lateralisation. Several studies have addressed this, one example being that of Netley and Rovet (1982), who gave Turner's and control girls a dichotic listening task. While the control females showed the expected right-ear (left-hemisphere) advantage, the Turner girls showed a left-ear advantage.

With regard to activational effects, Wisniewski (1998) considered evidence from individual differences in pubertal maturation rate in both sexes, and

---

[2] Despite a lack of clinically controlled double-blind studies as to its efficacy, DES was available in America for use by pregnant women to reduce the possibility of miscarriage or premature birth. Between 1938 and 1971 many millions of people were exposed to DES, either as a pregnant mother, or as a developing foetus.

menstrual cycle effects in females. In the former, Waber (1977) argued that sex differences in certain lateralisation tasks might be less dependent upon sex per se, but more influenced by the individual's rate of pubertal maturation. According to Waber, females typically enter puberty faster, and complete the process sooner than males (there is considerable individual variation though). Early pubertal maturation could be associated with reduced cerebral asymmetry, while later pubertal maturation could be associated with increased cerebral asymmetry. In support of this hypothesis, Waber (1977) did find that individuals who completed puberty at a later age (males and females) showed an increase in hemispheric specialisation as measured by a dichotic task. In a more rigorous study, Waber *et al.* (1985) conducted a longitudinal assessment of early- and late-maturing teenagers on dichotic performance and found support for the earlier hypothesis; however, studies by Vrbancic and Mosley (1988) and Meyer-Bahlburg *et al.* (1985) have been unable to confirm this 'maturation' hypothesis. As none of these studies conducted hormonal assays it is difficult to decide what if any role circulating pubertal hormones might have.

A second line of activational evidence comes from studies attempting to find relationships between the characteristic hormone profile of the menstrual cycle and cerebral lateralisation. The logic behind such studies reflects the fact that, at certain points of the cycle, levels of the hormones estradiol and progesterone are very low (menses), while at other points of the cycle levels of these hormones are very high (estradiol during the follicular and luteal phases; progesterone during the luteal phase). Chiarello *et al.* (1989) tested women during their menstrual, follicular and luteal phases on a visually presented lexical decision task. While accuracy appeared to be unaffected by menstrual phase, response criterion assessed by signal detection methods did show a relationship, the right hemisphere demonstrating a stronger response criterion than the left during the follicular and luteal phases (high estradiol), but a left hemisphere dominance during menses.

Similarly, Bibawi *et al.* (1995) tested women during menstruation and the midluteal phase (and a sample of men tested over the same time difference) on a chimeric[3] faces test. In their version, the same face was photographed with two emotions ('happy' and 'neutral') and participants were asked to identify the emotion displayed in the split-face. This task has been shown to exhibit a right-hemisphere advantage. They also conducted an object identification task (chairs) that within groups reveals no hemispheric advantage, while individuals (especially females) do display considerable variance in the hemispheric advantage associated with this task – possibly reflecting hormonal events. While performance on the object identification task showed

---

[3] Such tasks are named after the mythical Chimera, a monster composed of several different animals, and involve a split face consisting of the left half of one face and the right half of another.

no phase shift in males, performance by females did show such a shift, as the left hemisphere was more activated during the midluteal phase compared to menses. Performance on the chimeric faces task showed no such fluctuations in either sex. A key problem for these 'activational' studies is the lack of direct assessment of hormone concentrations, rendering any conclusions concerning hormone fluctuations and hemispheric asymmetry rather tentative.

### An explanatory model?

At a meeting in 1980 in which dyslexia[4] was being discussed, neurologist Norman Geschwind was surprised by the number of parents of dyslexic children who reported that their offspring were also plagued by immune system disorders (e.g. hay fever) and migraine headaches, and were described as being non-right-handed. His interest aroused, he collaborated with Peter Behan, and in a series of studies they demonstrated the then unexpected link between left-handedness and these disorders. In 1982 Geschwind and Behan published a paper that was only three pages long, but the implications of which have reverberated around psychology departments ever since. Their assertion caused such a stir because of the radical nature of their argument. In essence they proposed that cerebral lateralisation (the 'marker' they used for this was handedness) in adults was strongly associated with circulating levels of testosterone experienced during foetal life. In addition, the levels of this hormone also impacted upon the developing immune system (Geschwind and Behan, 1982).

Thus, they boldly attempted to link handedness, immune diseases like hay fever, migraine, and developmental disorders like dyslexia with the prenatal actions of testosterone. Your hormonal environment before birth could thus have a profound impact not only upon your neurodevelopment, but also on your physical health and well-being as an adult. Geschwind then collaborated with neurologist Albert Galaburda and the pair delivered several other (much larger) papers a few years later (Geschwind and Galaburda, 1985a, 1985b, 1985c), and they summarised the entire theory in book form (Geschwind and Galaburda, 1987). All in all, the theory became extremely complex and wide-ranging by linking a variety of biological/neurological characteristics, and the main exponents have provided numerous scientific reports in the form of peer-reviewed journal articles to back up their claims.

This was a bold hypothesis indeed, and not surprisingly it caused a great stir at the time. The theory became known as the 'GBG Model' (after the initials of the principal authors) and while its core concepts perhaps remain mysterious in the eyes of the general public, its key assertions have certainly entered the realm of assumed scientific 'fact' in that many are taken for granted. Thus, readers of popular magazines (and often scientific articles) are

---

[4] A broad term applied to individuals experiencing specific reading disabilities despite normal intellectual/sensory functioning.

provided with assertions such as 'left-handers are more likely to suffer from hay fever', or 'left handers make better tennis players, mathematicians or musicians because of their enhanced right hemispheric functioning'. The proof of the pudding of course rests in the eating, and like all 'grand theories' in the social sciences it has been attacked on numerous evidential and theoretical grounds. But first, what exactly did the theory propose?

The basic idea of the theory is that levels of circulating testosterone during the prenatal period slow development in certain cortical regions of the left hemisphere of the brain (in most people this hemisphere controls the processing of verbal information and the right side of the body), leading to the corresponding greater development of certain cortical regions of the right hemisphere (this controls non-verbal information processing, such as spatial/mathematical ability, and the left side of the body). Thus, high levels of testosterone may cause such retardation in the left hemisphere that certain functions (handedness, language processing) 'shift' to the right hemisphere. This then seemed to explain certain observations, for example that left-handedness is more common in males, as are certain developmental disorders (e.g. dyslexia). It also provided some rationale to observations that the spatially, numerically and musically 'gifted' may be more likely to be left-handed (e.g. Aggleton *et al.*, 1994; Benbow, 1988).

As the male foetus is typically exposed to higher levels of testosterone, the GBG model thus predicted that males will show enhanced right-hemisphere processing (enhanced spatial/mathematical/logical skills) but reduced left-hemisphere processing (impaired language/social skills) to such an extent that the individual may show a greater susceptibility to certain developmental disorders (e.g. autism, dyslexia, stuttering, etc.). A further consequence of this proposed alteration in left-hemisphere functioning is that it may lead to what Geschwind and Galaburda (1987) referred to as 'anomalous dominance', i.e. an increase in left-handedness.

A final key prediction of the GBG model suggests that testosterone will have an influence on the developing immune system via its actions on the thymus gland (a two-lobed organ located in the lower part of the neck and the upper region of the chest cavity). The prime function of this gland is to manufacture and release thymus cells (T-cells) into the blood that are then used by the immune system (alongside B-cells) to combat infections (Miller, 2002). Elevated levels of testosterone may thus impair the functioning of the thymus, leading to a greater likelihood of immune system related health problems. Since the original formulation of the theory, the authors have made some modifications; for example, Rosen *et al.* (1991) suggested that asymmetry does not result from a retardation of growth in the left hemisphere, but rather from enhanced growth in the right hemisphere. Thus, testosterone is assumed to have different effects, but the end result is the same.

According to Bryden *et al.* (1994) the GBG theory is not as straightforward as it first appears, and the evidence routinely cited in support of it may not be as strong as is often claimed. It is beyond the scope of this text to evaluate in detail all of the principal hypotheses of the model (one major association, for example, is argued to be between immune disorders and neural crest disorders) but I shall focus on those key relationships which directly involve testosterone. Perhaps the central claim of the model involves the effects of testosterone on anomalous dominance. Recall that most individuals are assumed to display a standard dominance pattern consisting of left-hemisphere dominance for verbal processing, right-hemisphere dominance for non-verbal processing, and right-handedness. Recall as well that the model assumes that as males are arguably exposed to higher levels of testosterone in the womb, they should be more likely than females to display anomalous dominance. The testing of such proposed relationships should thus be fairly routine, but, as we shall see, things are rather more complex than they first seem.

Bryden *et al.* (1994) first point out that the key measure used to ascertain anomalous dominance is that of handedness, probably because simply asking someone to describe which hand they use for various tasks is a quick and simple thing to do, and far easier (and cheaper) than obtaining detailed neuropsychological tests using highly specialised equipment (brain scans, etc.). The problem is that while handedness is most probably related to language lateralisation, it is by no means a very good predictor of it: right-handers may not always have language lateralised to their left hemisphere, and the majority of left-handers seem to have language lateralised to the left hemisphere (in direct contradiction to the model). While language dominance and handedness might well be related to one another, right hemisphere processing seems to be related to neither of them.

A key problem could be the diverse ways in which handedness has been assessed and defined: some studies use multiple-item questionnaires while others simply ask participants which hand they write with; in some cases people have been defined dichotomously as either left-handed or right-handed (the division being rather arbitrary), but in other studies linear scales, with extreme left-handers and extreme right-handers making up the end points and vague categories like 'mixed-handed' lying somewhere in-between, have been used. Nonetheless, males clearly display an increased incidence of non-right-handedness; for example, in a sample of 12,000 participants in seventeen different countries Perelle and Ehrman (1994) reported that males were much more likely to be described as left-handed, thereby confirming a key hypothesis of the model. The issue of definition also raises its head when assessing possible links between handedness and certain developmental disorders. Bishop (1990) pointed out that studies cited in support of the model have not confined the term 'developmental dyslexia' to the group that it is primarily aimed at, i.e. individuals who have reading problems but perform to a normal intellectual standard in other areas. In support of the theory, though, Bishop (1990) did find that the incidence of left-handedness was almost twice as high in a sample of dyslexics compared to a normal control group, a finding replicated by Obrzut and Atkinson (1993) in children with learning disabilities. With regard to testosterone and cerebral lateralisation, evidence has come from several different sources.

## Circulating testosterone and handedness

In a series of studies, Üner Tan has shown that individuals exhibiting the standard right-hemisphere dominance pattern had lower levels of circulating testosterone than those displaying 'anomalous dominance' (Tan, 1991a). However, in other studies the same author has reported that an increase in right-handed skill (left-hemisphere dominance) is associated with higher levels of circulating testosterone and thus contrary to the previous findings (Tan, 1990; 1991b). Moffat and Hampson (1996) pointed out two problems with these studies by Tan: first, they did not control for diurnal fluctuations in circulating testosterone levels; and second, it seems that individuals classed as 'anomalous' as regards dominance may actually have been right-handed. In their study Moffat and Hampson (1996) recruited forty male and forty female volunteers and conducted a precise measure of hand preference. Circadian fluctuations in testosterone and oral contraceptive use (in the females) were also controlled. Within both sexes independently, right-handers displayed higher testosterone levels than left-handers – a finding directly contrary to the prediction of the GBG model.

## Prenatal testosterone and lateralisation

Of course, a key problem with the studies just described is that they are relating handedness or hand-skill preference to circulating testosterone and not to prenatal testosterone as explicitly discussed in the GBG model. So, a second line of evidence considers prenatal testosterone and subsequent lateralisation indices. In one study (already discussed in this chapter), Grimshaw *et al.* (1995a) found that girls who had higher testosterone exposure at week 16 of gestation were more strongly right-handed and more likely to be left-hemispheric language processors than girls exposed to lower levels. In boys, higher levels of prenatal testosterone were associated with right-hemisphere processing for emotional material. As only a small number of left-handers were present in the sample, only the degree and not the direction of hand preference could thus be reliably assessed, but this study clearly seemed to refute the GBG hypothesis. The authors did note a key potential problem with their study (and others of a similar nature) in that testosterone levels were measured at sixteen weeks gestation in both sexes, the problem being that males and females have been shown to follow different developmental trajectories; for example, cortical development progresses at a faster rate in females (Levy and Heller, 1992). It is therefore possible that the authors sampled putative testosterone effects during a window of right-hemisphere development in boys, but left-hemisphere development in girls.

In a novel approach to the issue, Elkadi *et al.* (1999) used a sample of twins, arguing that a female foetus located in the same womb as a male twin might be exposed to higher levels of testosterone (secreted by the male twin) than a female sharing a womb with another female twin.[5] They compared hand preference in fifty-nine opposite-sex and sixty-one same-sex twins in adulthood. Measures of the strength of hand preference and the incidence of left-handedness in fact revealed no difference between opposite-sex and same-sex twins of either sex. In a more recent study, though, Cohen-Bendahan *et al.* (2004) assessed sixty-seven opposite-sex twin girls, sixty-seven opposite-sex twin boys and fifty-three same-sex twin girls in their performance of a dichotic listening task in order to measure functional cerebral lateralisation. Those girls who had gone through foetal development sharing a womb with a male co-twin (and thus perhaps having been exposed to higher levels of testosterone during that time) did indeed show a less feminine pattern of cerebral lateralisation compared to girls sharing a womb with another female.

Other studies have utilised 2D:4D, the putative marker of prenatal testosterone exposure. Thus, Manning *et al.* (2000) measured 2D:4D in 156 boys and 129 girls and assessed relative hand performance using Annett's peg-moving task (pegs are moved from one side of a board to the other as quickly as possible using left and right hands separately). The average time taken by the left hand was subtracted from the average time taken by the right hand to gain a measure of lateralised hand preference (LHP); the greater the LHP, the greater the tendency to perform faster with the left hand relative to the right hand. A lower (more masculinised) right-hand 2D:4D ratio in the sample as a whole was associated with a reduction in left-hand performance times (the left hand was faster), and hence provides some support for the GBG model.

More recently Fink *et al.* (2004) assessed hand skill in forty-five boys and forty-eight girls, using the 'Hand Dominance Test' which comprises several tests of manual dexterity, assessing both speed and precision. The score provides a ratio (D) which relates to a performance advantage of one hand relative to the other. The authors found that all correlations between test scores and left- and right-hand 2D:4D were significantly positive in right-handed participants in the sample as a whole. High prenatal testosterone was thus associated with increased left-hand skill, again in accord with the GBG model.

## An alternative theory

Evidence in favour of the GBG model thus appears to be inconclusive and somewhat contradictory. An alternative theory, which has been called the 'callosal hypothesis', was formulated by Sandra Witelson and colleagues.

---

[5] This supposition is well grounded in the animal literature as the intrauterine position has been shown to determine hormone exposure, with female foetuses lying adjacent to male foetuses experiencing physical and, arguably, behavioural masculinisation as a result of higher testosterone exposure (e.g. Vom Saal, 1989).

They have argued that cerebral lateralisation does not result from specific developmental effects occurring within the hemispheres, but instead reflects alterations to the large fibre bundle, the corpus callosum, which is vital for the functional integration of the two hemispheres. In particular, callosal axons are pruned during foetal and neonatal development; in part this pruning is mediated by the actions of testosterone (Witelson, 1991; Witelson and Nowakowski, 1991). Greater axonal pruning leads to greater lateralisation of function, and, in men at least, higher levels of prenatal testosterone should be associated with stronger cerebral language dominance and a stronger right-hand preference.

If the callosal hypothesis is correct then we should expect to identify clear differences between the corpus callosum in males and females. This large fibre tract undergoes marked changes in overall size during postnatal development and is so large that it is easy to locate and measure, not just in post-mortem bodies but (more conveniently) in live volunteers via brain scanning methods. Sexual (and racial) dimorphism of this structure was originally reported by anatomist Robert Bennett Bean in a survey of 152 brains of men and women of European and African descent. All brains (which had all been preserved using a variety of methods) were severed down the midline to reveal the corpus callosum and then Bean plotted the area of this fibre pathway against brain weight. The result showed a strong positive correlation, those of African descent having a smaller front portion (the genu) in relation to the posterior portion (the splenium) (Bean, 1906). Franklin Mall was sceptical of such claims, and conducted his own assessment of 106 brains, taking great care not to know beforehand the race or sex of the brain concerned. He found no variation in the genu or the splenium and noted that any group differences were obscured by large individual differences (Mall, 1909).

More recent techniques of establishing possible sex differences (the search for racial differences having been discarded) have focussed on statistical techniques like linear regression, but a bewildering number of methods by which the corpus callosum is 'split' into its different regions have been utilised, thus making comparison between studies problematic. The debate was kick-started again by the report of De Lacoste-Utamsing and Holloway (1982) in which they compared nine male and five female brains and declared that, while the overall area was almost identical, the splenium was significantly larger in the females (around 218 mm compared to 186 mm). The same difference was identified in foetuses from as early as twenty-six weeks of gestation, possibly indicating that hormonal influences on brain structure occur before this time (De Lacoste et al., 1986). An opposite sex difference was also found for the anterior region (the genu), which is sometimes reported to be larger in men than women. Allen et al. (1991) performed MRI scans of the corpus callosum in twenty-four age-matched children, and 122 age-matched adults. In adults, while they found no sex differences in terms of overall area of the corpus callosum, they did report a dramatic difference in the shape, with the splenium being more bulbous in females than in males. Similarly, in the children, the corpus callosum changed markedly in shape with age, the shape of the splenium being sexually dimorphic, though this was not significant.

These authors also criticised the methodology used in such comparative studies and pointed out that measurements have been performed in a variety of ways; there are clear age-related changes in the size and shape of the corpus callosum, but investigators have typically not used age-matched controls; the size and shape of the corpus callosum varies considerably between individuals, thereby requiring large sample sizes to demonstrate significant sex differences; and finally, post-mortem studies may be inaccurate because fixing techniques can affect size and shape.

In a meta-analytic review of forty-nine previous studies that had investigated the size and shape of the corpus callosum, Bishop and Wahlsten (1997) concluded that there were no significant sex differences in size or shape of the splenium. While MRI studies have shown that males have a larger corpus callosum they also demonstrate that males have bigger brains; when this factor is controlled for, then sex differences in relative size vanish. The authors also raise the point that even if there are minor variations in callosum size between the sexes, how this might relate to hemispheric specialisation is hard to understand, as the sexes do not appear to differ in axon size, or myelination (Aboitiz et al. 1992).

So, there appears little strong evidence for sex differences in the corpus callosum that might relate to functional differences. Note that this 'callosal' theory generates hypotheses very different from the GBG model, and the Grimshaw study previously cited does provide some support for it, though the callosal hypothesis does not specifically make predictions for females (as they are exposed to much lower levels of testosterone than males). It is of course possible that certain elements of both theories may be correct. Suggestive of this is the study by Gadea et al. (2003), who examined testosterone, handedness and linguistic lateralisation in adult females. Their sample of twenty-four left-handers and twenty-four right-handers provided saliva samples, had their hand preference measured, and conducted a dichotic listening task. Right-handed participants showed higher circulating testosterone levels (in accord with results by Moffat and Hampson (1996) and supporting the callosal hypothesis); in addition, however, higher testosterone levels were associated with a lesser degree of lateralisation for verbal material, which thus supports the GBG model. The methodological points raised by Bryden et al. (1994) thus seem all the more pertinent as we still seem a long way from teasing apart the possible contributions of testosterone to cerebral lateralisation.

# 8 **Reproductive/sexual behaviours**

Previous chapters have adopted a unidirectional stance outlining the presumed causal relationship between hormone secretion and physiological/ neurological differentiation. In chapter 3, however, remember that I raised issues of causality, and discussed the key difficulty facing behavioural endocrinologists in attempting to decide whether alterations in hormone levels influence a behaviour in question, or whether the onset or termination of a particular behaviour has a subsequent effect on hormone levels. Human behavioural endocrinological studies have tended to focus their attention on the former, and have thus mainly considered the effects of hormones on behaviour (van Anders and Watson, 2006a). With regard to reproductive behaviours (and the kinds of behaviours we will consider in subsequent chapters) it becomes increasingly obvious that we must also consider the reverse relationship – how behaviour may affect hormone levels.

One problem relates to defining what we mean by sexual behaviours; a further issue concerns how we may compare such behaviours between the sexes, and indeed between species. As regards the former, sexual behaviours are simply a set of actions with the primary aim of ensuring that the male sperm is delivered successfully to the female ova. The motivational force that drives individuals to seek out members of the opposite sex and copulate with them has been called 'sex drive' or 'libido'.[1] It is typically noted that in most species sex drive is stronger in males than in females, arguably because the two sexes have different pathways to reproductive success. Female eggs are 'expensive' to produce, and are limited in supply, while male sperm is 'cheap' to produce and in plentiful supply. Because of pregnancy and subsequent milk production, females invest significantly more in their offspring than males, and thereby enhance their reproductive potential by nurturing their current offspring at the expense of investing in future offspring. Males on the other hand enhance their reproductive success by seeking to mate with as many reproductively capable females as possible, and thus spend more time in seeking out novel mating partners. These behavioural specialisations into nurturing effort versus mating effort lead to

---

[1] A term first introduced by the Austrian neurologist and founder of psychoanalysis Sigmund Freud (1856–1939).

clear differences between the sexes, with females in most species providing considerably more parental investment (PI) than males (Low, 2000).

The extent to which human reproductive/sexual behaviours can be neatly explained in terms of differential parental investment, and compared to apparently similar behaviours in animals, is of course hotly debated. A key problem for researchers of human sexuality is that humans are notoriously private creatures when engaging in sexual activities, and thus researchers have to rely on self-report (subjective) accounts rather than observed (objective) behaviours (Symons, 1979). It is also true to say that human sexual behaviours are in many ways divorced from the basic sexual act: a whole host of activities can be described as 'sexual' but may not actually involve penetrative sex and fertilisation of the egg. This calls into question the validity of comparing humans and animals. However, it is obviously very difficult to conduct experiments on humans involving castration, hormone treatments or brain lesions, and so researchers have focussed on non-human subjects to conduct such studies, and derive hypotheses that may then be related to the human condition.

Ågmo and Ellingsen (2003) note that sexual behaviours in many species cannot simply be understood as behaviours subserving reproduction, as it is unlikely that any animal engages in such behaviours with that specific end in mind. Individuals engage in sex because the act of doing so produces a positive affect – people (and presumably animals) have sex because they enjoy it! According to Pfaus (1996), while the behaviours themselves may differ in complexity, it should be possible to draw direct comparisons between species, and derive a coherent theoretical framework within which different behaviours and their hormonal correlates can be understood. Indeed, Ågmo (1999) has considered internal (hormonal and physiological) factors and external (environmental and social) factors determining sexual motivation, and has formalised an 'incentive motivational model' of sexual behaviour that can be equally applied to human and animal sexual behaviours.

## Animal sexual behaviours

As pointed out by Mas (1995), working out the neurobiological mechanisms of goal-oriented behaviours such as sex is highly challenging because they stem from complex interactions between environmental/ hormonal/neural factors. For most animals, sexual behaviours occur in a sequence of fairly well-defined stages. At each stage the individual must be responding to both internal and external factors, each of which is having some influence on the current behaviour. Beach (1956) originally proposed a heuristic to attempt to define copulatory behaviours by separating sexual behaviour into 'appetitive' and 'consummatory' stages. This two-stage distinction has since been applied to other behaviours such as feeding, aggression and drug-taking behaviours in both animals and humans.

Appetitive behaviours are those which bring the individual into contact with the particular goal at hand, i.e. a sexually receptive female. They tend to be quite flexible, and are probably derived from learning and social experiences. For example, sexually naïve male rats will attempt to continue to copulate with a sexually satiated female rat, who will aggressively fend off their intentions. Sexually experienced male rats, however, will correctly interpret behavioural signals from the female that she does not wish further copulation, and leave her alone (Pfaus, 1996). Consummatory behaviours are those that are then performed when individuals are in contact with their primary goal, and they tend to be more highly stereotyped and species-specific, and are probably innate.

In the past, investigators have focussed their attention on rodents (principally rats and mice) as these species display a highly stereotyped pattern of sexual behaviours, enabling researchers to devise fairly reliable behavioural measures to assess the different behavioural components, and their possible hormonal underpinnings. Pfaus (1996) provided a detailed description of rodent sexual behaviours. He explained that, unlike in humans, rat copulatory behaviour is characterised by a series of interrupted encounters between male and female. Sexual encounters are initiated by sexually receptive females: after a period of mutual anogenital investigation, the female will begin to solicit contact from the male; she will wiggle her ears and run away from the male for short distances, jumping as she does so (hopdarting). She will then crouch down. As the male palpates her flanks she will assume the sexually receptive position called 'lordosis' (she flexes her spine, extends her hind legs and moves her tail to one side). The adoption of this position by the female is vital if successful copulation (i.e. penetration) is to occur as it serves to elevate the vaginal opening, without which penetration and ejaculation are impossible (Pfaff *et al.*, 1978). The male then mounts the female (but penetration does not necessarily occur) and she may dart away again. The entire process is repeated, with the male perhaps achieving intromission (penetration); after several bouts of intromission the male will ejaculate.

Ågmo (1997) was able to quantify such behaviours and described the techniques that have enabled researchers to derive useful behavioural indices that can perhaps be used to assess hormonal contributions. For example, the time from when a male and female are first introduced to when the first mount occurs is called 'mount latency'; the time from when they are first introduced to the first intromission is called 'intermission latency'. In both cases it is assumed that the shorter these latencies, the stronger the male/female sex drive. Normally around twenty mounts, with ten to fifteen intromissions, are seen prior to the first ejaculation; the time between the first intromission and ejaculation is thus called the 'ejaculation latency', which again is assumed to provide a motivational measure of sex drive.

Following ejaculation, the male enters a 'postejaculatory refractory period' for approximately five minutes before he is sexually interested in the female again. She shows a similar refractory period for only around one minute, after which she may solicit copulation again. It is assumed that the shorter this 'ejaculatory interval' then the stronger the sex drive, but Ågmo (1997) cautions that it varies independently of the mount latency, and responds differently to various experimental manipulations, and thus may not form a true measure of sex drive. As the number of intromissions and ejaculations increases, the female will solicit less and less, and display aggression to males who continue to attempt to mount her.

The above description focuses largely on the components of male sexual behaviours that can be quantified and measured. Beach (1976) provided a similar distinction for female sexual behaviours, conceptualising them as three different phases of copulatory activity. The first phase is called 'attractivity', which refers to the stimulus value of the female to a male; for example, if a male chooses to spend more time with a particular female then it is assumed that she is more 'attractive' to him than a female with whom he does not spend as much time. So what is it about the female that leads the male suddenly to find her more attractive? In some species there are obvious physical changes. For example, female primates clearly display their reproductive status by the swelling and colour change of the skin area around the perineum. In rodents, chemical stimuli appear to be important for sexual attraction; a female rat will rub her anogenital region against the ground and thus presumably provide some kind of chemical trace that allows wandering males to know of her whereabouts (Calhoun, 1962, cited in Beach, 1976).

In primates, scent marks may play an important role in the evaluation of potential mates by providing cues towards the age, health and reproductive potential of the individual (Snowden *et al.*, 2006). Murphy (1973) demonstrated the power of these chemical secretions by smearing immobilised male hamsters with vaginal secretions from an estrous female, and noting that other males attempted to mount these hapless males. Such behaviours were not seen towards immobilised males free from such chemical advertisements. Males also showed great interest in a bottle containing such secretions, but in this case did not attempt to mount the bottle! In the cotton-top tamarin, Ziegler *et al.* (1993) demonstrated that odours secreted by females during the periovulatory stage directly stimulated sexual arousal in males. Other attractant features consist of changes in female behaviour. For example, female rhesus monkeys who present their rear ends to males more frequently are more likely to be mounted by these males than females who present less often (Dixson *et al.*, 1973).

The second phase is called 'proceptivity' and is the extent to which a female will initiate sociosexual encounters with males, and thus reflects both her overt behaviours and her underlying motivational state. In many species this will entail the female moving from a state of disinterest in the male during anestrus, to a state where she becomes actively interested in males, and will approach a male and follow him around. She may then actively solicit the sexual attention of the male by adopting species-specific presentation behaviours and specialised gestures and movements (hop-darting and ear wiggling in the female rat, presenting her rear in primates, etc.).

The final phase is called 'receptivity' and is the state of responsiveness of the female to the sexual initiation of the male, i.e. will she allow the male to copulate with her? Such behaviours have been quantified and can range from a simple 'success ratio' (the percentage of all sexual attempts by the male which the female allows to culminate in a full mount) to a more complex quotient (i.e. the 'lordosis quotient' in rats). Note that proceptivity and receptivity are quite similar, and Beach himself admitted that they are arbitrary distinctions with no clear boundary between them.

## Hormones and sexual behaviours in male rodents

In male rodents, certain sexual behaviours are clearly linked to hormonal status. In mice, for example, males display low basal testosterone levels interspersed with pulsatile increases that reach levels around twenty times that of baseline levels. The presence of a female, or indeed the presence of only her urinary pheromones, is sufficient to trigger a testosterone surge within ten minutes; as levels of testosterone rise, male behaviour shifts from courtship to mating (James and Nyby, 2002). Researchers had not expected to find clear relationships between alterations in testosterone and specific reproductive behaviours, because it was assumed that testosterone exerted its neural effects via relatively slow genomic mechanisms, the finding that castrated males take several days to recover their libido following testosterone replacement (e.g. Smith *et al.*, 1977) being considered good support for this assumption. However, it is now clear that steroids can affect target tissues within seconds via non-genomic mechanisms (e.g. Sachs and Leipheimer, 1988), and of course we now understand that steroids can have direct effects within neural tissue (see information on neurosteroids in chapter 2).

James and Nyby (2002) therefore examined the possible rapid effects of testosterone on male reproductive behaviours. In their first experiment, sexually experienced male mice were first exposed to female urine or water, and then placed in a cage with an ovariectomised female who had been brought into behavioural 'heat' via estradiol and progesterone treatment. Pre-exposure to female urinary pheromones (both fresh and old) led to a significant reduction in mount latency compared to the water exposure. A problem with this is that exposure to female urine does not just affect testosterone, but also GnRH, LH, corticosterone, epinephrine and norepinephrine (Bronson and Desjardins, 1982; Maruniak and Bronson, 1976). In order to address this, in their second experiment, gonadally intact males were injected with either a high dose of testosterone or a neutral substance, and their latency to mount a sexually receptive female was recorded. Males receiving testosterone mounted females around 33% faster than those receiving the control substance. These experiments thus confirmed that reflexive testosterone release in response to a female or her urine leads to a rapid change in certain reproductive behaviours.

Similarly, Ågmo (2003) evaluated sexual motivation in male rats by introducing sexually inexperienced individuals to a choice of receptive females, non-receptive females or males, in a large open area. The males opted to spend their time in close proximity to the receptive females, and such preferences (assumed to reflect a stronger motivation) were abolished by castration, but subsequently restored with injections of testosterone propionate. However, such effects were influenced by sexual experience. For example, Matuszczyk and Larsson (1994) had two groups of castrated male rats, one group being sexually experienced prior to castration, the other group not being experienced. These individuals were then implanted with either testosterone or estradiol, or an empty tube, and compared with intact experienced and naïve males, on their preference for a sexually experienced male, a castrated male, a sexually receptive female or an ovariectomised female. The naïve animals (whether castrated or intact) showed no clear preferences, but the sexually experienced males (intact or receiving testosterone) showed a clear preference for the receptive female. More recently, Constantini *et al.* (2007) demonstrated that in Siberian hamsters castration prior to puberty abolished copulation in adulthood in all individuals lacking sexual experiences; however, some individuals that were sexually experienced prior to castration showed no reduction in sexual activity following castration. The authors suggested that the neural circuits mediating sexual behaviours were still able to operate without gonadal hormone stimulation, perhaps because they had been organised at puberty (or before).

It seems fairly clear, then, that testosterone serves as a 'trigger' for male sexual behaviours in appropriate environmental conditions (i.e. the presence of a sexually receptive female). However, the answer is more complex. Early studies had demonstrated that injections of estrogen could serve just as well as testosterone in promoting masculine sexual behaviours (e.g. Ball, 1937). This puzzle was solved following the discovery by Naftolin *et al.* (1975) that testosterone exerts its neurological effects after being converted into estradiol via aromatase, or following its conversion into DHT via 5α-reductase. The research spotlight was thus turned on to the role of testosterone metabolism in the activation of sexual behaviour.

For example, Beyer *et al.* (1976) first castrated a group of sexually naïve male rats. They then gave each a daily injection of testosterone over a three-week period and monitored their copulatory behaviours. The testosterone did induce sexual activity in most animals. The animals then received daily pre-treatments of antiestrogens and aromatase inhibitors before their injection of testosterone, and once more their copulatory behaviours were assessed. Daily treatment of various antiestrogens had no effect on the subsequent behaviours, though the very highest dose of one such compound did reduce sexual behaviours. One aromatase inhibitor (called aminog-lutethamide) completely abolished the sexual behaviours normally seen in response to testosterone treatment. This study thus demonstrates that at least some of the effects of testosterone on sexual behaviours in male rats are seen after testosterone is converted to an estrogen via aromatase.

More recent work on songbirds, however, has raised problems with this fairly simple steroid-metabolism approach. Ball and Balthazart (2006) reviewed several such studies and note that an emerging idea is that estrogenic metabolites of testosterone may be crucial for a general activation of masculine sexual motivation, but specific behavioural actions may require androgenic metabolisation. Thus there may be several layers of complexity over and above the simple notion that testosterone exerts its effects after conversion to estradiol.

The experiments described previously indicate that sex steroids produce their effects by acting upon brain regions controlling sexual behaviours. As we have seen in a previous chapter, an important brain region subserving sexually dimorphic behaviours is the medial preoptic area (mPOA) lying anterior to the hypothalamus. In rodents, lesions in this area generally abolish sexual performance, though sexual motivation remains intact. The mPOA contains dopaminergic neurons and treating male animals with lesions to the mPOA with the dopamine agonist lisuride temporarily restores sexual behaviours (Hansen *et al.*, 1982). In normal rats, injection of a dopamine agonist also facilitates copulatory behaviour, while adminis-tration of dopamine antagonists reduces sexual behaviours (Mas, 1995). However, social history can alter the effects of mPOA lesions. For example, young rats with mPOA lesions reared in social isolation never copulate as adults, but similar lesions have little effect when the rats are reared with others – presumably because social living elevates dopamine levels (Twigg *et al.*, 1978).

In rodents the olfactory system is important for reproductive behaviours, a key structure being the vomeronasal organ (VNO).[2] This auxiliary olfac-tory sense organ lies within the nasal septum and seems to be responsible for detecting specific large non-volatile molecules such as pheromones. It is con-nected to the accessory olfactory bulb via the vomeronasal nerves, and thence to the amygdala. The mPOA is also connected to the amygdala via the stria terminalis and the ventral amygdalofugal pathway, with damage to these pathways and to parts of the amygdala having similar effects as mPOA lesions. Removal of the olfactory bulbs prevents males from attempting to mate, especially in rats who are sexually naïve; destruction of the VNO in mice also prevents mating behaviours. Pfaff and Pfaffmann (1969) showed

---

[2] Also called 'Jacobson's organ', after the Danish anatomist Ludvig Jacobson (1783–1843) who discovered it in 1809.

that exposure to the odour of estrous females produced electrical activity in the olfactory bulbs and the mPOA, but mPOA activation disappeared following castration. Testosterone replacement therapy restored mPOA responsiveness. Autoradiographic studies have confirmed that receptor binding for testosterone is clearly seen in the mPOA, the bed nucleus of the stria terminalis and the corticomedial nuclei of the amygdala, showing that via dopaminergic neurons these structures play a key role on hormonally mediated reproductive behaviours (see chapter 4).

## Individual differences

Male sexual behaviour differs markedly, with some individuals showing great interest and others less so. This had been assumed to reflect individual differences in circulating levels of testosterone, animals with a 'high' sex drive being presumed to have higher levels of circulating testosterone than those with a 'low' sex drive (so called 'dud-studs'). However, Damassa *et al.* (1977) noted that findings were equivocal, because the standard method of implanting testosterone (subcutaneous injection) produced highly variable blood hormone levels that could not be accurately measured. With the development of specialised slow-release capsules, and radioimmunoassay, then studies could investigate more closely possible testosterone-dose–behaviour relationships. In their study Damassa and colleagues first weeded out a small group of 'non-copulators', animals that had failed to ejaculate on shaping tests of sexual behaviour, and in comparison to sixty 'copulators' they demonstrated significantly lower levels of testosterone. When provided with implants of testosterone, the 'non-copulators' receiving the highest doses began showing normal copulatory behaviour patterns.

So far so good: in animals with a probable hormone problem, normal behaviours can be restored following appropriate supplementation. In the 'normal' animals, though, the picture was slightly more complex: following castration the 'copulators' received testosterone-releasing capsules of different strengths, and they returned to their pre-castration copulatory behaviours even when the amount of testosterone they received was only 10% of normal levels. Higher doses did not increase copulatory behaviours, and there was no relationship between dosage and various behavioural coefficients. There thus appears to be a degree of redundancy in the testicular supply of androgens for maintaining sexual behaviours. However, the authors pointed out that while a small amount of testosterone is needed to maintain a reproductive behaviour, much higher amounts are needed to restore it once it has been completely extinguished by castration.

In any case, if serum testosterone levels do not differ between males with high or low sex drives this does not mean that there are no differences neurologically. Recall that androgens exert their effects at androgen receptors, or after conversion to estradiol (via aromatase) at estrogen receptors. Clark *et al.* (1985) placed intact male rats with receptive females in successive weekly tests to determine their basal levels of sexual activity, and separated them into those with a high versus low sexual responsivity. They then assessed nuclear estrogen receptor content and found that the sexually unresponsive rats demonstrated significant reductions in estrogen receptor levels within the mPOA. In support, Chambers *et al.* (1991) assessed serum testosterone, neural androgen metabolism and binding, and sexual behaviours in old and young male rats. In their first study, they found that old rats did not ejaculate during intromission, and, in comparison to the young males, demonstrated lower levels of serum testosterone, lower levels of androgen receptors, and reduced aromatase activity in the mPOA. In their second experiment they gonadectomised young and old males but then gave them equivalent testosterone supplementation so that their serum levels were comparable. In sexual behaviour tests, all of the young males ejaculated but only 25% of the old males did. Androgen receptor and aromatase activity was also comparable, suggesting that while testosterone is related to alterations in neural androgen binding and metabolism, it may not be related to certain sexual behaviours (though only one behaviour was studied).

More recently, researchers have been able to utilise more advanced techniques in order to assess the precise neurological actions underlying such behaviours – notably the respective roles played by the estrogen receptors ERα and ERβ in various brain regions subserving reproductive behaviours. 'Knockout' mice have been created which completely lack the ERα; the behaviours of these 'ERKO' animals can then be compared to 'wild-type' animals. For example, Ogawa *et al.* (1998) created male ERKO mice and compared their sexual behaviours with wild-type mice following gonadectomy and testosterone replacement. The ERKO males displayed normal mounting and intromission behaviours in response to the testosterone treatment; the provision of dihydrotestosterone propionate was also effective in restoring mounting behaviour (though it was more effective in the wild-type mice). However, neither testosterone nor dihydrotestosterone injections were able to restore ejaculation in the ERKO males, suggesting that the ERα may be responsible for the regulation by testosterone of consummatory behaviours, but not of motivational aspects of behaviour.

While progesterone is traditionally regarded as a 'female hormone' as it is crucially involved in a progestational role in maintaining pregnancy, evidence is mounting for its important role in male sexual behaviour. Progesterone seems to have antiandrogenic effects. For example, Diamond (1966) gave supraphysiological doses of progesterone to male guinea pigs on a daily basis and observed significant impairments in their sexual behaviour. This study was replicated by Connolly and Resko (1989) and they showed that daily injections of a synthetic progestin impaired sexual behaviour in intact males. However, the problem with such studies is that they are providing doses far higher than would ever be seen naturally; if more 'normal' dose levels are administered, then such effects are not seen (Erpino, 1973). These effects are probably due to the inhibitory effect of progesterone on testosterone, perhaps by decreasing the reduction of testosterone to its more powerful metabolite DHT (Stern and Eisenfeld, 1971). An alternative explanation is that progesterone may instead directly regulate androgen receptor expression or activity; in support, Connolly *et al.* (1988) showed that progesterone injections in male guinea pigs led to a significant decrease in androgen receptors whilst having no effect upon circulating testosterone.

## Hormones and sexual behaviours in female rodents

In many animal species sexually mature females clearly advertise their reproductive capability and availability at a time known as 'the rut', 'heat' or more scientifically 'estrus'.[3] The estrus cycle reflects the recurring physiological changes that are triggered by GnRH, FSH, LH, estrogen and progesterone, and that are associated with the fertile phase surrounding ovulation. The estrus cycle can be clearly differentiated from the period of 'anestrus', when these hormones are not being produced in high levels and sexual availability is not being promoted. In some species (humans, some primates, bats and shrews) the females instead have a 'menstrual cycle', the differences being that during the menstrual cycle the endometrium is shed as menstrual blood if the egg is not fertilised (in species displaying estrus the endometrium is absorbed), and that females are sexually active throughout the cycle, even if they are not about to ovulate (Feder, 1981).

Such characteristic behaviours are under the hormonal control of the ovulatory cycle, as natural selection has designed females to alter their mating behaviours in order to coincide with maximum fertility, thus ensuring successful fertilisation. As female reproductive behaviours are cyclical, and there are many hormonal changes involved in generating and regulating these cycles, it has been difficult to ascertain which hormones are acting in which phase, and having what effects. The development of non-invasive external markers that reflect ovarian activity greatly improved our understanding of the hormonal regulation of ovarian cycles. In the 1920s, Georgios Papanikolaou developed a routine analysis of vaginal cell samples in order to detect pre-cancerous processes (this method is now called the 'Pap test', or 'smear test'), but it also enabled changes in cellular content of the vagina to be matched with hormonal fluctuations. The role of estrogens in reproductive cycles was soon established: injecting ovarian extracts from slaughtered pigs into ovariectomised female mice produced physiological and behavioural changes associated with normal female mice (Allen and Doisy, 1923).

However, not all ovariectomised females responded to estrogen treatment, and it was realised that another substance must be involved. It was soon

---

[3] A rough translation from the Latin word 'oestrus', meaning 'gadfly' or 'in a frenzy'.

discovered that estrogen and progesterone act synergistically to cause physiological and behavioural estrus (Dempsey *et al.*, 1936). Progesterone in fact serves two functions in the rodent estrus cycle: first, in association with estradiol, it initiates sexual behaviours, but as the cycle continues and estrogen levels fall, the remaining elevated levels of progesterone then inhibit sexual behaviour.

It is possible to link hormonal changes with the various components of female sexuality as defined by Beach (1976). In terms of 'attractivity' it has been noted that estrogen levels enhance female attractiveness; for example, male rats show little interest in socially interacting with a female unless she is in estrus. Their behaviour towards her will then rapidly change, and they will show significantly more 'approaches', follow her around and attempt to copulate with her (Calhoun, 1962, cited in Beach, 1976). The strength of this motivation has been assessed by requiring males to traverse an electrified floor in order to reach the female, and such painful crossings were more frequent when the female in question was in estrus (Warner, 1927, cited in Beach, 1976).

Proceptive behaviours are much more likely to be seen during estrus (whether natural or artificially created), as female rats show a significant increase in approach behaviours, and ovariectomised females injected with estrogen and progesterone will show a marked increase in their bar-pressing behaviour when the reward is access to a male (French *et al.*, 1972). If ovariectomised estrogen-primed female rats are injected with different doses of progesterone then it has been noted that their receptivity follows a dose-related pattern: the higher the dose of progesterone, then the shorter the latency to return to the male following intromission (Fadem *et al.*, 1979). In many rodent species receptivity has also been strongly related to natural hormonal fluctuations, the females becoming maximally receptive during the phase of their cycle when estradiol secretion is at its maximum and progesterone levels are beginning to rise. The key signal of receptivity is the lordosis response, and the presence of estradiol is vital for this behaviour. For example, Kow and Pfaff (1975) reported that progesterone treatment alone does not induce lordosis in ovariectomised female rats; estrogen treatment does induce lordosis but to a lesser extent than when estrogen and progesterone are provided in the temporal pattern seen in normally cycling females. So, the estrogen surge acts to prime lordosis, and the subsequent rise in progesterone serves to facilitate it. However, an injection of estrogen followed by another injection of estrogen (but not progesterone) also led to a facilitatory effect on lordosis; however, higher doses of estrogen were required in such cases.

As with male mice, female ERKO mice lacking the ERα can be created and their reproductive behaviours compared to their female wild-types. In one such study, ERKO and wild-type mice were ovariectomised and then given injections of estradiol, followed by an injection of progesterone some hours later (to mimic the hormonal milieu of normal estrus) prior to the behavioural testing. The ERKO females failed to show the lordosis response, were deficient in displaying the proceptive behaviours that normally precede the lordosis response, and were extremely aggressive towards males who attempted to mate with them. This manipulation had no effect on female attractiveness, as male mice attempted to mate with both groups with equal frequency (Rissman et al., 1997). The authors concluded that the ERα within the hypothalamus is essential for sexual receptivity but admit that ERKO mice may also lack progesterone receptors and thus one cannot relate the behavioural deficiencies solely to the lack of estrogen receptors. Similarly, Musatov et al. (2006) created a virus vector that 'knocked out' ERα and the progesterone receptor within the ventromedial nucleus of the hypothalamus (VMH), a region critical for certain female reproductive behaviours. Silencing of the ERα led to a complete blocking of the lordosis response in female mice.

Other proceptive behaviours such as hop-darting and ear wiggling appear to be more dependent upon progesterone than estradiol: while low levels of such behaviours can be elicited by high levels of estradiol, several studies have demonstrated that progesterone within standard physiological limits is vital for such behaviours to occur (e.g. Whalen, 1974). However, these two hormones are closely related in terms of their genetic effects: once the molecules of hormone have bound to their receptors, the receptors change conformation and, in a complex process, lead to target genes altering their rate of transcription (Beato and Sánchez-Pacheco, 1996). Estradiol bound factors bind to the estrogen response element of the progesterone receptor gene and induce gene expression; therefore estradiol can have a profound impact upon the progesterone receptor gene, and transcriptional activity of such receptors can be enhanced by Steroid Receptor Coactivator-1 (Oñate et al., 1995). Molenda-Figueira et al. (2006) showed that infusion of antisense SRC-1 (this prevents gene expression) into the VMH decreased lordosis in rats treated with estradiol, while similar infusions during progesterone administration reduced ear wiggling and hop-darting.

Of course, if we are to attempt to link hormonal changes with behaviour then we also have to consider the role of the neurotransmitters in the brain, as manifestations of steroid induction of behaviour rely upon changes in neuronal activation and this can involve alterations in synthesis, release, reuptake and receptor-binding (McCarthy and Pfaus, 1996). All of the key neurotransmitters appear to be involved. For example, cholinergic antagonists inhibit lordosis in hormone-primed female rats, while cholinergic agonists facilitate sexual receptivity (Menard and Dohanich, 1994). Estradiol in combination with progesterone acts dramatically to increase norepinephrine within the VMH (Etgen et al., 1992). During estrus, females are more sensitive to dopamine agonists such as amphetamine, and such agonists can increase both proceptivity and receptivity, but there is also evidence that dopamine antagonists enhance only receptive components – the role of dopamine is thus clearly complex. Serotonin can act either to inhibit or to facilitate lordosis, depending upon which subtype of serotonin receptor has been activated (studies citied in McCarthy and Pfaus, 1996).

## Hormones and sexual behaviours in primates

It was initially assumed that hormones were not strongly related to female primate sexual behaviours (the majority of studies have been conducted on rhesus monkeys) because females who had been ovariectomised showed a willingness to mate, intact females displayed no consistent cyclical patterns to their sexual behaviours, and specific measures of female sexual behaviour such as 'presenting' do not vary with the cycle (Eaton and Resko, 1974; Rowell, 1972). As females thus appeared to be constantly receptive it was assumed that hormones (as they are cyclical) played little role in triggering or mediating sexual behaviours. However, it has been pointed out that this misperception may have arisen as a result of the reliance upon a standard laboratory technique in which mating behaviours were analysed. Wallen (1990) noted that such studies often consisted of a single female being paired with a single male in a small enclosure over a lengthy time period. Her choice in whether or not to accept the male as a mating partner was thus removed, and may have given the false impression that she was sexually receptive at all times.

Since the 1970s, rhesus monkeys have been studied in large groups living 'free' in outdoor enclosures, conditions better replicating their natural social environment. Studies that followed then began to demonstrate clearer links between the female ovulatory cycle and her sexual behaviours. For example, Wilson et al. (1982) described the copulatory behaviour of free-living female rhesus monkeys. In this species, copulation is normally restricted to a two-week period in the year; during that time copulations are discrete but occur daily with fairly high frequency. They monitored the copulatory behaviours of sixteen females over a three-hour period during each day for a four-month period. Blood was collected three days per week before mating had begun to establish baseline levels, and then once the female had begun to mate it was collected on a daily basis and assessed for estradiol, progesterone and testosterone. The mean duration of mating activity was found to be around sixteen consecutive days. During this period significant relationships were established between hormone levels and sexual activity.

During the early follicular phase estradiol levels were low, and no copulations were recorded. During the late follicular stage, levels of estradiol rose and this was associated with the onset of copulatory behaviours. During these phases progesterone levels remained low. In the late luteal phase mating behaviours reduced, and this decrease was associated with a gradual rise in progesterone in the face of gradually reducing levels of estradiol. An analysis of progesterone on the last day of observed copulations compared to the next day when no mating occurred revealed a significant rise in progesterone concentrations. On a daily basis, individual differences in copulation could be associated with daily changes in serum estradiol, but not with changes in progesterone or testosterone. However, this was not a dose-related effect, as once estradiol levels had reached a certain threshold, then further increases did not lead to a further increase in copulation. This study clearly demonstrated that the occurrence and frequency of female mating behaviours was associated with clear changes in the endocrine system. The onset of mating was associated with a rise in estradiol while the termination of such behaviours was related to a rise in progesterone.

It has been established that gonadotropin-releasing hormone (GnRH) agonists prevent ovulation and lead to low levels of estradiol, and Wallen *et al.* (1986) focussed on the possible role of such a GnRH agonist in the sexual interest of rhesus monkeys. In their study, six intact females living in a large outdoor group received the agonist or no treatment. During this period their sexual behaviours were recorded over four days per week. Following fifteen days of GnRH agonist treatment ovulation was suppressed and estradiol levels dropped, and the frequency with which females initiated proximity behaviours and copulated with males showed a gradual decline during the treatment.

In terms of Beach's stages, an observational study of free-living male chimpanzees showed that they never mounted the females whose sex skin (around the buttocks and genitals) was unswollen, but showed a clear preference for approaching and mounting females whose skin was swollen (this indicates that she is in estrus). If ovariectomised female rhesus monkeys are injected with estrogen, their attractivity, as measured by the 'acceptance ratio' (the proportion of female invitations that result in a mounting attempt), showed a clear increase (Dixson *et al.*, 1973). Johnson and Phoenix (1976) ovariectomised twelve female rhesus monkeys and then, using a repeated-measures design, injected them with estradiol, estradiol plus testosterone (in differing doses) or a control substance, and evaluated their attractivity, proceptivity and receptivity behaviours when paired with eight different males. Males were more attracted to females during estrogen treatment, and small amounts of testosterone in conjunction with estradiol further enhanced their attractiveness. However, higher doses of testosterone significantly reduced this attractiveness. Proceptive behaviours were enhanced by estradiol and testosterone, but receptive behaviours were stimulated by estrogen but not by testosterone.

The most common measure of proceptivity is the extent to which females will attempt to gain and maintain contact with other males. For example, Bonsall *et al.* (1978) utilised an operant conditioning paradigm in which nine females and seven males were placed in adjacent cages separated by a partition. In order to raise the partition, the female was required to press a lever 250 times within 30 minutes; a behavioural test lasting for one hour was then instigated. High estradiol levels at mid-cycle were associated with shorter latencies to complete the required lever presses by females, a greater mount rate, and shorter ejaculation latencies in the males. High progesterone levels on the other hand were associated with longer lever pressing latency times and longer ejac- ulation times; fluctuations in testosterone did not appear to be related to any female behaviours. Zehr *et al.* (1998) focussed on the possible role of estradiol in triggering female sexual motivation behaviours in five ovariectomised and five intact rhesus monkeys within a large social group. The ovariectomised females were treated with estradiol implants and these led to a significant increase in female-initiated interactions with males compared to the untreated group. These changes were independent of male sexual interest or activity.

As regards receptivity, studies have revealed that, as with proceptivity, measures of male ejaculation times showed a similar peak when estrogen levels were at their highest. For example, Wallen *et al.* (1984) observed sexual behaviours in nine intact group-living female rhesus monkeys across an ovulatory menstrual cycle. As estradiol levels began to peak, the females approached males and initiated contact with them, and these approach behaviours declined as estradiol levels dropped. Male mounts, intromissions and ejaculations peaked when estradiol levels reached their highest point, and then declined completely. Ejaculations in fact did not occur outside of a range of four days before and five days after this peak.

## Human sexual behaviours

The physiological and psychological components of human sex drive and behaviour still remain poorly understood, with the majority of clinical studies focussing on individuals with hormone abnormalities or physiologi- cal problems. Unlike rodents, where sexual behaviours are described in terms of sex drive and sexual activity, human sexual behaviour has been conceptu- alised in terms of three types of behaviours (Regan, 1996).

First, 'sexual desire' is a subjective psychological state in which the individual displays an interest in sexual stimuli, and is motivated towards seeking out sexual activities, though may not necessarily be sexually aroused. Measurement of this facet of behaviour is normally conducted via diary records, questionnaires, surveys, etc., and is notoriously prone to misreport- ing; sexual thoughts/feelings, for example, may be over- or underemphasised because of the social embarrassment inherent in such research, and the resulting data can thus be questioned in terms of their reliability and validity.

Second, 'sexual arousal' is regarded as a two-part process: the first reflects physiological – genital sexual arousal, and the second is the subjective awareness that one is genitally and/or physiologically aroused. Certain physiological facets of male sexual arousal (erection, ejaculation) are remark- ably similar in rats and humans, particularly in their neuroanatomical, neuroendocrine and neurochemical regulation (Meisel and Sachs, 1994). It is thus possible to define such measures and record them objectively via physiological recording techniques such as heart rate and blood pressure monitoring, latency to achieve orgasm, etc. (Meston and Frohlich, 2000; Pfaus, 1996). The key method in males is the measurement of penile erection via a penile plethysmograph[4] or a strain gauge. In females similar techniques can be used to assess temperature or lubrication changes in the genitals. Recording such events while individuals watch erotic material is possible if not a little impractical, but such studies have taken place. The possibility that individuals might show very different physiological/hormonal changes through stress/embarrassment remains a particular methodological problem, as we shall see. Indeed, while physiological measures of sexual arousal and subjective reports of arousal show quite close correlations in males, in women the two are often uncorrelated (Meston and Frohlich, 2000).

Thirdly, 'sexual activity' relates to any overt behaviour involving the sex organs and includes autoerotic activities (masturbation) and sexual intercourse. Unlike rodents, however, human sexual activities cannot easily be defined in terms of characteristic behavioural components: humans mate in a variety of positions, sexual encounters may not always be genital to genital, and sexual behaviours may not always incorporate another person. It is also the case that the occurrence of sexual activity does not necessarily imply a desire for such activity, and the absence of sexual activity does not suggest that desire is lacking. Pfaus (1996) points out that it is almost impossible to study human copulatory behaviours because of ethical restrictions and the reluctance of most individuals to volunteer for such research. Most of our knowledge thus comes from surveys and questionnaires. There are now several examples of studies involving consenting adults engaging in sexual activities, during which physiological and hormonal indices are being recorded, though the extent to which results from such individuals may generalise remains open to question.

The human sexual response can be viewed as an increase in sexual excitement and arousal, a plateau during which sexual stimulation is being experienced, orgasm, and then a refractory period, though researchers differ considerably on the precise timing and definition of these stages. Both males and females exhibit the same set of responses, but except for pelvic thrusting, human copulatory behaviours show marked differences from those seen in animals, being less sexually dimorphic, and more likely to be learned. Unlike rats, human females do not display a characteristic sexual response akin to lordosis, and there is no animal model for female sexual arousal and orgasm.

---

[4] The original design for this contraption was a volumetric air chamber. When placed over the penis the volume of displaced air could be ascertained as the penis became enlarged. It was designed in the 1950s by sexologist Kurt Freund (1914–96) in an attempt to prevent young males from avoiding military service by pretending to be homosexual – the device was placed over their penis and they were shown erotic heterosexual material, the subsequent air displacement thus 'proving' their manliness to fight!

So, while methodological problems and ethical considerations remain a considerable barrier to teasing out hormone–behaviour interactions in terms of human sexual behaviours, it should be possible to make some inroads into this issue.

## Hormones and male sexual behaviours

It is assumed that sexual behaviours begin to appear at puberty, but Friedrich *et al.* (1991) noted that sexual behaviours occur throughout childhood, usually consisting of exploratory and self-stimulatory activities. Many prepubertal children engage in sexual behaviours with other children, but they do not appear to experience such behaviours in the same way that pubertal and postpubertal individuals experience them. Needless to say, research on this rather taboo topic is sparse, and the possible role of hormones in the development and maintenance of such behaviours in children remains mysterious. When it comes to adolescents/adults, however, there is a lot more information, and evidence typically comes from several sources.

### Testosterone replacement in hypogonadal males

Hypogonadal males are so described because their testes fail to produce sufficient levels of testosterone (a male producing a normal amount is referred to as being 'eugonadal'). This clinical condition (caused by various pathological states which can make the interpretation of certain findings difficult at times) can thus form a useful means by which to assess sexual functioning and behaviours in comparison to eugonadal males. In a carefully controlled repeated-measures double-blind experiment, Davidson *et al.* (1979) injected six hypogonadal men with either 100 mg of testosterone, 400 mg of testosterone or a placebo, over a five-month period. During this time the men were asked to keep a daily log of their erotic thoughts and sexual behaviours and activities. Androgen treatment was significantly associated with rapid increases in erection frequency and coitus, such effects being dose-dependent. As there was no change in self-reported mood, the authors concluded that the effects were related to testosterone fluctuation alone.

Similarly, Kwan *et al.* (1983) studied six hypogonadal males and six control males, and asked them to keep daily logs recording their sexual feelings and activity; in addition the volunteers were monitored throughout the night, and various psychophysical measures were recorded, including penile tumescence. The effects of 200 mg, 400 mg and a placebo were compared using the standard double-blind, cross-over method. With testosterone administration, three of the hypogonadal males showed increased frequencies of sexual thoughts, activities, orgasms and spontaneous erections, with reductions in nocturnal penile tumescence and spontaneous daytime erections being seen in the placebo condition. However, erectile responses in response to visual erotic stimuli within a daytime laboratory setting did not show this relationship.

Carani *et al.* (1995) also examined the effects of testosterone supplementation on erectile responses during sleep, and during the presentation of visual erotic materials in hypogonadal and control males. After a baseline phase (no medication), nine hypogonadal males received their usual androgen supplements, and after three months erectile responses were measured in both groups. In response to androgens, nocturnal penile tumescence in the hypogonadal males showed a significant improvement relative to baseline, in terms of both penis circumference and rigidity (not to the same extent as the control males). Penile responses did not, however, differ from those seen in the control males during visual erotic exposure, and did not increase in response to androgen replacement. These studies thus perhaps suggest that there are two erectile systems – a nocturnal mechanism seemingly dependent upon androgens, and one in response to visual stimuli while awake, and seemingly not dependent upon androgens. An alternative (and theoretically simpler) explanation could of course be that the lack of physical reactions in the daytime laboratory setting reflects the undoubted increase in embarrassment typically experienced in such situations.

Wang *et al.* (2000) compared two methods of testosterone administration – transdermal patches applied to the skin, and gel (called 'AndroGel') rubbed on the skin (three doses of gel being utilised). In their large study, 227 hypogonadal males were randomly assigned to one of the treatments (a placebo was employed for the gel but not for the patches) and received their supplementation for six months (a cross-over occurring at three months). At specified time points throughout the testing the volunteers completed detailed questionnaires concerning a range of sexual behaviours and incidence of sexual thoughts/desires, etc. Testosterone administration (in either gel or patch form) was associated with significant increases in sexual function, desire and motivation within thirty days, and such benefits were maintained throughout the treatment period. As there was no dose-related response, the authors concluded that once a threshold of serum testosterone has been achieved (around the low normal range) then this was sufficient to normalise sexual function and motivation). Increasing testosterone levels to the high normal range had no additional effect on sexual behaviours. This raises the interesting point that normal males appear to secrete more circulating testosterone than they actually need for the maintenance of normal sexual function (Bancroft, 2005), this echoing similar findings in rodents outlined previously (Damassa *et al.*, 1977).

In individuals not diagnosed with hypogonadism, but rather with the more vague term 'pubertal delay', associations between hormone supplementation and sexual behaviours are less clear-cut. Finkelstein *et al.* (1998) studied twenty-six male adolescents classified as having constitutional delay of puberty. In a randomised, double-blind, placebo-controlled, cross-over trial, the participants received either testosterone (in three doses approximating early, middle and late typical pubertal exposure), or a placebo for a three-month period, the treatment regimes alternating over the twenty-one-month testing period. During these treatments the volunteers were asked to complete a version of the 'Udry Sexual Behavior Questionnaire' (the individual describes his sexual thoughts, feelings and behaviours). The effects of testosterone administration seemed to be rather limited, as only the incidence of nocturnal emissions and the touching of other individuals showed significant increases.

## Hormone administration in 'normal' males

Studies involving hypogonadal males thus indicate that the provision of testosterone to deficient individuals restores certain sexual behaviours to within 'normal' levels. What then if androgens are administered to individuals with normally functioning gonads and normal levels of circulating testosterone? As we have just seen in the hypogonadal studies, provided that a baseline level of serum testosterone is achieved, then sexual behaviours are restored to normal levels, but additional testosterone seems to have little effect. One would thus perhaps predict that providing additional testosterone to males who are already at or above this baseline should have little noticeable effect.

Anderson et al. (1992) recruited thirty-one healthy adult males, and, using a single-blind, placebo-controlled design, gave one group 200 mg of testosterone enanthate on a weekly basis for eight consecutive weeks. The other group received a placebo for the first four weeks and then 200 mg of testosterone for the remaining four weeks. During that time, the men were asked to complete the 'Frenken Sexual Experiences Scale', a test consisting of four scales covering various aspects of sexual motivation and experience; they also kept a daily log of the incidence of sexual desires, erections, masturbation and intercourse. The testosterone enanthate led to around a 50% rise in plasma testosterone compared to baseline, and a significant increase in one of the scales was observed (the extent that the individual will seek out auditory or visual sexual stimuli) in the group receiving testosterone. Other behavioural measures (e.g. masturbation, sexual intercourse, etc.) showed no differences between the groups.

In a more complex study, Bagatell et al. (1994) used a GnRH antagonist called 'Nal-Glu' to create an acute but reversible state of hypogonadism in a sample of fifty healthy males. Once androgen suppression was achieved, they were then able to administer testosterone in two doses – the lower dose returning testosterone levels to around half that of baseline, and the higher dose approximating baseline levels. As testosterone might exert its effects after being converted to estradiol, in one condition the males also received 'Teslac', an estradiol antagonist, in addition to the testosterone supplement.

Over a six-week assessment period the effects of these pharmacological manipulations on self-reported sexual behaviours and functioning were recorded. In those who received 'Nal-Glu' alone, the severe testosterone deficiency manifested itself in reductions in the frequency of sexual desires, fantasies, intercourse and masturbation, with a near-significant effect on the incidence of spontaneous erections; these effects, however, did not become apparent until four to six weeks of treatment. Those receiving 'Nal-Glu' plus testosterone showed no change in their sexual behaviours/functions, and the estradiol antagonist had no effect; in human males, then (in contrast to male rodents), testosterone is not having its effects after conversion to estradiol. When serum testosterone levels returned to baseline levels then the incidence of reported behaviours also returned to normal. Once more, this study confirmed that low levels of circulating testosterone are sufficient for the maintenance of normal sexual behaviours.

Similarly, Bhasin *et al.* (2001) assessed the effects of five different doses of testosterone enanthate in sixty-one eugonadal males who were concurrently receiving a GnRH agonist. You may be feeling some confusion here, as what I have just described appears to be contradictory – recall that the Bagatell *et al.* (1994) study used a GnRH antagonist to reduce serum testosterone levels while Bhasin *et al.* (2001) used a GnRH agonist. Surely these will have opposite effects? Not quite. Recall that in chapter 2, I explained the feedback loop concerning GnRH and gonadal steroid production. Normally this is a positive loop in that GnRH stimulates the release of the gonadotropins from the anterior pituitary, which in turn stimulates steroid production in the gonads (a GnRH agonist should thus enhance steroid production). However, the release of these steroids feeds back to the hypothalamus to prevent further GnRH production, as well as stopping production of the gonadotropins from the anterior pituitary (a negative feedback loop). Thus, a GnRH agonist can also serve as a 'blocker' to steroid production. Anyway, Bhasin *et al.* (2001) rendered their sample hypogonadal, and then restored them with varying doses of testosterone while assessing various physical parameters and sexual functioning. The scores for sexual activity and sexual desire showed no significant changes at any dose.

Alexander *et al.* (1997) assessed the effects of a high dose of testosterone supplementation (200 mg) that would cause serum levels to be in the high – very high normal range, in ten healthy males. A control group of twenty males received no supplementation. The behavioural measures consisted of self-reported sexual arousal, and sexual enjoyment in response to auditory erotic material (a female voice describing sexual activities between males and females), and selective attention to the same sexual stimuli (assessed by a dichotic listening task). The group receiving testosterone supplementation showed a significant increase in their self-reported arousal to the auditory material. In addition their selective attention for the sexual stimuli also increased. No such changes were seen in the control males.

O'Connor *et al.* (2004) pointed out that previous studies had tended to use frequent injections of short-acting testosterone esters such as testosterone cypionate or testosterone enanthate. These induce rapid and highly variable levels of circulating testosterone, and may thus lead to inconsistencies in observations of hormone–behaviour relationships. In their study, they described a new compound called testosterone undecanoate, which is normally delivered in large doses that maintain circulating testosterone levels in a stable pattern within the normal physiological range for eight to twelve weeks. They recruited eighteen healthy males, and their partners (where possible) to provide some confirmation of the self-report evidence provided by the males. Each was randomly assigned to receive either 1000mg of the compound for eight weeks, or a placebo; after a wash-out period they received the alternate substance. A weekly log of the occurrence of daily sexual behaviours and experiences was kept, along with various behavioural questionnaires including mood, aggression (their data concerning aggression will be discussed in chapter 10), self-esteem and irritability.

The testosterone treatment led to a significant rise in serum testosterone and estradiol, and a suppression of gonadotropins, but no significant effects of treatment regime were noted for frequency of sexual intercourse, sexual desire, satisfaction with their sexual experiences, or masturbation frequency. The authors suggest that a key difference between their study and previous ones reporting significant effects of exogenous testosterone on sexual arousal (but not sexual behaviours) may be that these studies focussed on cognitive aspects of sexual behaviour (motivations, arousal, etc.) and thus testosterone may simply have an effect on cognitive/attentional processes which are involved in sexual perceptions and motivations, but not on actual sexual behaviours (such as intercourse or masturbation).

A final line of evidence concerns the role of progesterone. One early study by Heller *et al.* (1958) had demonstrated the profound negative effects of progesterone on male sexual behaviours by reporting that sexual libido showed a significant decrease in four males receiving injections of a progesterone compound. Similarly, Money (1970) reported the case of a transvestite with paedophilic homosexual tendencies who showed almost complete remission of his sexual urges and behaviours over a three-year period of medroxyprogesterone (MPA)[5] treatment.

In a famous landmark legal case in 1984 (*State of Michigan v. Gauntlett*) the judge ruled that a convicted chronic sex offender must receive such compounds as an alternative to being imprisoned (the Court of Appeal later ruled that this judgement, and therefore the use of MPA, was illegal). This led to a flurry of similar offenders agreeing to 'chemical castration' by progesterone compounds to avoid incarceration, and Cooper (1986)

---

[5] This compound is now known as 'Depo-Provera', and is a commonly used female oral contraceptive, acting to raise progesterone and decrease testosterone.

reviewed the outcomes of such studies covering around ninety individuals. While there were few trials which included adequate placebo controls, clinical observations did seem to indicate that such techniques were highly effective, especially when used in conjunction with other therapeutic methods. For example, Cordoba and Chapel (1983) treated a prolific paedophile sex offender with MPA for 500 days. During treatment his circulating testosterone fell to levels almost to within the normal female range, and there was a significant reduction in his libido with no recurrence of his sexual offences, but the focus of his sexual attentions (children) remained unaltered.

## Testosterone replacement in elderly males

As males age there is a steady decline in androgen levels, with serum testosterone decreasing steadily to levels below the typical eugonadal range. In a large-scale longitudinal study involving 1632 males aged forty to seventy, Travison *et al.* (2006) measured libido (as indicated by self-reported frequency of sexual thoughts and desires) and serum testosterone at three time points over the course of fifteen years. While libido and serum testosterone displayed a significant positive association, the difference in serum testosterone between those with a low libido and those with a high libido was extremely small (an average of around 3.4 ng/dl).

We have already seen that restoring testosterone levels to within the normal range in younger hypogonadal males appears to correct certain physical sexual parameters (such as impaired sexual motivation and function), so what happens in elderly males? In one study, Seftel *et al.* (2004) recruited over 400 males with a mean age of around fifty-eight, all of whom had one or more symptoms of low testosterone (reduced libido, reduced erectile functioning). The men were split into four independent treatment groups and received either a placebo or testosterone supplementation in the form of a patch or a gel (50 mg or 100 mg), the patch and 50 mg gel being roughly equivalent in terms of testosterone dosage. Before treatment (baseline) the males kept a daily log of sexual desires and sexual behaviours, and these records were maintained throughout the ninety-day experimental assessment, with evaluations taking place on days 30 and day 90. Comparison between baseline and these assessment days revealed a significant increase in nighttime erections, sexual intercourse and improvements in sexual desire, but only in the 100 mg gel condition. The other testosterone treatments showing no difference from placebo. Kaufman *et al.* (2004) argued that while aging in males is accompanied by a decrease in sex drive and potency, 80% of males aged over sixty remain sexually active, and the levels of testosterone required to sustain sexual activities is rather low (below the normal reference range in younger males). The most frequent causes of impotency and other sexual problems are non-hormonal.

## Circulating hormone levels in normal adults

The previous lines of evidence have of course been interventionist, i.e. they have involved the administration of some compound or other, and such studies can be problematical (ethically) for psychological researchers. The evidence in this section relates more to correlational studies, which have fewer ethical issues and can thus be more easily conducted by psychologists. Typically, however, they still involve blood/saliva sampling at some point. In an early study Fox *et al.* (1972) compared blood testosterone levels in a single individual just before and five minutes after orgasm during coitus, masturbation and non-sexual conditions. Testosterone levels were significantly higher during and immediately after sexual intercourse than in the control and masturbation conditions, though peak values of testosterone appeared to have no relationship to sexual activity. This finding was not, however, replicated by Lee *et al.* (1974) in a study involving five individuals and a broader range of time scales.

In a somewhat larger study, Kraemer *et al.* (1976) recruited twenty males to assess the possible relationship between morning testosterone levels and daily frequency of certain sexual behaviours over a two-month period. A within-subjects comparison showed that higher levels of testosterone were associated with elevated rates of sexual activity, but between-subjects analysis actually revealed a negative relationship between testosterone level and sexual activity (the higher the testosterone, the lower the activity). A possible confound is that sexual activity involves some degree of physical exertion (that might also influence hormone levels), and so van Anders *et al.* (2007b) assessed relationships between circulating testosterone and sexual activity compared to cuddling and physical exercise in young women. Salivary testosterone was found to be higher before and after sexual intercourse than the control conditions. There also appeared to be relationships between testosterone and orgasm, sexual desire and relationship commitment.

Udry *et al.* (1985) and later Halpern *et al.* (1993) both reasoned that the effects of androgens in males undergoing puberty might be analogous to androgen supplementation in hypogonadal adults; circulating levels of testosterone in prepubertal males are very low (akin to those of hypogonadal males) and during puberty these levels rise to reach adult levels (like the supplementation in hypogonadal males). The former study reported that free testosterone was a strong predictor of sexual motivations and behaviours in 102 adolescent boys, with no additional effects of age or pubertal development being noted. In the latter study, Halpern and colleagues predicted that if testosterone was acting as a biological substrate for sexual interest and behaviours, then these should show a positive correlation with rising testosterone levels during puberty. They tracked around 100 adolescent males for a three-year period, from the onset of puberty until a stage when serum testosterone levels approximated those of an adult. Questionnaires addressing sexual motivations and behaviours were regularly conducted. An initial data point as the males entered puberty was related to sexual interest at later time points, and did predict the transition to sexual intercourse. However, the authors urged caution in assuming that this represented clear support for a hormone–behaviour relationship because over the subsequent three years there was little relationship between testosterone and sexual behaviours. In fact pubertal development (including both physical and social changes) was more closely related to sexual behaviours.

## Prenatal hormone relationships

There has been a rapid growth in studies assessing the possible prenatal (organisational) effects of hormone levels on subsequent behaviours, using the putative proxy of the second to fourth finger length ratio (2D:4D). Some studies have focused on this putative indicator of prenatal testosterone levels and indirect measures of sexual behaviours. For example, Hönekopp *et al.* (2006) reported two studies looking at 2D:4D in males and their number of reported sexual partners. In student volunteers in Germany and Austria they found a significant negative relationship between 2D:4D and number of reported sex partners, such that a lower ratio (higher prenatal testosterone exposure) reflected a greater number of sex partners. This relationship was independent of circulating levels of salivary free testosterone.

So, if prenatal testosterone exposure is related to number of sex partners, it remains unclear as to how this might operate. Does it influence physical attractiveness, masculinity, personality factors such as dominance or confidence, sex drive, or some other behavioural characteristics? Other studies using this measure have shed some light on this issue. Russell (2006) showed that 2D:4D was not associated either with self-perceived attractiveness (in males or females), or with the attractiveness judgements made by others on photographs of the same individuals. This echoed results from a study conducted by myself and colleagues. We found that while male 2D:4D was not associated with female ratings of their attractiveness, judgements of masculinity and dominance were negatively associated with 2D:4D – the lower the finger length ratio, the higher the ratings of masculinity and dominance (Neave *et al.*, 2003).

However, Roney and Maestripieri (2004) did find that lower male 2D:4D was associated with higher attractiveness ratings from women who were engaged in actual social interaction with the men (rather than simply rating their photographs). These males also showed more courtship-like behaviours than males with higher 2D:4D.

## The effects of sexual behaviours on hormone levels

Thus far the data from human males suggest a dose–response relationship between testosterone and sexual interest at levels below the normal range (as seen in clinical populations) but no consistent relationships associated with variability in serum testosterone once a normal adult range has been achieved. We can, of course, also address the converse relationship, i.e. the effects that sexual behaviours might have on hormone levels. Some animal studies had indeed indicated a reciprocal effect of sexual behaviour on the endocrine system, the mere exposure of a male to a female being followed by a rise in the male's blood levels of testosterone irrespective of whether copulation occurred or not (e.g. Macrides *et al.*, 1975; Pfeiffer and Johnston, 1992; Rose *et al.*, 1972).

A famous letter to the journal *Nature* (Anonymous, 1972) provided an interesting inroad to this question. The individual concerned had indicated that the anticipation of sexual intercourse could lead to increases in testosterone (measured by increases in beard growth) but this is not easy to confirm. Hellhammer *et al.* (1985) measured salivary testosterone levels in twenty healthy males shown various films, two of which contained erotic material. Measurements were taken ten minutes before, during and fifteen minutes after viewing the film. As hypothesised, salivary testosterone showed a rapid and significant increase from baseline following the two erotic versions, a decline following a stressful movie, and no change after a neutral or an aggressive movie.

Stoléru *et al.* (1993) replicated this study in a cross-over design in which they measured LH pulsatility along with testosterone in nine undergraduates in response to both an erotic and a neutral film. Around three hours before the presentation of the stimuli, the monitoring began, with blood being sampled at ten minute intervals. One hour before the film, the participants were informed of its content, and a strain-gauge loop was fitted to record penile tumescence. The film lasted for around ninety minutes and blood continued to be collected for around five hours afterwards. Mean plasma testosterone levels were significantly higher just after the content of the film had been announced, and after ten minutes of the start of the erotic film compared to the neutral film. This suggests that plasma testosterone is changing in response to anticipated sexual arousal, and this mirrors a similar rise after actual sexual stimulation; the authors hypothesised that this initial rise was a central preparatory mechanism serving to facilitate sexual behaviours, and repeated increases may then contribute to maintain neural/ peripheral effectors of sexual behaviour.

Dabbs and Mohammed (1992) measured salivary testosterone in male and female couples on nights in which they had sex and nights in which they did not. They found that testosterone increased on the evenings when intercourse took place and decreased on evenings when it did not, in both males and females. As early evening measures did not differ between control and intercourse conditions, this therefore indicates that it was sexual activity producing a rise in testosterone, and not the other way round. The authors suggested that the lack of an anticipatory increase could be due to the fact that the couples were in a long-term relationship and their sex had become routine.

In a similar study Krüger *et al.* (1998) continuously investigated a range of hormone parameters in ten healthy males during a session containing neutral visual material and a pornographic film, after which they were required to masturbate to orgasm. Levels of epinephrine rose significantly just before masturbation and norepinephrine rose during this activity; cortisol levels dropped; prolactin showed a significant peak after orgasm and remained elevated thereafter; testosterone levels remained unaffected throughout the study. This postorgasmic prolactin response seems to reflect sexual satiety, and the rise in this hormone is stronger after penile–vaginal intercourse than after masturbation (Brody *et al.*, 2006). These findings suggest that previous studies focussing on hormone changes induced by masturbation may not be providing a true window into hormonal events resulting from actual sexual intercourse.

Of direct relevance to the animal literature described in the opening paragraph of this section is a study by Roney *et al.* (2003). They asked male students to engage in a short conversation, either with another male or with a female. These males provided saliva samples before and after the conversation, and had their behaviours (specifically, the degree to which they appeared to be interested in the other person, and if they tried to impress them) rated by their conversational partner. In the 'female' condition, a significant rise in testosterone was observed, especially in males who had experienced recent sexual intercourse and in those who were rated as having directed more courtship-type behaviours towards their female partner.

## Hormones and female sexual behaviours

Recall from chapter 2 that the gonadal steroids estradiol, progesterone and testosterone vary throughout the cycle in characteristic patterns that can be objectively recorded. These natural fluctuations can then be associated with various behavioural indices. Wallen (1990) made the excellent point that the ability and apparent readiness of human females to copulate throughout their menstrual cycle has been seen as evidence that complex human behaviours are divorced from their possible hormonal underpinnings. It was assumed, then, that human females (unlike female rats, for example) do not require ovarian hormones to trigger or modulate certain sexual behaviours. However, as described in a previous section, Wallen notes that such a conclusion misses the point that the ability to engage in sex needs to be distinguished from the motivations to engage in sex. The primate studies previously discussed showed that the two can easily be confused if the research methodologies are not carefully thought out. So, in order to attempt to understand the possible role of hormones in human female reproductive behaviours, we must differentiate the hormonal underpinnings of desire/motivation from those subserving actual copulatory behaviours. It is thus useful once more to focus on the conceptualisation of female sexual behaviours provided by Beach (1976), and determine to what extent human females can be placed within such a framework.

## Attractivity

The animal literature seems to demonstrate convincingly that females at their most fertile phase of the estrus cycle are more 'attractive' to males, this attraction apparently being governed by physical (e.g. skin colouration changes), physiological (e.g. pheromonal signals) or behavioural alterations (e.g. acceptance of the male's attention). It was assumed that human females did not emit such signals and that ovulation was concealed or 'cryptic' (Burley, 1979), but studies have begun to demonstrate that in certain conditions human males may be able to detect female ovulation, and show changes in their responsiveness to females. In general we would predict that certain hormone-dependent characteristics may reflect 'honest' signals that males can focus on in order to make judgements concerning sexual attractiveness. For example, it has been found that males prefer higher-pitched female voices over lower-pitched ones; individuals with higher-pitched voices display higher circulating levels of estrogen (Abitbol et al., 1999). Similarly, Jasieńska et al. (2004) found that women with the most attractive body shape (large breasts combined with a low waist-to-hip ratio) had higher estrogen levels than women with a less attractive shape. In addition, progesterone was specifically associated with waist-to-hip ratio, the lower ratio being associated with higher progesterone during the luteal phase.

As regards skin colour, van den Berghe and Frost (1986) reported that female skin colour changes in tone across the menstrual cycle, becoming lighter around the ovulatory phase and darker during non-fertile stages. It is also darker in women using the contraceptive pill. These authors proposed that such subtle changes may serve as a means by which males can differentiate between more fertile or less fertile females. Skin condition in general reflects the ratio of the gonadal steroids (especially estrogen and testosterone): women who have higher than average levels of circulating testosterone, for example, have more acne and facial hair (Lucky, 1995). To my knowledge, studies assessing alterations in skin colouration in females over the course of the menstrual cycle (taking objective hormone measurements) and male perceptions of these females have yet to be conducted, but one might predict significant relationships between estrogen or progesterone, skin colouration, and male ratings of attraction. One study has reported that males do not in fact rate lighter skin tones as being more 'attractive' (Fink et al. 2001) but this did not assess possible relationships between hormones and such perceptions.

One study that has begun to address this issue is that of Roberts et al. (2004). They took photographs of the same forty-eight women during the follicular and luteal phases of their cycles. Males and females were then asked to select which one of the pair of photographs was more attractive, and both sexes showed a clear preference for the photograph taken during the fertile phase. More recently, Law Smith *et al.* (2006) investigated the possible relationships between circulating levels of gonadal hormones in fifty-nine females, and male perceptions of their attractiveness, healthiness and femininity. Once photographed, composite pictures were created utilising the faces from females with the highest estrogen levels and the lowest estrogen levels – these composites were then rated by the males on those attributes just described. The faces representing females higher in estrogen were indeed viewed as being more feminine, attractive and healthy than those represent-ing females with lower estrogen levels, but the fact that males were not actually rating faces of 'real' women individually differing in circulating estrogen reduces the ecological validity of this study.

As regards body scent, Singh and Bronstad (2001) persuaded seventeen normally cycling women, not using an oral contraceptive, to wear a T-shirt for three consecutive nights during the follicular and luteal phases of their menstrual cycle. The shirts were frozen and then thawed, before fifty-two males were asked to sniff each shirt and rate it for odour 'intensity', 'pleas-antness' and 'sexiness'. Regression analysis revealed that the phase during which the shirt was worn significantly predicted its rating of pleasantness and sexiness. Using shirts from a smaller sample of four females, the authors then found that shirts worn during the fertile phase were rated as being significantly more pleasant and sexy than shirts worn during the non-fertile phase.

It is clear that our current understanding of possible relationships between circulating hormone levels and female attractiveness remains limited. From the animal literature we would expect that males would rate ovulating females as being more attractive (human studies now show some evidence for this), would wish to spend more time in their company (no evidence as yet), and would perhaps themselves show physiological or behavioural changes when in the company of ovulating females compared to non-ovulating females (no evidence as yet).

## Proceptivity

Recall that Beach (1976) admitted that the distinction between receptivity and proceptivity is often difficult to distinguish, and this certainly appears to be the case for human females, not least because precise assessments of cycle phase and measurements of intrinsic sexual state are not easy (Slob *et al.*, 1991). I will attempt to maintain as clear a boundary as possible: in this section I focus on behaviours that do not include an overt sexual element (sexual desire/moti-vation); I shall address overt sexual behaviours (e.g. copulation/masturbation) in the next section. The evidence from animal studies indicates that females will show much more interest in males during the most fertile phase of their cycle (whether this represents an increase in positive motivation, or a decrease in negative motivations – e.g. avoidance behaviours – remains to be ascertained), and show an increase in certain sexually motivated behaviours. In contrast to the previous section, there is rather more information concerning possible hormonal effects on proceptivity in human females.

In terms of stated preferences for the opposite sex, several studies have now shown that female perceptions of males do not remain stable, but instead fluctuate over the menstrual cycle. Penton-Voak *et al.* (1999), for example, asked thirty-nine females not using an oral contraceptive to select from a range of male faces (not 'real' faces, but composites manipulated to be masculinised or feminised by varying degrees) the most 'attractive' face, during follicular and luteal phases. During the most fertile phase (hormonal assays were not used to confirm this) the females showed a greater preference for the more masculinised male faces compared with the less fertile phase. In a second experiment, females could arrange male faces along a continuum ranging from feminised to masculinised, and select the most preferred face for a long-term or short-term relationship. For a sexual encounter, the preference was for a more masculinised face when tested during the follicular phase.

In a follow-up study, Penton-Voak and Perrett (2000) presented the different versions of the male faces in a popular magazine and asked female readers to select the face they found most attractive. After removing contraceptive pill-users from the sample, they were left with 139 females whom they could split into 'high conception risk' and 'low conception risk' on the basis of their answers to a menstrual cycle questionnaire. Once again, the high-conception group showed a clear preference for the more masculinised face compared to the low-conception group. A similar study by Koehler *et al.* (2002) assessed female preferences for male faces differing in symmetry, a preference for more symmetrical male faces being argued to reflect an adaptive mechanism whereby females gain indirect genetic benefits for their offspring, as physical asymmetry in humans is associated with genetically based disorders (references in Koehler *et al.*, 2002). They asked twenty-nine non-pill-using females to rate the attractiveness of various male faces differing in symmetry, during menses and the follicular phase of the cycle. A control sample of pill-using females was also included. Both groups showed a general preference for symmetry, but, in contrast to predictions, there was no effect of menstrual cycle phase on symmetry preferences.

In another variation on this theme, Jones *et al.* (2004) focussed on female preferences for the apparent health displayed in male faces; again, this is thought of as being an advertisement of a male's genetic qualities (e.g. his heritable immunity from infection). They predicted that preferences for health might also show a shift across the menstrual cycle, and in a large sample of 639 females did indeed find (unlike previous studies) that ratings given to faces manipulated to display better apparent health were higher during the less fertile phase, compared to the most fertile phase. In subsequent experiments they showed that such preferences were stronger in pregnant women, and in women using an oral contraceptive. The consistent factor here was assumed to be progesterone (higher in the luteal phase, in pregnant women, and in females using the pill) and the authors thus suggested that raised progesterone level is associated with an increased attraction to facial cues associated with indirect genetic benefits. More recently, Jones *et al.* (2005) have conducted a similar study addressing relationship satisfaction and face preferences. In ninety-three partnered women they found that estimated progesterone levels were positively related to preferences for femininity in male faces, and women in a stage of high estimated progesterone showed more commitment to their relationships. However, once more the faces used were not 'real' faces, and actual levels of progesterone, or any other hormone, were not directly ascertained.

In terms of sexual arousal, self-reports of female-initiated behaviours show an increase during the midcycle (e.g. Sanders and Bancroft, 1982), but sexual arousal when measured within a laboratory setting revealed no such increases at midcycle (e.g. Schreiner-Engel *et al.*, 1981), though, as previously mentioned, such studies are often compounded by high levels of stress and embarrassment. Matteo and Rissman (1984) pointed out that contextual factors are important in human sexual encounters, especially the influence of the male demanding sex and the use of the contraceptive pill which removes the fear of pregnancy. Indeed pill-users typically show little variation in their sexual activity during the cycle. In their study they examined sexual desires in lesbian couples free from male demands or the fear of pregnancy. Seven couples kept a log of their desires for fourteen consecutive weeks; peaks in sexual thoughts and fantasies peaked post-menstrually.

Slob *et al.* (1991) studied temperature changes in the labia of the vagina, and subjective sexual and genital arousal, in twelve pill-using women and twelve non-pill-using women whilst they watched an erotic movie. Participants were tested twice, once during the follicular phase and once during the luteal phase (progesterone assays provided an objective assessment of cycle phase). Women tested for the first time during the fertile phase showed higher levels of sexual arousal (both subjective and objective) than those tested for the first time during the non-fertile phase. So, menstrual cycle phase during the first assessment determined their initial response, and this appeared to affect the magnitude of the response during the second test. Slob *et al.* (1996) suggested that this might reflect a cognitive or conditioning response, and replicated this unexpected finding. Once more, women first tested in the follicular phase reported more subjective sexual arousal in response to an erotic movie. Precisely why this should be so remains uncertain, and as yet no authors have offered a convincing theoretical explanation of it. At the very least it means another potentially confounding variable to be considered in future studies.

Alexander and Sherwin (1993) reasoned that pill-users might be a good sample in which to assess possible associations between testosterone and sexual desires because secretions of estradiol and progesterone are suppressed, and thus remain low and stable throughout the cycle; testosterone on the other hand, while low, can still be quite variable. They asked nineteen pill-users who were not currently living with a regular partner to record their daily sexual desires and activities. Free testosterone was significantly positively related to sexual thoughts, sexual desires and the anticipation of sexual activity, though the degree of sexual enjoyment showed no such relationship. Gangestad *et al.* (2002) asked non-pill-using females to complete questionnaires concerning their sexual desires and their partners' behaviour just before ovulation and again during the non-fertile phase of their cycle. Women's sexual attraction to and fantasy about males other than their partner increased when they were in their fertile phase. In response to this, males increased their mate retention and vigilance behaviours (e.g. phoning them more often, looking through their personal belongings, etc.) when their partner was in her most fertile phase. In a follow-up to this study Haselton and Gangestad (2006) confirmed that, near ovulation, women showed heightened interest in attending social gatherings where they might meet men; women in relationships also admitted to flirting with men other than their current partner at this time.

There is thus some evidence that female perceptions of males, and their reported sexual interests, change over the course of the cycle, and perhaps differ as regards fertile versus non-fertile phases. However, the evidence is often contradictory, and is clouded by the fact that most studies rely upon self-report measures, and do not routinely confirm suspected changes in cycle phase with objective hormone measures. Indeed, Regan (1996) concluded that if there is a single cyclical pattern reflecting hormonal fluctuations that does characterise female sexual desires, then it is likely to be obscured by various methodological problems.

### Receptivity

Adams *et al.* (1978) measured female-initiated sexual behaviours in thirty-five married women who were split into those using and not using an oral contraceptive. In the non-pill group the women showed a clear increase in self-initiated sexual behaviours (masturbation and coitus) at their most fertile phase; the pill-using females did not show such changes, and in fact their sexual activity was very low. As estrogen levels show a clear peak at ovulation the authors linked such a surge to the greater sexual receptivity in the non-pill-users. They also speculated that the effects of the contraceptive pills on reducing estrogen and raising progesterone might explain the suppression of sexual activity seen in the pill-using group. Bancroft *et al.* (1980) reasoned that such effects might be due to hormonal effects (perhaps to reductions in androstenedione), but also possibly to alterations in mood, or to psychological reactions to fertility control. They recruited a group of pill-using women who had reported 'sexual problems' that they had attributed to their pill use, and a group of pill-users who had experienced no sexual problems. The hormone profiles of both groups were remarkably similar, but frequency of sexual thoughts correlated highly with plasma testosterone levels in the 'no problem' group but not in the 'problem group'. Androstenedione supplementation over a two-month period (using a double-blind, placebo cross-over design) had no effect on any of the variables assessed in either group.

Harvey (1987) asked sixty-nine normally menstruating females to keep a daily record of their sexual experiences over two or three consecutive menstrual cycles. A significant effect of cycle phase was observed, with masturbation and female-initiated sexual intercourse both peaking in the ovulatory phase, and progressively declining during the luteal and premenstrual phases. This suggests that women do initiate and engage in sexual activities during their midcycle, but the data for male-initiated sexual activities also showed the same pattern, thus hinting that males were able to deduce a partner's most fertile phase. Of course, whether this reflects the fact that the males were picking up hormonally mediated physical signals from their partners or were simply responding to her alterations in behaviour remains difficult to decide. Such complex interactions will not be understood by simply asking people to complete a few questionnaires.

Alexander *et al.* (1990) focussed on the possible role of fluctuating testosterone levels on female sexual behaviours in a sample of fifteen pill-users and eighteen non-pill-users. They first reviewed previous studies that had found few consistent relationships, and noted that such experiments had only measured levels of total testosterone from plasma. Recall that only free testosterone (which is not bound to sex hormone binding globulin) is thought to exert biological effects, and so Alexander and colleagues made sure they assessed SHBG, total testosterone, free testosterone and progesterone during all phases of the cycle; the women were asked to complete records of their sexual desires and sexual activities over the cycle. There were no major group differences in terms of sexual activities, though the oral contraceptive users reported a greater increase in sexual interests and activities during the premenstrual period, and made more attempts to initiate sexual activities with their partners. In terms of hormonal differences, non-pill-users displayed higher levels of free testosterone during the postmenstrual and midcycle phases and they also showed a greater drop in testosterone levels from midcycle to the menstrual phase. There were no correlations between changes in testosterone levels and the average frequency of sexual activity or levels of sexual desire in either group. However, there was a significant relationship between the decrease in testosterone from midcycle to menses observed in the non-pill-users, and the decline in their sexual desires at the same time.

In a larger study Bancroft *et al.* (1991) assessed relationships between plasma and free testosterone and various measures of sexual behaviour and attitudes in fifty-three non-pill-users and fifty-five pill-users. Only in the pill-users did they find a relationship between high levels of free testosterone and arousal by erotic imagery, and more frequent sexual activity with a partner. The authors admitted, though, that there are possibly numerous psychosocial factors that need to be considered when assessing possible relationships between circulating androgens and female sexual behaviours.

Van Goozen *et al.* (1997) took blood samples from twenty-one young women who were split into groups depending upon whether they reported experiencing premenstrual complaints or not. The two groups were asked to keep a diary of their sexual interests and behaviours over a single menstrual cycle. It was found that the groups in fact differed in their levels of estradiol and in the ratio of estradiol/progesterone, with those not reporting premenstrual complaints experiencing higher levels of both hormone parameters. In addition, this group reported a clear peak in sexual interest during the premenstrual phase, while the group experiencing premenstrual complaints reported a peak during the ovulatory phase. The authors suggested that fluctuations in androgen levels might underlie these group differences, though the groups did not actually differ in levels of this hormone. The study does clearly demonstrate that there is possibly another confounding variable, in the form of subjective ratings of premenstrual complaints (associated with objectively different hormone profiles), that perhaps needs to be considered in the future.

An additional point to consider was made by Wallen (1990), who argued that sexual behaviour might be found to be completely unrelated to hormonal mechanisms in females in long-term stable sexual relationships, as such women are comparable to female primates studied in small enclosures with a single male – they may engage in sexual behaviours for various reasons other than sexual desire. Alternatively, we might expect to see a much closer relationship between hormones and sexual activity in young sexually active females in whom mate selection and courtship are important, especially in those without a regular partner. Currently there appears to be a dearth of such studies. Of those studies mentioned in this section all have relied upon women currently in a relationship; around 65% of the sample in Harvey's (1987) study were single, though relationship status was not explicitly considered in the data analysis.

If it is assumed that females are more likely to engage in sexual activity around ovulation, then one might expect them actively to seek out prospective sex partners during that phase or engage in other behaviours that might attract a potential partner. Haselton *et al.* (2007) suggested that changes in female sexual motivations might manifest themselves in changes in self-ornamentation (e.g. clothing, grooming, etc.) and such changes might reflect hormonal fluctuations. They asked thirty young women (not using oral contraceptives) to pose for a full-body photograph during the follicular and luteal phases of their menstrual cycle. For once, cycle phase was confirmed by hormonal assays. The two photographs were then presented to both male and female judges, who were asked to select the one of the pair in which the person was trying to look more attractive. Both male and female judges showed a significant agreement that the photograph taken during ovulation was the one where the woman was trying to look more attractive – the nearer to ovulation, the stronger the effect. Qualitative judgements indicated that the women wore clothing that was more fashionable, nicer and displayed more skin during ovulation.

However, there is another possible issue to consider – the potential danger of becoming impregnated by an undesirable male. Chavanne and Gallup (1998) asked 300 female college students to keep a log of their activities; the focus was on sexual risk-taking behaviours, so, for example, watching TV at home was considered to be 'low risk', while walking alone in a dimly lit area was considered 'high risk'. Responses were then analysed in terms of which phase of the menstrual cycle participants appeared to be in during completion. In females taking the contraceptive pill, there was no variation in risk-taking behaviours as a function of menstrual cycle phase. However, those not using the contraceptive pill showed a significant decrease in their risk-taking behaviours during their most fertile phase (this was irrespective of general activity levels). In a replication of this study, Bröder and Hohmann (2003) also asked females to complete a questionnaire of their risk-taking behaviours once a week for four weeks. During the fertile phase women showed a reduction of 'risky' activities and an increase in 'non-risky' activities. The same effect was not seen in contraceptive pill-users.

## The menopause, and hormone replacement

Following natural or surgical menopause there is a marked drop in circulating levels of estrogen and progesterone. The effects on androgens are much less clear, with some evidence that androgens derived from the ovaries begin to fall several years before natural menopause, but then may actually rise again following the menopause, because estrogen-induced negative feedback is removed, and SHBG levels also decline (studies cited in Bancroft, 2005). Other authors point out, however, that there is a major reduction in testosterone levels after the menopause because the ovaries cease to produce androstenedione, a key precursor of testosterone (Miller, 2001).

Sexual behaviours have been reported to show a clear decline throughout the menopause. For example, Dennerstein et al. (1997) asked 201 women in the early stages of the menopause to complete a questionnaire on sexual functioning across the menopause and found that sexual functioning significantly declined with age. The obvious assumption has been to link this decline with the reduction in ovarian steroids, but supporting evidence for such an assumption has not been overwhelming. For example, Myers *et al.* (1990) conducted a double-blind study involving forty naturally menopausal women in which they received daily treatments of either estrogen, estrogen + progesterone, progesterone + testosterone, or a placebo, for ten weeks. Hormone treatment had no effect on self-reported mood, sexual behaviour or psychophysically measured sexual arousal, though the progesterone + testosterone group did report more satisfaction from masturbation. In contrast, Dennerstein *et al.* (2002) tracked 438 women aged forty-five to fifty-five from early to late menopausal transition, and found that while 42% of the sample reported a decline in sexual behaviours during the early phase, this rose to 88% during the later stages. In a subsample of this group (226 women) they also recorded hormone levels, and found that low estradiol was associated with lower scores on the sexual behaviour questionnaire during the early stages; as estradiol dropped further then so did scores on the questionnaire. No relation between androgen levels and sexual behaviours was found.

Other studies have focussed on women experiencing surgical menopause (removal of the womb and/or ovaries) and the effects of various hormone replacement therapies. Using a prospective, double-blind, crossover design, Sherwin *et al.* (1985) assessed the effects of three different replacement therapies (estrogen only, testosterone only, estrogen + testosterone, or placebo) in fifty-three women undergoing surgical menopause. A group of women who had received hysterectomies, but whose ovaries remained intact, were also included as a control group. Those receiving testosterone, on its own or in combination with estrogen, showed an enhancement of sexual desires and sexual fantasies, though the levels of testosterone may have reached supraphysiological levels, and it is thus not clear that normal levels of androgens in menopausal women would have the same effects.

Shifren *et al.* (2000) recruited a sample of women who had already undergone surgical menopause and who had all been referred (and treated with oral estrogen) for impaired sexual functioning. Following a baseline assessment, the women received transdermal patches containing either 150 μg or 300 μg of testosterone or a placebo for a twelve-week period. While the placebo group also showed a significant response, those receiving the higher testosterone dose reported a significant improvement in the frequency of their sexual activities and degree of sexual pleasure, but no alteration in sexual arousal. Bancroft (2005) concludes that as regards testosterone the evidence remains inconclusive because there are possibly other psychological factors (e.g. mood, well-being) that need to be considered.

As regards estrogen/progesterone, Sherwin (1991) studied the effects of various doses of estrogen and progestin on sexual behaviours in forty-eight menopausal women. After baseline assessments the women were assigned to one of four treatment groups for twelve months. Two of the groups received combinations of estrogen + progesterone (in two different doses), with the other groups receiving estrogen + placebo (again in two different doses).

Irrespective of group, ratings of sexual desire and arousal were highest during the first two weeks of treatment compared to weeks when no hormones were being administered. In his careful analysis of this paper, Bancroft (2005) notes that the graphs indicate that the group receiving the high doses of estrogen in addition to progesterone had much lower levels of sexual interest at baseline. They thus appeared to show a substantial improvement in sexual arousal with treatment, suggesting that higher doses of estrogen may be more beneficial. This issue remains to be adequately addressed.

## The role of oxytocin

While the primary emphasis has been on gonadal steroids, researchers have now begun to assess the possible roles played by other hormones (in tandem with the gonadal steroids), and also the interactions between these hormones and various neurotransmitters. One of the most researched substances is oxytocin,[6] a nonapeptide (it consists of nine amino acids) produced mainly within the supraoptic (SON) and paraventricular nuclei (PVN) of the hypothalamus and released into the CNS, periphery, brain stem and spinal cord in a pulsatile fashion via the posterior pituitary gland. It is chemically very similar to vasopressin (also called antidiuretic hormone), a substance produced in the same structures and released in the same manner. In the rat brain, oxytocin receptors have been located in various regions in the CNS but are particularly dense in the ventromedial hypothalamus (VMH), bed nucleus of the stria terminalis (BNST), amygdala, olfactory nuclei and lateral septum (cited in Carter, 1992). Interestingly, the same locations host androgen and estrogen receptors, and several aspects of oxytocin action seem to be regulated in part by the steroid hormones (Freund-Mercier *et al.*, 1987). Oxytocin is also produced within the male reproductive organs and these structures also contain oxytocin receptors attesting to the local effects of this peptide (Thackare *et al.*, 2006).

Oxytocin is a powerful hormone, producing contraction effects within smooth muscles such as those found in the breasts and in the uterus. During labour it is released in pulses and serves to contract the uterine muscles to expel the foetus and the afterbirth; indeed the word 'oxytocin' derives from the Greek term meaning 'quick birth' and analogues of it are used to induce labour and trigger breastfeeding as it stimulates milk ejection from the nipples (Gimpl and Fahrenholz, 2001). In males, a burst of oxytocin is released at orgasm and this acts to stimulate contractions within the reproductive tract that facilitate the release of sperm from the testes (Thackare *et al.*, 2006). The role of oxytocin in sexual behaviours remains

---

[6] Discovered in 1953 (alongside arginine vasopressin) by Vincent de Vigneaud (1901–78), an accomplishment that won him the Nobel Prize for Chemistry.

yet to be clarified, but in female rats oxytocin stimulates the lordosis response (Arletti and Bertolini, 1985), while injections of an oxytocin antagonist directly into the mPOA inhibit lordosis (Caldwell *et al.*, 1994). In male rats it enhances copulatory performance by shortening the ejaculation latency and the postejaculatory interval (Arletti *et al.*, 1985); it also induces a dose-dependent increase in penile erections, and yawning(!) (Melis *et al.*, 1986), though high doses serve to inhibit the same function (Argiolas and Gessa, 1991), thus suggesting that this hormone also plays a role in satiety of sexual behaviours.

In humans, an early study indicated that milk ejection (presumably dependent upon oxytocin release) could be triggered following orgasm (Campbell and Pedersen, 1953). Carmichael *et al.* (1987) measured plasma oxytocin levels before, during and after masturbatory orgasm in males and females, and found that levels of oxytocin rose significantly during sexual arousal in both sexes compared to baseline. Similarly, Blaicher *et al.* (1999) reported that the highest levels of circulating oxytocin were measured during or shortly after orgasm in women. Anderson-Hunt and Dennerstein (1994) described the case of a women who had been prescribed a synthetic oxytocin compound (via a nasal spray) in order to facilitate breast feeding. Milk production was indeed improved, but she reported that several hours after two sprays she felt an intense sexual desire and copious vaginal lubrication. More recently, Salonia *et al.* (2005) monitored plasma levels of oxytocin in thirty normally cycling young women, some of whom were taking an oral contraceptive. Oxytocin was found to fluctuate significantly throughout the menstrual cycle, being lower during the luteal phase than during the follicular and ovulatory phases (values did not differ between pill-users and non-pill-users). A questionnaire assessment of sexual function was also administered, and there were some significant positive correlations between oxytocin levels and certain items on the questionnaire, relating to sexual arousal and genital lubrication.

In her review, Carter (1992) suggested that oxytocin plays a significant role in the mediation of the sequential neurological/physiological events underlying sexual behaviours. Initially oxytocin in small amounts primes preorgasmic sexual activity, and simultaneously triggers a pulsatile release of central and/or peripheral oxytocin, this larger burst then playing a key role in the experience of orgasm, and the physiological events that follow on from this larger pulse may then contribute to sexual satiety.

# 9 Attachment/parental behaviours

Uvnäs-Moberg (1997) proposed that basic problems related to survival and reproduction (e.g. giving birth, lactation, infant socialisation, etc.) have led to physiological, psychological and behavioural adaptations in the form of social/attachment bonds. These bonds are formed during certain key reproductive events (sexual interaction, social interaction, birth, lactation, etc.) and the kinds of behaviours associated with such bonds are species-typical and highly individualised (Carter, 1998; Mason and Mendoza, 1998). These bonds are distinct from sex drive, which, according to Fisher (1998), may have evolved simply to motivate individuals to seek sexual activity with a range of partners.

In many diverse species it has been confirmed that individuals do form strong, long-lasting, yet flexible attachment bonds that seem to serve initially to facilitate reproduction, and then provide a sense of security, and reduce feelings of anxiety and stress (Carter, 1998). Mammals in particular display complex social relationships in which pairs, or a number of individuals, form a cohesive social group held together by social bonds and certain social affiliative behaviours (e.g. grooming). Forming an attachment bond to a specific individual must entail both perceptual, cognitive and emotional elements; and the similarity of the differing types of emotional bonds suggests some basic core biological process is at work. Mason and Mendoza (1998) suggest that newborns are equipped to form dynamic neurobiological representations called 'action schemata' that guide their behavioural responses to their environment. Via experiential processes, such schemata develop into strong attachment bonds for specific individuals (typically the primary caregivers). In adults, similar mechanisms could come into play when maternal and paternal attachment bonds are being formed with their offspring, and perhaps when adults form friendship and romantic bonds.

Crews (1998) notes that great diversity exists among animal species in terms of their reproductive/social behaviours and the hormonal mechanisms underlying them. Studying such differences may provide some insights into how such mechanisms evolved. Not surprisingly, many researchers have attempted to discover the possible role of the endocrine system in the establishment and maintenance of such behaviours.

## Adult pair-bonds

The first type of attachment bond to be considered concerns those that are commonly observed between unrelated adults forming reproductive relationships ('heterosexual attachment'). These initial social bonds then develop to form longer-term attachment bonds in order to motivate two individuals to remain together in order to facilitate parental duties.

### Social bonds in animals

'Monogamous' is the term given to species that display long-term social bonds between adult males and females that exist independently of the breeding season; this term also refers to the fact that the sexes will display sexual exclusivity, and that males will engage in parental duties and avoid incestuous relationship with the offspring (Kleiman, 1977). These characteristics are not seen in polygynous species, where the sexes do not form such strong social/reproductive bonds (amongst mammals, polygyny is much more common than monogamy). A popular model for assessing the biological bases of such social behaviours has been the vole, a small rodent found in the United States and Canada, which conveniently displays both types of mating behaviour. Three closely related species, the prairie vole (*Microtus ochrogaster*), the montane vole (*Microtus montanus*) and the meadow vole (*Microtus pennsylvanicus*), have been the object of much research attention because, while prairie voles are monogamous, both montane and meadow voles are polygynous. Male and female prairie voles form lifelong pair bonds and share all parental duties, even joining together to repel intruders aggressively from their territory; in stark contrast, males and females from the other species only get together for sex, and then actively avoid one another, the male playing no part in the rearing of the offspring (Carter and Getz, 1993).

The reproductive physiology of the monogamous prairie vole appears to be governed by social cues, jointly mediated by the olfactory and endocrine systems; thus, pheromones secreted by a non-related male trigger norepinephrine and LH-RH in the female within minutes, leading to LH release, and thence the secretion of estradiol and progesterone from the ovaries. Attention thus first focussed on the possible role of the gonadal steroids in the formation of social bonds in this species. Estradiol was found to be elevated in female prairie voles during estrus, but as this pattern was also seen in the polygynous vole species, it seemed unlikely to be the crucial factor. Alterations in progesterone, however, appeared more interesting. In the prairie vole, this hormone begins to rise several hours after the first sexual encounter and remains elevated; males and females continue to engage in bouts of mating, and when not mating they remain in close social contact. In the non-monogamous species, progesterone is released very shortly after the onset of mating but then drops;

mating is then discontinued, and the sexes do not stay in close social contact. In fact they may become overtly aggressive towards one another (studies cited in Carter and Getz, 1993).

A key factor is social and sexual experience. Williams *et al.* (1994) reported that a young female prairie vole entering estrus for the first time would develop a strong preference for a male if she was allowed to cohabit with him for a minimum of twenty-four hours. While mating was not essential for a partner preference to be established, those pairs that had mated within six hours of first meeting were much more likely to display a subsequent pair bond. The same process appeared to be happening in the males. Insel *et al.* (1995) noted that, after mating, male prairie voles showed an increase in affiliative behaviours towards the female and selective aggression against male intruders. In an initial experiment they tested males on various behavioural measures after twenty-four hours of either mating, social exposure (not including mating) or no social contact. Following the mating condition (but not the other two conditions) males showed typical affiliative and aggressive behaviours; in addition, they showed increased exploratory behaviours of an open-arm maze (taken to indicate a reduction in fearfulness). In a subsequent study, these authors attempted to determine the minimum amount of mating necessary for the formation of these social bonds; while only one hour of close social contact (including mating) was associated with an increase in social behaviours, the full repertoire was only seen in males given a day's access to the female. The polygynous montane vole showed no such behaviours over the same time span.

## Hormones and social bonding in animals

So what could it be about these intimate encounters that made the formation of a long-term pair bond more likely? Various hormones are released during sexual intercourse, with vasopressin and oxytocin perhaps being the most important. These are small peptides that are chemically similar to one another, and are produced within the supraoptic and paraventricular nuclei in the hypothalamus. Molecules of each are then transported to the posterior pituitary, where they are stored, before being released into the bloodstream; in addition both are secreted directly into the CNS. Within the CNS, receptors for oxytocin and vasopressin are found within the olfactory system, limbic-hypothalamic system and ventral forebrain, and in the brainstem and spinal cord, though there are large species differences in this distribution pattern (Insel and Young, 2000). The density and distribution of oxytocin binding (but perhaps not vasopressin) can be strongly influenced by estrogens, progesterone, androgens and glucocorticoid activity (studies cited in Carter, 1998). In rats, developmental experiences have been shown to alter adult gene expression for both oxytocin and vasopressin receptors, and thus we have here an excellent example of how individual experiences can influence adult social behaviour via hormonal mechanisms (Ostrowski, 1998).

The first stage of social bonding is the formation of social familiarity. In rodents this depends predominantly on pheromonal olfactory cues detected by the Vomeronasal organ and transmitted to the accessory olfactory bulb and thence to the amygdala (Keverne, 1999), these structures being rich in oxytocin receptors. When two individuals are first introduced, they engage in mutual sniffing, and as they become more familiar these olfactory investigations decrease. Such behaviours show a marked increase when another stranger is introduced. Such characteristic and easily observed behaviours are thus used as a quantitative assessment of social recognition memory. The administration of vasopressin seems to enhance social memory, while oxytocin administration to male rats can either facilitate or inhibit social memories (Benelli *et al.*, 1995). Ferguson *et al.* (2000) compared a strain of normal wild-type male mice with mutant male mice lacking the oxytocin gene, on social memory formation (the investigation of a novel ovariectomised female mouse). While the wild-type mice displayed normal social memory (a decrease in olfactory investigations), the mutant mice failed to develop social memory. This was not due simply to a problem in the olfactory system as the mutant mice performed normally in olfactory detection tasks. Treatment with oxytocin but not vasopressin enhanced social memory in the mutant mice, while treatment with an oxytocin antagonist produced social memory deficits in the wild-type mice.

Once these initial bonds have been formed, individuals then form stronger affiliative/sexual bonds. As discussed in the previous chapter, oxytocin increases during physical contact, grooming, vaginal stimulation and breast stimulation, and shows a marked increase during the orgasmic (ejaculatory) phase in diverse species (Carter, 1992). Williams *et al.* (1994) implanted slow-releasing oxytocin pumps[1] into ovariectomised adult female prairie voles. They were then housed with a novel male for six hours, after which a preference test was conducted (the female is allowed free choice between two compartments housing the male she was previously partnered with or a strange male). Compared to a group who received a control substance, the females treated with oxytocin showed a significant preference for the familiar male over the new male. Oxytocin administered peripherally had no such effect, and the administration of a selective oxytocin receptor antagonist inhibited the behavioural effect of central oxytocin administration. Similarly, in males, intracerebrovascular treatment with oxytocin also has a facilitatory effect on partner preference formation (Cho *et al.*, 1999).

In male prairie voles vasopressin rather than oxytocin appears to play the more important role, with several studies demonstrating that infusions of vasopressin (both long and short term) facilitate partner preference formation, and selective aggression towards intruder males (Cho *et al.*, 1999; Winslow *et al.*, 1993). The injection of a vasopressin antagonist eliminates

[1] These deliver oxytocin directly into the CNS via the ventricles. Oxytocin cannot be given intravenously because, as it is a peptide, it cannot cross the blood–brain barrier.

this increase in attacks directed towards intruder males following mating, and vasopressin infused directly into a male when accompanied by his female partner triggers an increase in hostility towards new males (studies cited in Carter and Getz, 1993).

Thus, the behavioural effects of both oxytocin and vasopressin are mediated by their receptors (OTR and V1aR respectively) in a gender-specific manner. While it has been established that both receptor types are widely distributed throughout the brain, the region of the ventral forebrain has been assumed to be especially important in pair-bond formation. Within this region, an injection of an oxytocin receptor antagonist directly into the nucleus accumbens blocks the formation of partner preferences in female prairie voles (Young et al., 2001). Similarly, injections of a V1aR antagonist into the ventral pallidal region block partner preferences in male prairie voles (Lim and Young, 2002, cited in Lim et al., 2004b).

However, establishing precisely which brain regions express OTR and V1aR has been problematic, but Lim et al. (2004b) carefully compared receptor binding in adjacent brain regions using autoradiographic techniques. They confirmed the presence of oxytocin binding in the nucleus accumbens, and vasopressin binding in the ventral pallidum, with males showing a greater density of vasopressin fibres than females (no sex differences were found for oxytocin). These brain regions are closely connected to one another, and both are related to the brain's reward system, specifically in limbic system aspects of motivation and reward, and in reinforcement-driven motor behaviours. The possible role of dopamine must also be considered. Both regions are key parts of the mesolimbic dopamine reward pathway: dopamine is released into the nucleus accumbens during mating in rats, and it also appears necessary for pair-bond formation (studies cited in Lim et al., 2004b).

One might thus expect to find differences in the oxytocin and vasopressin receptor genes, differences in number and location of the receptors, or differences in actual levels of these hormones between the monogamous and polygynous species. As the central infusion of vasopressin into polygynous voles does not affect their social behaviours, actual levels of vasopressin are unlikely to be important (Young et al., 1999). Lim et al. (2004a) suggested instead that the specific location of the V1aR within brain regions modulates pair-bonding behaviours. In support, Insel et al. (1998) have reviewed a series of studies demonstrating marked species differences in the distribution of oxytocin and vasopressin receptors. In the prairie vole, for example, oxytocin receptors are found predominantly in regions associated with reward and reinforcement, while in the montane vole the same receptors are more densely housed in the lateral septum.

In a different vein, Pitkow et al. (2001) have reported that the V1aR gene is structurally different in the male prairie vole compared to the polygynous males; the receptor also displays increased levels of expression within the ventral pallidum. Similarly, Young et al. (1999) discovered a small expanded sequence (this is called a microsatellite polymorphism) on the V1aR gene in the prairie vole which is absent in the montane vole, and this sequence could therefore be responsible for pair-bonding in the monogamous species. Lim *et al.* (2004c) were then able to insert the variant of this gene directly into the ventral pallidum of male meadow voles, whereupon vasopressin receptors were triggered, and these formerly antisocial males began to display social characteristics more akin to their monogamous cousins. Interestingly, Hammock and Young (2002) found considerable individual variability in the distribution of the V1aR within the brain of prairie voles, which could well explain individual differences in the ease with which pair-bonds are formed, and their duration when formed.

The assumption then is that the behavioural effects of oxytocin and vasopressin are regulated via their particular receptors. However, the explanation may be more complex than that. These peptides are very similar to one another (they only differ in two amino acids) and thus they may have the capability to influence one another's receptors either antagonistically or agonistically (Carter *et al.*, 1995). Indeed, Cho *et al.* (1999) have shown that while oxytocin and vasopressin are sufficient on their own to increase social contact in prairie voles, the administration of both combined is necessary to facilitate partner preferences completely. De Wied *et al.* (1993) have suggested the existence of an additional receptor system that is capable of recognising both peptides.

## Hormones and social bonding in humans

It is interesting to speculate on the possible genetic–hormonal basis of human social behaviours and this of course remains a highly controversial field of research, as there is undoubtedly a wealth of additional social and experiential factors to consider when looking at how complex human social bonds are formed and maintained. Nevertheless, researchers are beginning to make firm inroads into this area. There are several lines of evidence:

### Individuals with social deficits

Autism is a neurodevelopmental condition first described by child psychiatrist Leo Kanner, though the term 'autistic' ('autos' is the Greek word for 'self') was first used by Eugen Bleuler to describe the extreme social withdrawal seen in adults with schizophrenia. Autism is characterised by a lack of social responsiveness, lack of empathy, lack of eye contact, an intense dislike of change, excellent rote memory for meaningless material, obsessive interests, and behavioural, physical and linguistic repetition (Kanner, 1943).[2] More recently autism has been conceptualised as a triad of impairments (often

---

[2] Hans Asperger (1906–80) provided further insight concerning 'autistic psychopathy', by noting that the parents of autistic children often displayed similar traits, though not to the same severe degree as their children (such individuals were often diagnosed with what has since been termed 'Asperger's syndrome'), thereby hinting at a genetic cause.

called 'Wing's triad' after the researcher Lorna Wing who first proposed them), the key deficits being in socialisation, communication and imagination, and it is also clear that it is a complex neurodevelopmental disorder involving several possible mechanisms (genetic, hormonal and environmental).

Hammock and Young (2006) have recently speculated that oxytocin and vasopressin systems may contribute to the kinds of social deficits seen in autism. They described one study showing that levels of oxytocin in the blood plasma of autistic boys were lower than those found in a group of age-matched controls. Within the control group there were significant positive associations between oxytocin levels and measures of social behaviour; however, the opposite was found in the autistic sample, in that those with the more 'normal' levels of oxytocin displayed poorer social behaviours (Modahl *et al.*, 1998). A similar study has reported lower levels of vaso-pressin in the blood plasma of autistic children (Al-Ayadhi, 2005), but as yet there is no clear theory to explain such findings. More recently Hollander *et al.* (2007) administered oxytocin or a placebo to fifteen autistic adults and assessed their performance on comprehension of emotional speech. While all showed an initial improvement, those receiving the placebo reverted to baseline performance after a delay, while those receiving oxytocin better retained the ability to assign correct emotions to speech information. Some genetic studies are beginning to cast some light on this issue, with one study reporting a relationship between autism and the oxytocin receptor gene (Wu *et al.*, 2005) while another has found anomalies in the vasopressin V1a receptor gene (AVPR1a) in individuals with autism (Kim *et al.*, 2001). Clearly, links between these peptides and conditions like autism remain to be fully evaluated.

Other evidence has instead focussed on possible hormonal influences in the development of autistic disorders, or behaviours that could be described as 'autistic-like', e.g. antisocial behaviours. While we have seen that oxytocin/vasopressin may serve to enhance social behaviours in animals, testosterone has been strongly implicated in antisocial behaviours (in humans and animals) and may act to antagonise the effects of oxytocin/vasopressin. In support of this notion, males have higher levels of testosterone, and tend to display less prosocial behaviours then females (Baron-Cohen, 2002). In addition, in both males and females Harris *et al.* (1996) have shown that low levels of testosterone are associated with prosocial personality charac-teristics. Several studies have assessed relationships between levels of testos-terone in amniotic fluid and subsequent aspects of social behaviour. For example, Lutchmaya *et al.* (2002a) note that autism is characterised by a lack of eye contact, and this is noted in early infancy; eye contact is regarded to be of key importance in normal social development. They correlated amni-otic testosterone levels with rate of eye contact between the infants (aged one year) and their parents during play sessions. Female infants made significantly more eye contacts, and a quadratic relationship was found between eye contact and foetal testosterone in the whole sample, and in the sample of males. Thus, low and high levels of testosterone were associated with reduced eye contact, while medium levels were associated with more eye contact.

Similarly, Manning *et al.* (2001) suggested that autism may in part arise as a result of testosterone exposure during the prenatal period. In their study they compared 2D:4D in male and female children diagnosed with autism or Asperger's syndrome; those with autism displayed a significantly lower 2D:4D compared to control children, indicating that the autistic children had been exposed to higher levels of testosterone prenatally. Interestingly, the parents of the autistic children also showed the same lower pattern of 2D:4D. In a normal sample of children, Williams *et al.* (2003) reported that females with a lower (more masculine) 2D:4D displayed more hyperactivity, greater problems with social cognition, less prosocial ability and poorer peer relationships compared to girls with more feminine finger length ratios.

If higher levels of prenatal testosterone somehow predispose an individual to autism then one might expect that individuals exposed to very high levels (as in certain disorders – see chapter 6) might also show a greater predisposition to autism. In congenital adrenal hyperplasia (CAH) individuals of both sexes are exposed to high levels of adrenal androgens during the prenatal period. Knickmeyer *et al.* (2006) tested sixty CAH individuals and forty-nine of their unaffected relatives on the 'Autism Spectrum Quotient' (AQ), a fifty-item questionnaire measuring the extent to which a person displays traits associated with autism. In normal individuals this test reveals a clear sex difference, as males score higher than females. Their results provided some support to their theory, as female CAH patients demonstrated a significantly higher AQ score, and higher scores on the subscales measuring social skills and imagination. However, none of the CAH females displayed a score that would be indicative of a clinical diagnosis of autism, and the authors concluded that while prenatal androgens may contribute to autism-like traits, additional factors are clearly also involved.

## Bonding behaviours in 'normal' individuals

In individuals with no developmental disorders there is also increasing evidence that hormones play a role in behaviours associated with social bonding. A key aspect of normal prosocial behaviour is that of empathy – the identification with, and understanding of, another's feelings and motives (this is sometimes referred to as 'theory of mind'). A basic form of empathy is thought to be the ability to mimic another individual, especially facial expressions. In tasks where the individual observes the facial expressions of other individuals, those diagnosed with autism, or who display psychopathy, show a distinct lack of empathy via their lack of facial mimicry. Hermans *et al.* (2006) sought to establish the effects of testosterone administration on facial mimicry behaviours in normal young women. In a placebo-controlled, double-blind experiment, women viewed movie clips of faces changing from a neutral state to an emotion of anger or happiness after receiving a dose of testosterone or a placebo. Electromyograms[3] were taken from their facial muscles while they watched the movies to ascertain the extent of their facial mimicry. Results showed that testosterone administration led to a significant decrease in facial mimicry, and this arguably reflected a decline in empathetic behaviour.

Smiling is an innate, culturally universal human prosocial signal formed by flexing the muscles around the eyes and mouth, and is regarded as a gesture of pleasure, amusement, affiliation and appeasement. As there is a well-established sex difference in smiling, in that females smile more than males under both natural and experimental social conditions (LaFrance *et al.*, 2003), it has been suggested that testosterone to some extent determines the degree of smiling. This is assumed to be a consequence of the increased male preoccupation with their social status, and a selection pressure for males to exhibit and communicate more competitive, and fewer affiliative social gestures (Ellis, 2006).

Several studies have now demonstrated that testosterone is indeed related to smiling. For example, Dabbs *et al.* (1996) reported that male college students who had higher circulating levels of testosterone smiled less frequently than those with lower circulating levels. In females, Cashdan (1995) also found that women with higher levels of testosterone demonstrated less frequent smiling during group discussions. Finally, Dabbs (1997) took photographs of 119 males and 114 females in both smiling and non-smiling conditions, and measured their salivary testosterone. Within the male participants only, the smiles of high testosterone individuals were judged to be less friendly and more dominant than those of low testosterone individuals. The smiles of these males showed less crinkling around the eyes, and less upward and outward movement of the corners of the mouth.

Zak *et al.* (2005) argued that a key aspect of human social encounters is that of trustworthiness, and predicted that one might expect to see relationships between levels of oxytocin and trustworthy behaviours. In their study participants were placed into pairs and each received a monetary amount. One of the pair was then asked how much of that amount they would like to transfer to the other person (they were not allowed to communicate with the other person). Both were aware that whatever sum was transferred from one to another would be tripled; the second person could then nominate a sum to be transferred back to the first ('intention of trust' condition). In a different condition, the judgement of how much could be transferred was made at random. Immediately following their decisions, blood samples were taken and levels of peripheral oxytocin assessed. Oxytocin levels were significantly higher in the 'intention' condition in the second individual (who

---

[3] EMGs provide a graphic record of the electrical activity of the muscles.

was responding to the trustworthy gesture of the first person); there were no relations between oxytocin and the gesture made by the first individual. Thus, oxytocin appears to be related to the response to trust, rather than the act of trust itself. This of course does not tell us whether higher levels of oxytocin in the second individual led to this trustworthy response, or whether the trustworthy response led to higher levels of oxytocin. However, the authors argued that, as the individuals did not meet, it is more likely that higher oxytocin levels are influencing trust rather than the other way round.

Kosfeld *et al.* (2005) took this research one stage further by assessing the effects of intranasal administration of oxytocin on trusting behaviour, using the same game. They hypothesised that, compared to placebo, those receiving oxytocin would show higher money transfers to the second member of the pair (again the two did not meet), i.e. they would show more trusting behaviours. Indeed, oxytocin administration led to a significant increase in trust by the investors, with 45% of the sample making the maximum transfer compared to only 21% in the placebo group; this was not due to a general tendency in the oxytocin group to take more risks. Note that this result contradicts that of Zak *et al.* (2005), who found that oxytocin was associated with the response by the 'receiver'. In the Kosfeld *et al.* (2005) study it is associated with the initial transfer by the investor, and no relationship was found for the response by the receiver. However, as the experimental paradigms were clearly different this may not be surprising. Both studies raise the intriguing possibility that human trust is associated with certain hormone levels, and can perhaps be manipulated by hormonal intervention.

## Heterosexual pair bonding

Love is usually defined along the lines of a subjective, strong, intense and passionate affection for a single person, and is undoubtedly a complex emotion as it usually contains cognitive, erotic, emotional and behavioural components (Hazan and Shaver, 1987). Until fairly recently the emotion of love has been the sole preserve of artists, poets and philosophers; however, evolutionary biologists have argued that behaviours are simply adaptations to the physical and social environment, and reproductive behaviours (including emotional states such as love) can be explained along similar lines. It has been suggested that brain mechanisms underlying courtship attraction in animals are essentially the same as those seen in humans experiencing the emotion of love (Fisher *et al.*, 2006). In animals, courtship attraction is usually brief (lasting from minutes to weeks), but in humans Marazziti *et al.* (1999) proposed that the intense early stage of romantic love lasts around twelve to eighteen months. However, the behavioural traits associated with human romantic love (an increase in energy, euphoria, focussed attention on the other individual, obsessive behaviours associated with the other individual, affiliative behaviours, craving to be with the person, and possessive behaviours) are all observed in mammalian courtship attraction (Fisher *et al.*, 2006).

Several studies have now assessed neurological correlates of romantic love. For example, Bartels and Zeki (2000) recruited seventeen females who described themselves as 'truly, deeply, and madly in love' and conducted brain scans while they viewed a photograph either of their romantic partner or of a friend of the same sex as their partner and whom they had known for a similar amount of time. When viewing their loved one, brain activity showed two distinct areas of activation: the middle insula in the left hemisphere and the cingulate cortex – regions long associated with emotional processing and with euphoric states. More recently, Fisher *et al.* (2005) conducted the same kind of study on seven males and ten females and reported that brain activation was localised to the ventral tegmental area (VTA). This region is rich in dopaminergic neurons, and forms a key part of the brain's reward system that plays a role in arousal, pleasure, focussed attention and the motivation to seek rewards (Martin-Soelch *et al.*, 2001). Notably, the brain regions that show activation to one's loved ones do not overlap with those regions subserving sexual arousal, indicating that these two experiences are fundamentally distinct (Diamond, 2004).

These studies of course did not consider possible hormonal correlates of this behavioural state. However, Marazziti and Canale (2004) collected blood samples from twelve males and twelve females who had recently fallen in love, and from the same number of matched controls. The group that had fallen in love showed significantly higher levels of cortisol than the control group, perhaps reflecting the greater arousal and higher stress levels typically reported in new lovers. In addition, males who were in love had significantly lower testosterone levels and FSH levels, but the opposite was true for females in love, as they displayed significantly higher testosterone levels. Interestingly, hormonal measures were repeated twelve to eighteen months later in sixteen of the participants who no longer reported being 'obsessed' by their partner. Their hormone profile now showed no differences from the control group. This suggests that the early stage of love can be related to state-dependent and reversible hormonal fluctuations, possibly associated with some physical or psychological characteristics associated with this emotional state.

It has been suggested that variation in testosterone levels may be a reflection of, and an influence on, the amount of behaviour devoted to mating versus parenting efforts, with testosterone increasing when males are seeking new mating partners, and then decreasing when relationships are established (Gray, 2003). In the early stages of a romantic relationship the kinds of social behaviours needed first to attract, and then to retain a mate may be facilitated by testosterone. I will discuss the possible role of testosterone in human aggressive/dominance/competitive behaviours in the next chapter, but at this point it is sufficient to state that key components of mating effort (notably male to male competition, and mate seeking) are facilitated by testosterone, with testosterone seemingly of key importance in human social dominance encounters (Mazur and Booth, 1998). High levels of testosterone might not, however, be conducive to a stable long-term relationship possibly involving parental duties (see later section in this chapter). For example Booth and Dabbs (1993) assessed marital relationships in over 4000 male military veterans and found that those with lower levels of testosterone were more likely to marry; those with higher levels who did marry were much more likely to get divorced.

We might thus predict that males in a committed long-term relationship may display lower testosterone levels than single males. In support, Burnham *et al.* (2003) compared testosterone levels in 122 males in a variety of relationships; males who were 'paired' had testosterone levels 21% lower than males not currently in a relationship. Marital status did not appear to be important here, as unmarried males in long-term relationships had similar levels to males who were married. Similarly, Gray *et al.* (2004) measured testosterone (at two time points during the day) in 107 male undergraduates, all of whom were unmarried, but some of whom were in committed long-term relationships. As in the previously described study, males in committed relationships had lower testosterone levels than single males (this was only found between samples taken later in the day). An additional factor concerned whether or not a male had previous experiences of being in a committed relationship – males who were single but had such experience demonstrated significantly higher testosterone levels than single males lacking such experience. The authors suggested that variation in testosterone levels may be associated with mating effort, higher levels being associated with enhanced mating success.

If this is the case then we might expect that individuals in so-called 'polyamorous' relationships (they are involved in multiple sexual relationships) should be expected to show even higher levels than individuals who are single, and certainly more than those in stable monogamous relationships. Van Anders *et al.* (2007a) were able to track down such individuals (twelve males and seventeen females) and compared their testosterone levels with a group of singletons (eleven males, thirteen females) and a group with one partner (eleven males, six females). As expected, partnered males had significantly lower levels than single males, and the polyamorous males had the highest levels (though they did not quite differ significantly from the single males). The polyamorous females, however, did display significantly higher levels than single women and partnered women.

The issue of causation remains a problem here. Is it the case that males with lower testosterone levels are better able to retain a mate and settle into long-term relationships, or does the act of being in a long-term relationship serve to reduce his testosterone levels? The answer, of course, would be to conduct longitudinal studies, taking a group of single men and assessing their testosterone levels on a regular basis and then tracking these same males as they enter into relationships. Owing to the time constraints and financial costs, such studies are rare. In one such study, Mazur and Michalek (1998) followed a group of male Air Force veterans and found that those who were married had lower levels than those who were single. During a divorce testosterone levels were high, but if the male remarried then his testosterone levels showed a corresponding decline. This then indicates that the relationship status determines testosterone level.

In another longitudinal study, van Anders and Watson (2006b) also tracked testosterone levels over time (over a much shorter period though) and monitored relationship status in both heterosexual and homosexual individuals. Participants initially completed a questionnaire concerning their relationship status and provided a saliva sample. The first hundred were then contacted once per month in order to monitor their relationship status, and additional testing sessions were arranged around six months after the baseline session. The authors found that single heterosexual males had significantly higher testosterone levels than partnered heterosexual males; interestingly the homosexual males showed no such differences. In females, while heterosexual women showed no differences with respect to partner status, single homosexual women had significantly higher levels than partnered homosexual women.

Thus, individuals with a preference for female partners appear to show differences in testosterone with respect to partner status. In terms of the longitudinal aspect, those individuals who maintained their relationship status (partnered or unpartnered) showed no differences in testosterone levels (these remained high); however, individuals who were single at baseline, but who were then in a relationship at the second assessment, showed a significant decline in their testosterone levels. Importantly, single individuals with lower testosterone were more likely to enter into a relationship than were single males with higher testosterone. These results thus indicate an influence of testosterone on partnering, rather than an influence of partnering on testosterone (as shown by Mazur and Michalek, 1998).

A possible confound has recently been suggested by van Anders and Watson (2007a), who noted that previous studies have not differentiated between individuals in long-term relationships who live near to their partner (i.e. in the same city) or those who conducted long-distance relationships (the partner lived in a different city). They argued that if being in a relationship per se is crucial, then testosterone levels should not differ between individuals whose partners live nearby or far away: both groups should display lower levels than single people. Conversely, if relationship status is important, then testosterone might be higher in individuals whose partners live far away (and be more comparable to single people), compared to those whose partners live nearby. To assess this, they recruited males and females who were either single, had partners living in the same city or had partners living in a different city. Women in same-city relationships demonstrated significantly lower testosterone levels than single women, but the same-city group did not differ from women whose partners lived in a different city. In males, single men had significantly higher testosterone levels than long-distance partnered males, and showed a trend for higher levels compared to males in same-city relationships. The same-city and different-city males showed no differences in testosterone levels. Thus, the female data better fitted what they called the 'relationship status' hypothesis, while the male data best fitted the 'relationship orientation' hypothesis. As their sample sizes were not that large such sex differences remain speculative. Clearly much more research of a longitudinal nature taking into account such possible confounds is required.

For the moment then we can only guess at the causal relationship between testosterone and mating versus parenting efforts. Dabbs (2000) described testosterone as a mixed blessing as regards relationships: on one hand higher levels are useful for attracting a mate and fending off potential male rivals, but if those same high levels are maintained during a relationship, then the relationship may well suffer. It is perhaps most likely that there is a reciprocal relationship, with testosterone affecting mating behaviour, and the outcomes of those behaviours then affecting testosterone (this certainly seems to be the case for dominance encounters – see next chapter).

There are also likely to be individual differences, perhaps reflecting different social experiences or different genetic/physiological factors. Recently, McIntyre et al. (2006) have considered the possible role of extrapair sexual interest as a moderator of the effects of relationship status on male testosterone. They predicted that males in committed relationships who were interested in pursuing short-term sexual relationships with women other than their partner might not show a drop in testosterone levels in comparison to males in a relationship who show no such interests. In two studies involving undergraduate males, they took salivary samples, measured the willingness of a person to engage in casual sex outside of a relationship, and also asked whether such behaviours had taken place. In the first study, in males in a relationship, higher testosterone levels were associated with higher scores on the sociosexuality index (a measure of the willingness to engage in sex outside of a relationship). In the second study, they confirmed that single males had higher testosterone levels then males in a relationship. In addition, in males in a relationship, interest in extrapair sexual encounters significantly predicted testosterone levels – the higher the interest, the higher their testosterone. Thus, males in committed relationships who remained interested in new sexual encounters maintained high testosterone levels. This was irrespective of relationship length or stated depth of commitment.

## Offspring–parent attachments

A second bond is that between offspring and parent. Infants in a wide variety of species display very strong attachment bonds with their primary caregivers ('filial attachment'). Developmental psychologist John Bowlby speculated that such behavioural responses were an evolved mechanism designed to keep infants in close proximity to their caregivers in order to max-imise their survival, and such responses are clearly seen in human children (Bowlby, 1982). This bond is very strong, and a key feature of it is the obvious signs of agitation and distress manifested when the individual is removed from the carer to whom he/she is strongly attached. The separation of the infant from the caregiver leads to extreme feelings of distress, and is referred to as 'separation anxiety'. It has been speculated that this initial attachment mechanism was then co-opted for the purpose of keeping mating partners together in order to enhance the survival chances of their offspring (Hazan and Zeifman, 1999).

If an infant becomes separated from the primary carer, then this separa-tion is associated with a variety of physiological and behavioural changes. A key behavioural response is a dramatic increase in vocalisation, and the nature and duration of these vocalisations are often used as a marker for the degree of distress felt by the infant, and thus used as an indirect measure of attachment (Panskepp *et al.* 1997). The principal physiological change is associated with an increase in the secretion of glucocorticoids, especially cor-ticosterone and cortisol, and so levels of both hormones are also used as an indicator of separation anxiety.

Animal models of the effects of separation anxiety on behavioural and neuroendocrine responses suggest that even very limited periods of separa-tion in infancy can lead to significant impairments in both domains. For example, McCormick *et al.* (1998) showed that while a single episode of sep-aration caused no obvious ill effects, one hour of separation per day from postnatal day 2 through to postnatal day 8 led to a significant increase in cor-ticosterone in infant rats. Interestingly, Knuth and Etgen (2007) confirmed this stress response in as few as six consecutive one-hour isolation sessions, and then demonstrated that, when tested as adults, these animals displayed increased anxiety responses to standard testing situations (elevated maze and open-field tests), though their stress responses appeared to be normal.

The effects of maternal separation are bidirectional in that mothers sepa-rated from their infants also display similar behavioural and neuroendocrine abnormalities (Macri and Wörbel, 2007). Similarly, Boccia *et al.* (2007) com-pared the effects of long (three hours) versus short (fifteen minutes) maternal separation for twelve consecutive days in rat mothers. When their offspring were weaned, the mothers had to undergo a forced swim test for fifteen minutes on one day and for five minutes the next day (a standard test of behavioural and physiological stress). Mothers who had been separated from their pups for the longer duration showed a clear increase in anxiety behaviours (the authors argued that the behaviours were so marked that they described them as reflecting 'depression'). These mothers also showed a significant reduction in pup-licking – a behaviour known to influence the stress response in offspring.

As oxytocin and vasopressin have been so closely related to the formation of social bonds in adults, it is not surprising that investigators have assessed their possible role in filial attachment behaviours. For example, Insel and Winslow (1991) showed that distress vocalisations in infant rat pups could be dramatically reduced following central treatments of oxytocin. Winslow and Insel (1993) then demonstrated that the same reduction was seen following central vasopressin administration. Variations in maternal care have also been associated with neurological changes to oxytocin receptor density in the amygdala, mPOA, and paraventricular nuclei of the hypothalamus (Francis *et al.* 2002).

In humans, assessing links between early life experiences and alterations in the neuroendocrine system is not straightforward because it is impossible to conduct controlled studies. Researchers have to rely on retrospective assessments of early life experiences, or conduct costly and time-consuming longitudinal studies. In addition, there is of course a wide range of additional social/developmental/environmental factors that have to be taken into consideration. Nevertheless, adverse childhood experiences such as early parental separation or bereavement have been shown to influence the stress response (Luecken and Lemery, 2004). In addition, such experiences have been assumed to form major risk factors in adult mental health problems such as depression, anxiety and personality disorders (e.g. Agid *et al.* 2000); such problems can be ameliorated by the experience of positive social relationships (House *et al.* 1988).

As it has been reported that levels of urinary oxytocin are decreased in children who have experienced maltreatment and abuse (Fries *et al.* 2005), Meinlschmidt and Heim (2007) assessed the possible role of oxytocin in adults with varying childhood experiences. Their novel method was to use an intranasal spray to administer oxytocin (or a placebo) to nineteen males, nine reporting childhood experiences of being separated from their primary carer, and ten reporting no such adverse experiences. Following oxytocin administration, those males who had experienced maternal separation showed a marked decrease in cortisol; males lacking such negative experiences showed no such effect. The authors suggested that this reflects an alteration in central sensitivity to oxytocin (perhaps by alterations in receptor density or function), presumably in those same brain regions identified in animals, and arguably caused by their early childhood experiences. Such intriguing speculations remain, as yet, unproven.

## Parent–offspring attachments

The third type of bond is between parents and offspring ('parental attachment') and a common assumption is that parents form bonds with their offspring that are similar in intensity to the bonds that offspring form with them. However, Mason and Mendoza (1998) caution that this is not necessarily the case. They point out the great diversity in patterns of parental behaviour among different species and note that the formation of an attachment bond between parent and offspring does not automatically imply a strong emotional attachment, and conversely that poor parenting does not imply that an attachment bond has not formed. For example, titi monkeys make perfectly adequate parents, but neither parents shows any sign of forming close emotional bonds with their offspring. They display no obvious behavioural signs of distress when the offspring is removed, and show no preference for their infant over strange infants. In contrast, macaques form strong attachments to their offspring within a few weeks. They then carefully monitor the offspring, retrieve them at the first sign of danger, and show great distress when their offspring are removed from them.

## Maternal behaviours

Over the years a wide range of maternal behaviours has been described across species. While many of the hormonal and neural mechanisms that underpin the formation and maintenance of such behaviours show considerable similarities, there are many between-species differences. Some examples are as follows.

### Birds

Birds show great diversity in their patterns of parental care. Some are brood-parasitic (they lay their eggs in other birds nests, and provide no parental care, a good example being the European cuckoo); in a few species (e.g. the jacana) it is the male that provides the bulk of parental care. In around 90% of bird species, however, the sexes form monogamous relationships and both contribute substantially to their offspring (nest building, incubating the eggs, collecting food, protecting the chicks, etc.). Early advances in our understanding of the role of hormones in maternal and paternal behaviours came from studies of the ring (or ringneck) dove (*Streptopelia risoria*). This species has long been domesticated, and demonstrates a highly consistent pattern of courtship, mating and parental behaviours, which make it an excellent research tool. Both sexes share in the nest building, incubation and feeding of the offspring (called a squab) as both sexes possess a specialised exocrine gland called the 'crop sac' which is the source of protein- and fat-rich 'milk' (technically it is more like curd than milk).

In her review, Silver (1978) summarised research addressing the role of hormones in parental behaviours in this species. In terms of incubation, she described that ovariectomised female doves treated with estrogen followed by progesterone (as occurs naturally when they are fertilised) displayed nest-building and egg incubation; those injected with only estrogen or progesterone (or a control substance) did not display these behaviours. During incubation, prolactin is secreted by the anterior pituitary gland, and this triggers growth of the epithelial cells in the crop sac in such a predictable manner that crop growth has long been used as a reliable bioassay for prolactin (crop weight varies from around 0.5 g at the start of courtship, to around 4.5 g after hatching). A simple linear relationship between prolactin secretion and crop sac development was thus predicted, but Cheng and Burke (1983) demonstrated that this was not quite the case. During the early phase of incubation, crop weight showed a delayed response to prolactin secretion and the two events were not correlated. During midincubation, however, a strong positive correlation between prolactin secretion and crop weight was observed; when the eggs hatched and prolactin reached a peak, there was no correlation with crop weight.

A characteristic feature of maternal behaviour is some bird species is 'broodiness', a collection of vocalisations, nesting, incubation and protective behaviours. For example, a hen lays only one egg every day or two and she will not begin to incubate them until the whole clutch is laid. She will then sit on the clutch with her wings slightly spread for around three weeks, and will 'growl' and peck if disturbed; she will only leave the nest once a day to eat, drink and defecate. Riddle et al. (1935) reported that increased levels of prolactin were associated with increased broodiness. However, as prolactin levels also rise in brood-parasitic species during egg-laying, but they do not display broodiness, it is probably not levels of prolactin per se, but rather an increase in neural sensitivity to it. We now realise that the neuroendocrine control of broodiness is extremely complex. Sharp et al. (1984) reviewed this topic in hens, and confirmed that the neurotransmitters serotonin and dopamine were of key importance. They suggested that the preovulatory surge of LH is mediated by a temporary decrease in the inhibitory action of serotonin and dopamine on the secretion of LH-RH. Serotonin is also directly involved in the release of prolactin, as drugs that act as serotonergic agonists also stimulate the release of prolactin. As there do not appear to be any receptors for serotonin in the anterior pituitary, an additional releasing-factor is probably involved. The authors suggest that vasoactive intestinal polypeptide (VIP) is the likely candidate – it acts to stimulate prolactin release, especially after estrogen-priming (as would be seen at ovulation).

## Mammals

Broad et al. (2006) point out that key evolutionary developments in mammals were placentation, and enhanced post-birth care. As the female bears the biological burden of carrying the infant to term, and then providing vital sustenance in the form of milk, it is not surprising that the bond between mother and infant is assumed to be stronger than that between father and infant (it is also the case that as males can never be certain that the offspring they are helping to raise are biologically 'theirs', they should be less likely to show strong offspring bonds). How such maternal bonds become established and how they are then maintained have thus formed key research questions.

Interestingly, it is now clear that the developing infant is no passive backseat passenger during the development and maintenance of this set of complex biological/social behaviours. Heap (1994) revealed that the placenta contains trophoblast cells which are formed during the first stage of pregnancy from the embryo and mediate the implantation of the foetus into the placenta. Once established, they produce and secrete steroids, peptides and growth factors, that not only determine the growth of the foetus, but that also enter the mother's bloodstream and influence her metabolism, physiology and behaviour. The presence of the foetus then provides a neuroendocrine trigger to activate such behaviours, probably to ensure that its birth will coincide with optimum maternal milk availability and care.

## Precocial mammals

In grazing animals such as cattle, sheep, goats, horses, etc., offspring need to be well advanced at birth in order to keep in close contact with the herd and avoid predation. The young of these species are referred to as 'precocial' and are relatively independent from birth, being able to maintain their own body temperature and stand/move around. To ensure the rapid maturation of their offspring, mothers produce a large quantity of high-quality milk which is reserved solely for their offspring (non-related individuals trying to access this resource are quickly rejected). In sheep, separation of the lamb from the mother triggers a set of characteristic 'anxiety' behaviours in both individuals (distress calls and hyperactivity); as this species is easy to keep and maintain, and clearly displays strong social bonds between mother and offspring, it has formed a useful research tool in order to assess the role of hormones in maternal bonding behaviours. A key aspect in the initiation of this bonding mechanism is the initial process of birth and the subsequent suckling of the offspring, both processes releasing oxytocin and endogenous opioids.

For example, Keverne et al. (1983) injected non-pregnant ewes with estrogen and progesterone to mimic the final stages of pregnancy, and tested their maternal responses when presented with newborn lambs. Half of the group received vaginal stimulation for five minutes prior to presentation of the lambs to mimic the birth process, while half did not. Oxytocin levels in the stimulated ewes showed a big rise, and 80% of them showed maternal responses, but only 20% of the non-stimulated ewes showed a maternal response. Similarly, Krehbiel et al. (1987) compared maternal behaviours in first-time and experienced mothers who received an anaesthetic (the animal feels no vaginal stimulation), either at the first signs of birth or just before expulsion. The introduction of a late anaesthetic had little effect on maternal behaviour (compared to controls) but severe deficits in maternal behaviours were noted in ewes receiving an early anaesthetic; this was especially noticeable in first-time mothers. Lévy et al. (1992) then went on to demonstrate that the administration of an anaesthetic during birth prevents the release of central oxytocin and thus inhibits maternal behaviours. Infusion of oxytocin into anaesthetised ewes during birth then triggers the onset of maternal behaviours. Clearly, then, in this species oxytocin is vital for the onset (though not necessarily for the maintenance) of maternal behaviours.

*Rodents*

Rodents produce young described as 'altricial', i.e. the infants are completely helpless in that they are blind and deaf, have little motor control, and cannot regulate their body temperature. They thus depend upon their mother not only for suckling, but also to keep them warm and retrieve them should they fall out of the nest. It has been assumed that (like sheep), the hormonal changes associated with pregnancy and the birth process should be associated with the onset of maternal behaviours, and a key role was assumed for oxytocin. Indeed, central administration of oxytocin triggers the onset of maternal behaviours in virgin female rats within a short period of time, and treatment with oxytocin antagonists inhibits the onset of maternal behaviours. Such effects are likely to be associated with interactions with the gonadal steroids and/or the dopaminergic system (Pedersen, 1997; Fahrbach *et al.* 1985).

Female adult rats do not, however, make naturally good mothers as they display considerable aversion towards pups that are not their own. Fleming (1986) has hypothesised that one way in which hormones could induce maternal behaviour in this species would be to reduce the mother's normal aversive responses towards pups. This theory is supported by findings that the onset of maternal behaviours in female rats can be facilitated by tranquilliser treatment (Hansen *et al.* 1985), that mice lacking oxytocin receptors display higher levels of anxiety (Mantella *et al.* 2003) and that centrally administered oxytocin antagonists increase anxiety in female rats (Neumann *et al.* 2000). This anxiety-reducing effect of oxytocin may therefore indirectly facilitate maternal behaviours (Uvnäs-Moberg, 1998). Hormones may thus prepare first-time mothers to accept their offspring just before the end of pregnancy. In experienced mothers such hormonal actions may not be necessary, as those that have given birth show no such avoidance behaviours. It thus seems that certain hormones during pregnancy and the birth process may act to prime mothers for postpartum maternal behaviours, but are perhaps less important for their maintenance (Stern, 1989).

Lactation and suckling may play an important two-way function in the bonding process. Lactation (the ability to produce milk) is dependent upon the release of oxytocin, and also involves an increase in the production of vasopressin, prolactin and endogenous opiates, and a concurrent reduction in the HPA stress axis (Carter and Altemus, 1997). The milk itself also contains oxytocin and prolactin, which may then influence the offsprings' attachment behaviours, perhaps by interacting with their ability to cope with stress (studies cited in Carter, 1998). In turn, suckling by the infant releases endogenous opiates in the mother, partly perhaps to alleviate the discomfort caused but also perhaps to strengthen the reward process. In addition, oxytocin is released, which may have a similar affect (Kinsley and Lambert, 2006).

Pregnancy and motherhood are associated with neurological alterations, especially in the mPOA of the hypothalamus, a region rich in steroid receptors and which has been associated with various sociosexual behaviours. For example, Keyser-Markus *et al.* (2001) reported that cell bodies within the mPOA of late-pregnant and estradiol/progesterone-treated rats were significantly larger than cell bodies in ovariectomised and diestrous (the short period of sexual quiescence between two estrus periods) individuals. These cells displayed an increase in somal area (this indicates an increase in cellular activity) and dendritic branching indicative of an enhancement of information-processing capability. These presumably contribute to alterations in maternal behaviours.

### Non-human primates

Understanding possible relationships between hormone states and caregiving in non-human primate mothers is considerably more complicated than that in rodents, because caregiving behaviours displayed by primate mothers are not confined to pregnancy and lactation. Indeed, maternal responsiveness has been assumed to reflect experiential, cognitive and social factors. (e.g. Benedek, 1970). This perception possibly came about because early studies using single isolated female primates failed to demonstrate associations between hormone levels and female responsiveness to infants (e.g. Holman and Goy, 1980). An additional complicating factor is that the extent of hormone involvement in primates appears to be considerably wider than that seen in rodents, and so ascertaining clear hormone–behaviour relationships has been difficult. However, there are now several useful primate models all of which typically rely upon the assessment of group-living animals.

Marmosets, for example, show a characteristic hormone profile during pregnancy (levels of estradiol and progesterone rise sharply just before birth; estradiol levels then drop around twenty days prior to the birth), which makes them good research subjects. Using an operant paradigm, Pryce *et al.* (1993) correlated levels of these hormones with the number of bar presses made by four pregnant common marmosets to gain access to infant sensory reinforcement. As the ratio between estradiol and progesterone reached its maximum, levels of bar-pressing showed a corresponding peak. The authors then demonstrated that administration of the same hormones to three non-pregnant females produced a pattern of bar pressing similar to that seen in the pregnant females.

Similar results were obtained by Maestripieri and Zehr (1998). In their first study, hormones were monitored throughout pregnancy in eight female pigtail macaques, and levels correlated with maternal behaviours directed towards young infants of other mothers. The mean rate of infant-directed interactions increased in the last eight weeks of pregnancy, and were significantly predicted by higher levels of estradiol, and also by the estradiol:progesterone ratio (high estradiol to low progesterone). In their second study, five ovariectomised rhesus macaques were treated with estradiol, and their behaviours compared to non-pregnant females and untreated ovariectomised females. Estradiol-treated females showed a significant increase in their infant-directed behaviours: such behaviours increased in the first week of treatment and showed a clear decrease shortly after termination of the treatment. Infant-directed behaviours in the non-pregnant and untreated females remained low but were still present, indicating that pregnancy hormones are not fully necessary for such behaviours to be shown.

In red-bellied tamarins, Pryce *et al.* (1988) assessed relationships between urinary estradiol levels during pregnancy and postpartum infant-directed behaviours. The pregnant mothers were split into two groups, one group having previously demonstrated good mothering skills, and one group having displayed poor mothering skills (determined by infant survival rates). Around four to five weeks before birth, estradiol levels remained constant in the good mothers, but showed a significant decline in the poor mothers. At one week before birth, the good mothers had significantly higher estradiol levels. During a two-hour period after the birth the good mothers spent more time cleaning and carrying their infants than the poor mothers, and the infants of poor mothers were more likely to die through neglect.

Baboons also provide a good model because the characteristics of the baboon menstrual cycle are very similar to those seen in human females and the pattern of estrogen and progesterone secretion are almost identical. Bardi *et al.* (2004) measured gonadal and adrenal steroids in eighty-nine group-living female baboons during pregnancy and early infant care. They found that cortisol was associated with the quality and quantity of infant-directed behaviours. For example, mothers who had higher levels of cortisol after birth showed less infant-directed behaviour, but mothers who had higher cortisol before birth showed more infant-directed behaviours. The authors suggested that higher cortisol levels before birth (high levels are typically seen in primate mothers, partly created by indirect stimulation from estrogen) may reflect modifications to the adrenocortical system to ensure increased maternal attentiveness to the newborns. Normally, levels of cortisol drop after the birth, but if high levels are maintained then this may trigger anxiety and fear reactions to the infant. Such effects may be particularly evident in inexperienced mothers.

However, other studies have shed doubt on these apparently clear links between steroids and maternal behaviours in non-human primates. For example, Bahr *et al.* (2001) were unable to find relationships between levels of estradiol, progesterone and the estradiol:progesterone ratio (assessed from their metabolites in urine) during pregnancy, and subsequent maternal behaviours in gorillas. Similarly Maestripieri and Megna (2000) measured ovarian hormone levels during early lactation and found no link between these levels and individual differences in mothering styles in rhesus macaques. Fite and French (2000) actually found that marmoset mothers with higher levels of prepartum estradiol were more likely to have offspring who died early in infancy (apparently partly through neglect).

Fite *et al.* (2005) considered the potential role of testosterone in one aspect of maternal behaviour – the decision whether to maintain one's investment in current offspring, or devote one's attention to future offspring. As we have already seen, circulating testosterone in males may mediate the trade-off between investing in current or future offspring, higher levels of testosterone seemingly acting to inhibit parental effort, but increase mating effort. In other (non-primate) species, testosterone has also been related to suppressed responsiveness to offspring (e.g. Juárez *et al.* 1998), and a decrease in testosterone associated with the onset of maternal care (examples cited in Fite *et al.*, 2005). In the Fite *et al.* (2005) study, urinary testosterone excretion was measured in female marmosets and their maternal caregiving behaviours recorded. Those females that had conceived while they were still carrying their current offspring showed higher levels of testosterone and displayed a dramatic reduction in caregiving behaviours. In females that conceived when they were not still heavily involved in caring for their current offspring, testosterone levels remained low, and they showed no changes in their caregiving. Such females are thus able to make trade-offs between current and future offspring, especially when current demands are high. This may be mediated by testosterone.

As with birds, the hormone prolactin has been implicated in infant caregiving by male and female parents and allo-parents. Soltis *et al.* (2005) measured prolactin in groups of squirrel monkeys. Adults (including non-mothers) living in a group that included infants displayed significantly higher urinary levels of prolactin compared to adults living in groups lacking direct contact with infants (they were able to see, hear and perhaps smell them but not touch them). In addition, there was a positive relationship between prolactin levels and the proportion of time spent caring for infants. So, physical contact appears to be necessary for the alterations in prolactin levels – in this instance the environment is having an influence on hormone levels.

In primates such as rhesus monkeys, the activity of the endogenous opioids appears to be very important for caregiving behaviours, with this system being activated during pregnancy and suckling, simultaneously to promote positive affect and to decrease anxiety. Studies have shown that, in comparison to placebo-treated mothers, treatment with opiate receptor antagonists such as naloxone leads to a significant reduction in attachment and caregiving behaviours. These mothers neglected their offspring, failed to groom them, and did not attempt to retrieve them when they wandered away (Martel *et al.* 1993; 1995).

Finally, the role of oxytocin in establishing maternal behaviours in primates was demonstrated by Holman and Goy (1995). In their study, two female rhesus monkeys who had never been pregnant were injected with oxytocin or saline, and their behaviours towards infants monitored. Oxytocin administration led to an increase in infant-directed activities such as touching, observing and lip-smacking, and a decrease in agonistic behaviours directed towards the infants.

*Humans*

A starting point for considering hormone–maternal relationships concerns so called 'maternal personality', i.e. the stated interest in children, and the attitudes and motivations concerning pregnancy and child-rearing. Thus far this aspect has been rather underresearched, which seems somewhat surprising as human breeding behaviours must be much more sensitive to individual/personal factors than equivalent behaviours in animals.

One line of evidence has come from those females who have experienced atypical hormone exposure during development. Thus, females experiencing some degree of physical (and presumably psychological) masculinisation as a result of CAH (see chapter 6) have been asked about their interest in infants and their nurturing tendencies. Several studies have indeed reported that adult CAH females show less interest in motherhood than control females (Dittman *et al.* 1990) and CAH girls showed less interest in infants (as rated by their parents) than their sisters (Leveroni and Berenbaum, 1998). Helleday *et al.* (1993) noted that twenty-two adult CAH females scored significantly lower on a 'detachment' subscale of a personality test (this is argued to reflect distance in social relations, and thus perhaps forms an indirect measure of affiliation motivation and maternal intimacy). Finally, when such females are observed interacting with dolls, they display fewer parenting 'rehearsal-type' behaviours (Ehrhardt and Meyer-Bahlburg, 1981). Despite the methodological issues raised by such patient studies (see chapter 6), and the fact that the studies described above can be criticised on the means by which 'maternal' attitudes and behaviours were assessed, it seems that early hormonal exposure may impact upon subsequent maternal motivations.

A second line of evidence has come from a single study correlating maternal personality and desire for offspring with circulating levels of testosterone. In this, twenty-seven adult females completed the Bem Sex-Role Inventory and a series of questions assessing maternal personality and reproductive ambition. Salivary testosterone was significantly negatively correlated with the BSRI item 'loves children' and self-rated 'broodiness'. To my knowledge this issue has not yet been addressed using markers of prenatal hormone exposure (such as 2D:4D).

As regards the expression of parental behaviours during pregnancy or following the birth, the picture is complicated by several issues. First, hormones appear to be neither necessary nor sufficient for the appearance of parental behaviours. Thus we find that adoptive parents, siblings, relatives and unrelated caregivers grow attached to infants in similar qualitative and temporal ways as the biological mother. Secondly, unlike rats, human mothers do not show stereotypical maternal behaviours and there appears to be no single set of behaviours that characterise human maternal behaviours. In different cultures, maternal responsiveness can be measured in a variety of ways and caregiving behaviours directed towards the infant also shows great variability.

Finally, a key ethical and methodological issue concerns the taking of hormone samples (normally from blood or via amniocentesis) in pregnant women. Such invasive techniques for purely research purposes are rarely welcomed by pregnant women, and thus studies tend to be conducted on fairly small samples. However, there are some similarities in that human mothers show characteristic responses to their infants shortly after birth, and it is assumed that mothers show strong motivation to interact with their infants. It is also the case that salivary sampling has removed some of the problems associated with invasive testing, though this technique does not always permit the analysis of certain key hormones.

In their review of human maternal responsiveness, Fleming and Corter (1988) suggested that, for the first-time mother, the endocrinological events during pregnancy and the birth serve to 'sensitise' her to the physical and emotional challenges of motherhood; once she has begun caring for her infant, though, endocrine parameters will cease to be important as experiential, emotional and social factors will assume greater prominence. As there are large fluctuations in various hormones throughout pregnancy and just after the birth, it was expected that such alterations would be mirrored in emotional and behavioural responses towards infants. While mothers do indeed display heightened responsiveness to offspring during the latter stages of pregnancy, it has proved difficult to link such changes with fluctuations in endocrine status.

Fleming et al. (1987) had reported a significant linear relationship between levels of cortisol and the intensity of the mother's contact behaviours with her infant on the third day after birth. This relationship was strongest in those mothers who had previously expressed positive attitudes towards their pregnancy and to their infants. The authors speculated that a cortisol rise occurs just after birth in order to produce a certain level of arousal in the mother, so that she attains an appropriate degree of maternal responsiveness. If the mother is 'positive' then her responses to the infant will also be positive. However, it might be predicted that in mothers approaching the birth with negative attitudes, then high levels of post-birth cortisol might trigger more avoidance behaviours towards the infants. This of course cannot be tested experimentally (it would be unethical to create negative attitudes in pregnant mothers) and so we have to rely upon correlational data to test this prediction. The wide range of additional confounding factors (e.g. social and environmental circumstances of the mother and the characteristics of the infant) render such predictions almost impossible to evaluate clearly.

Corter and Fleming (1995) reported no significant relationships between changes in maternal feelings during pregnancy and fluctuations in levels of estradiol, progesterone or cortisol. In a later study of 667 women in varying stages of pregnancy, Fleming et al. (1997) showed that while hormonal fluctuations during pregnancy did not relate to attachment feelings during this period, the pattern of change in the ratio of estradiol to progesterone throughout pregnancy was related to feelings of attachment towards the infant following the birth. A problem with such studies, though, is that they typically use self-report questionnaires, and then correlate the answers with hormone levels; such methods may not be sensitive enough to reveal significant relationships, as associations between self-report and actual behaviours are not always strong. Using a more objective technique, Fleming *et al.* (1990) assessed endocrine correlates of maternal attitudes and behaviours. The behavioural responses of new mothers to their infants was measured by video taping their activities, which were split into affectionate behaviours (e.g. cuddling), vocal behaviours (e.g. singing), approach behaviours and caregiving activities (e.g. nappy changing). There were no relationships between hormone levels and maternal responsiveness as measured by self-report questionnaire. However, levels of cortisol were positively associated with approach behaviours, especially in those mothers who had reported more positive maternal feelings during pregnancy.

We have already seen in female animals that the actual physical process of birth is vital for the onset of maternal behaviours, vaginal stimulation being associated with a release of oxytocin which then seems to influence maternal behaviours. It is interesting to speculate that those human mothers not receiving vaginal stimulation during the birth process (i.e. they receive a caesarean section) may thus not receive a central oxytocin boost, and hence may not display the full repertoire of mothering/attachment behaviours. Several unpublished studies and conference presentations provide equivocal evidence for this idea, and there appears to be a dearth of experimental studies on this issue. Nissen *et al.* (1996) provide some interesting evidence as they compared hormonal patterns in women delivering infants by vaginal or by caesarean routes. In response to breastfeeding, the women experiencing a vaginal birth showed significantly more oxytocin pulses during the first ten minutes of breastfeeding, and a significant rise in prolactin twenty to thirty minutes after the onset of breastfeeding. This suggests that mothers experiencing a caesarean section have an altered pattern of oxytocin release. Whether this is due to the missing vaginal stimulation or to the fact that such mothers are often denied skin-to-skin access to their infants shortly after birth (due to lengthy medical procedures) remains to be confirmed. As these authors did not explore any differences in maternal attachment between the two groups, links between delivery type and subsequent mother–infant bonding remain speculative, but on the basis of the animal literature one would perhaps expect such relationships to be seen.

As endogenous opioids have been found to be important in primate maternal behaviours, researchers have also assessed their possible effects in humans, with the particular focus of mothers dependent upon heroin. Despite the fact that such studies are complicated by a host of confounding variables, it would be hypothesised that heroin addicted mothers might show impairments in their caregiving behaviours, as heroin occupies the same opioid receptors, thereby blocking the actions of the endogenous opioids. Indeed Lejeune *et al.* (1997) reported that, compared to matched controls, a significant proportion of mothers addicted to heroin had been referred to child protection agencies for neglecting, abandoning or abusing their offspring. This, of course, may be related to a host of other factors, but Mikhail *et al.* (1995) revealed that, compared to non-drug-using mothers, heroin-addicted mothers maintained on methadone reported a diminished maternal–foetal attachment score during their pregnancy.

## Paternal behaviours

As some male birds and mammals demonstrate high levels of parental care, we could predict that hormonal relationships would also exist for paternal behaviours. Some evidence is as follows.

### Birds

Initial studies in ring doves strongly suggested a hormonal component to paternal behaviours, as castrated males do not display incubation behaviours, even if they have been paired with a female during the courtship/nesting process. Feder *et al.* (1977) measured circulating testosterone in male ring doves over the course of the reproductive cycle, and noted that within a few hours after initial pairing, levels rose. During the courtship and copulation stages, levels continued to rise, but then showed a gradual decline, so that, by the onset of incubation, levels were once more at baseline. Supplementation of estradiol to castrated male ring doves restored certain reproductive behaviours (such as nest soliciting), suggesting that testosterone is exerting its effects after conversion to estradiol via aromatisation. Steimer and Hutchison (1981) showed that in castrated males the conversion of testosterone to estradiol was markedly increased if the males received testosterone supplements. Increased aromatase activity was observed in the preoptic area, and thus in male birds at least certain male courtship behaviours are strongly influenced by the action of this metabolite in a specific brain region.

### Rodents

Reburn and Wynne-Edwards (1999) compared two species of dwarf hamster – one of which shows little direct paternal involvement (*Phodopus sungorus*) and another which shows high levels of paternal involvement (*Phodopus campbelli*). Blood samples were taken from males of each species before mating, during their partners' late gestation and during early lactation, with levels of prolactin, testosterone and cortisol being measured. Compared to premating levels, the paternal species displayed higher levels of cortisol before the birth, and higher levels of prolactin during lactation, than the non-paternal species. Thus, as in females, elevations of prolactin and cortisol appear to be involved in the expression of parental behaviour. Both species showed a significant drop in testosterone around the birth, and the authors argued that this represents a testosterone-mediated decrease in aggression to avoid harming the pups, but testosterone rises again during lactation perhaps to facilitate defence of the pups.

Links between testosterone and parental behaviours could reflect the breeding history of the animal. Trainor and Marler (2001), for example, suggested that in species characterised by postpartum estrus (the female becomes fertile whilst current offspring still require considerable attention) males may display behaviours characteristic of parental involvement, and also behaviours related to renewed reproductive effort (aggression, territoriality, mate guarding, etc.). The extent to which we can begin to unravel the possible hormonal underpinnings of these mutually exclusive behaviours remains open to debate. However, Trainor and Marler (2001) suggest that in such species testosterone may not necessarily act to inhibit parental behaviours.

Other studies have failed to find clear relationships between hormones and parental behaviours. For example, Lonstein and De Vries (1999) castrated a group of male prairie voles and compared their subsequent responses to pups with a group of intact males. Both groups in fact displayed parental behaviours towards the pups with little behavioural differences being noted; the implantation of estrogen pellets directly after castration had no effect. Analysis of vasopressin fibre density in the lateral septum revealed no differences between the two groups; in a subsequent study, however, analysis of the same fibres eight weeks after castration revealed a significant reduction in fibres in the castrated group. Such changes were not associated with behavioural differences, and the authors concluded that parental behaviour in this species appears to be divorced from neuroendocrine activity.

In some species of mice and gerbils, castration reduces parental behaviours, while castration plus testosterone supplementation serves to maintain parental behaviours (studies cited in Trainor and Marler, 2001). In order to determine the precise role of testosterone, Trainor and Marler (2001) conducted two studies assessing the effects of various therapies following castration on parental behaviours in male California mice. In their first study they revealed that castrated males displayed higher levels of paternal behaviours following testosterone or estradiol supplementation, compared to males receiving dihydrotestosterone or a control treatment. In a second study they showed that the effects of testosterone were mediated by estrogen receptors – testosterone is thus exerting its effects after being converted into estradiol via aromatase.

The expression of paternal behaviour may not even be dependent upon reproductive/parental experiences. Male adult prairie voles, for example, can display high levels of parental behaviour even if they are sexually naïve. Similarly, male rats show an increase in the frequency of their parental behaviours the longer they are housed with non-related infants. In female rodents lacking sexual experience, one trigger for the onset of maternal behaviours is signals from the pups themselves. Exposure to pups leads to a rise in prolactin and thence maternal behaviours (studies cited in Brown and Moger, 1983). These authors explored this relationship in male rats, hypothesising that pup-exposed males would display an increase in prolactin with increased pup exposure. Indeed, the longer that males were exposed to pups then the greater the likelihood that they would display the full repertoire of paternal behaviours. Males exposed to pups had significantly lower levels of prolactin than males housed without, but these levels were independent of exposure time. There were no differences in testosterone levels. However, prolactin and testosterone levels were correlated with the frequency of parental behaviours, and the authors suggested that this might reflect individual differences – those males that react most positively to pups may also show the greatest hormonal response.

In rodents, then, a complex picture emerges, with neuroendocrine activity, paternal responsiveness, breeding strategy and life experiences all being inter-related. In some species there seem to be no clear links between hormone parameters and paternal behaviour; in others gonadal steroids may play a role before birth, but afterwards prolactin may assume greater importance. In yet others, testosterone appears to be playing a dual role. First it acts via androgen receptors to promote reproductive behaviours, and during a slightly different (but often overlapping) time frame it acts via conversion to estradiol to facilitate parental behaviours. This explains why paternal behaviour can be induced and maintained in an animal which is also demonstrating high testosterone levels.

*Non-human primates*

A key problem for investigating neuroendocrine–paternal behaviour associations in primates is that in most species fathers display very little parental involvement. In some species (notably tamarins and marmosets), however, fathers do provide extensive parental care after birth, and so these species have provided the bulk of the evidence to date (Maestripieri, 1999). An initial focus was on prolactin, with Ziegler *et al.* (1996) examining relationships between urinary prolactin and parental care in the male cotton-top tamarin. Data were collected in eight males for two weeks prior to the birth of their offspring, and for two weeks after the birth. A group of non-parental males served as a control. Prolactin levels demonstrated a significant rise before the birth, and levels remained high during the postpartum period in all fathers. Levels in those individuals who had previous experience of fatherhood was higher than in those individuals lacking such experiences. Levels of cortisol just after the birth in experienced fathers was also lower than that in non-experienced fathers.

Initially, it was assumed that testosterone levels were divorced from paternal behaviours, as Ziegler and Snowdon (2000) showed that male cotton-top tamarins displayed high levels of paternal behaviour from birth, despite maintaining high levels of circulating testosterone. However, it is likely that such relationships are complicated by parental experience. For example, Nunes *et al.*

(2001) measured hormone levels in male black tufted-ear marmosets across various significant parental events. Males who showed higher rates of paternal involvement with their offspring (as assessed by changes in carrying behaviour) had lower levels of urinary testosterone, estradiol and cortisol than those which showed lower rates of paternal behaviour. Paternal experience was found to be a key factor, with testosterone levels being significantly lower in males who were raising their second batch of offspring (as such males were only a few months older than those raising infants for the first time, the authors ruled out age as a possible confound). Males experiencing fatherhood for the first time showed a significant increase in cortisol directly after the birth, but males experiencing their second batch of infants showed a decline in cortisol levels.

There are clear species differences, however, which make it difficult to draw general conclusions from these primate studies. For example, Schradin *et al.* (2003) compared prolactin levels before and after birth in fathers and non-fathers in three different monkey species. There was a clear difference in prolactin levels between father and non-father titi monkeys, though this species did not show a rise in prolactin after birth. Goeldi's monkeys displayed an increase in prolactin during the period that they were carrying their infants, but fathers did not have higher levels than non-fathers. In the common marmoset, fathers had higher levels of prolactin than non-fathers, and new fathers showed a clear increase in prolactin after the birth.

*Humans*

Human males can be counted amongst the approximately 5% of mammals that form long-term pair-bonds and provide considerable parental care. There are, however, considerable cross-cultural variations in pair-bonding behaviours and patterns of paternal care that make generalisations difficult. Anthropologists use the term 'couvade' to refer to a variety of customs and rituals performed in non-industrialised societies by males before, during and after the birth of their offspring. These rituals include food taboos, mimicking the act of childbirth, and even the existence of psychosomatic symptoms similar to those seen in their pregnant partners. Numerous sociological and anthropological theories have been proposed to explain the existence of the couvade, but for the purpose of this chapter the biological ones seem more pertinent. It has been suggested that the couvade may be an adaptive physiological and psychological mechanism designed to prepare the father to become emotionally attached to the developing infant, and ensure his presence and commitment after the birth (Elwood and Mason, 1994).

As we have seen, there is good (though not unequivocal) evidence for a neuroendocrine component to the onset and maintenance of parental behaviours in a variety of animal species. It is not surprising then that researchers have turned their attention to human males, who typically (though not always) display considerable parental involvement. In fact, in many ways the search for hormonal correlates of paternal behaviours is more straightforward than the equivalent search in human females, because the added complication of extreme hormonal fluctuations throughout pregnancy are absent.

Storey *et al.* (2000) recruited thirty-four couples attending antenatal classes and asked them to provide blood samples before and after the birth of their child. Before the birth, expectant fathers had high levels of prolactin and cortisol, and after the birth showed reduced levels of testosterone (a 33% reduction compared to males tested during the late postnatal period). Males who responded the most to infant-related stimuli (they were asked to hold baby dolls and listen to taped infant cries), and who demonstrated couvade symptoms, showed the highest prebirth prolactin, and lowest postbirth testosterone. The authors argued that increasing levels of prolactin coupled with decreasing levels of testosterone serve to prime males for parental responsiveness. Interestingly, male hormone levels were strongly tied to those of their partner; the authors argued that male hormone levels are triggered by pheromonal changes in the woman as her hormone levels change through pregnancy.

In a similar study, Berg and Wynne-Edwards (2001) regularly measured estradiol, cortisol and testosterone in twenty-three fathers pre- and postnatally, and in fourteen non-fathers over the same time period. Overall, compared to the non-fathers, the fathers demonstrated significantly lower testosterone and cortisol; the presence of estradiol was detected in a significantly higher proportion of the father sample than in the non-father control group. Within the males becoming fathers, testosterone levels were lowest immediately after the birth (arguably in preparation for paternal caring duties) and cortisol levels were highest in the week prior to the birth (possibly related to the increased stress experienced at this time).

Fleming *et al.* (2002) exposed new fathers, experienced fathers and non-fathers to infant cries, and measured their affective and endocrine responses. Overall, fathers displayed lower testosterone levels than non-fathers but the groups did not differ in terms of cortisol. Experienced fathers displayed significantly lower levels of testosterone and cortisol than first-time fathers in general; in response to the stimulus of an infant's cries, these experienced fathers demonstrated a greater affective reaction, and showed an enhanced prolactin response combined with a reduced cortisol response. Fathers with lower testosterone demonstrated less sympathy, but a greater emotional response to infant crying, and those with higher levels of prolactin reported feeling more positive. The authors pointed out that the interplay between hormones and behaviour in this context is complex, as not only did the sound of infants crying lead to alterations in fathers' endocrine status, but endocrine status prior to hearing the crying also influenced the behavioural and emotional response to the crying.

In a longitudinal study Delahunty *et al.* (2007) asked twenty-one couples to give two blood samples just before birth, and at two to three weeks and then two months after the birth. Nine of the couples then repeated the study around the births of their second babies. Between each blood test (separated by thirty minutes), the couples were exposed to infant cries and fathers held their babies while the mothers held a doll. Prior to the birth of their child, male prolactin levels decreased following exposure to the infant stimulus; following the birth, prolactin levels also decreased after men held their first newborn, but increased after holding their second newborn. These changes showed great individual variation however, with variables such as experience of fatherhood and emotional reactivity being related to alterations in prolactin responsiveness in association with hearing an infant crying or holding an infant. The authors cautioned that while paternal responsiveness has a neuroendocrine basis, it is flexible and heavily dependent upon the social context.

In animals, the role of testosterone in the trade-off between mating and parenting effort has been discussed. Gray *et al.* (2002) measured evening salivary testosterone in fifty-eight males who were either unmarried, married without children or married with children, to see if the same trade-off was occurring in humans. The prediction would be that married men with children would have lower levels than married men without children, and unmarried males would be expected to show the highest levels. These predictions were confirmed. Amongst the married men those scoring higher on a 'spousal investment' measure (the degree to which an individual invests in his partner as opposed to investing in himself), and who elected to spend more time with their wives, had the lowest levels. The authors suggested that lower testosterone levels may facilitate parental care by decreasing the likelihood that a father will engage in competitive/mating behaviours. Similarly, Gray *et al.* (2006) examined testosterone and marital/fatherhood status in 126 Chinese males. Both morning and evening levels of salivary testosterone were significantly lower in fathers than in non-fathers (whether married or single). In light of testosterone's assumed role in mating versus parenting effort, the authors expected that levels would be lower in those fathers who had children less than four years of age (these were presumed to be displaying greater paternal investment). This prediction was not however upheld.

## Summary

Despite the species differences, the evidence presented in this chapter strongly supports the notion that the neuroendocrine system plays a powerful role (along with social and sexual experience) in initiating and maintaining social attachment bonds. In the initial stages of forming any social bond, it seems that oxytocin and vasopressin may facilitate such actions by modulating the dopamine reward pathways in the nucleus accumbens and ventral pallidum. In these regions, dopamine activity is thought to mediate the pleasurable sensations associated with reinforcing stimuli (the individual to whom one is attached). More recent theories have put forward a slightly different interpretation in that dopamine may be involved in cue saliency, in calculation of costs/benefits or just perhaps as a generalised modulator of behavioural drives (Salamone *et al.* 2005).

Once a bond has been formed, the neuroendocrine system may then function to ensure homeostasis. Mason and Mendoza (1998) speculated that key neuroendocrine components were the limbic system, hypothalamic–pituitary–adrenal (HPA) axis, the autonomic nervous system and the immune system. They argue that these systems are integrated to fulfil two main functions – first to prepare the individual to respond adaptively in harmful circumstances, and second to restore normal functioning when the perceived threat has passed. The removal of the attachment figure would trigger the first set of neuroendocrine responses, while its return would trigger the complementary responses.

In terms of maternal/paternal attachment, the steroid and oxytocin systems (along with endocrine stimulation from the foetus acting via the placenta) may act to 'maternalise' the brain during pregnancy and parturition. After the birth, the infant's survival depends to a larger or smaller extent (depending on the species) on the formation of a close bond with the mother, and this bond appears to be formed via the oxytocin system acting in parallel with the glucocorticoid/serotonergic/endogenous opiate systems, to reduce the normal anxiety and aversion associated with new offspring (Carter, 1998). In many species this process is short-lived: after weaning, the parents begin to devote their energies to the next batch of offspring and their attachment bonds for their current offspring weaken. In primates, however, the parent–offspring bonding process is much more complex and long lasting, and involves more diverse neuroendocrine and brain mechanisms. Broad *et al.* (2006) speculated that there was an evolutionary progression away from neuroendocrine-dominated aspects of parental behaviours, towards greater activation of the emotional reward-related systems involving dopaminergic/opioid activity in the ventral striatum, as well as greater involvement by the frontal cortex. In humans, the steroid hormones during pregnancy may be redundant in that maternal care can and does take place without pregnancy and birth, and in our species infant bonds extend beyond the immediate parents to encompass siblings, and the wider family. However, the pregnancy hormones may well prime the oxytocin and dopaminergic systems to predispose the parents to form social bonds from birth.

Precisely how, then, does this complex series of hormonal/neurotransmitter/opioid interactions actually influence our motivations, responses and perceptions towards our loved ones? For example, is it the case that these systems influence the way the brain processes sensory stimuli such that new social relationships or new infants appear less threatening or more appealing? Or is it that associating with new friends/lovers/offspring somehow becomes much more rewarding? Evidence concerning the influence of hormones in the limbic system emotional centres and the dopaminergic reward centres certainly suggests that this may well be the case. Exactly which brain regions are influenced, how, and for how long, still remains deeply mysterious.

# 10 Aggressive/competitive behaviours

In the animal kingdom, aggression is viewed as a biological set of behaviours, adaptive and intentional, and necessary for the survival of the individual. It has been defined as 'overt behaviour with the intention of inflicting damage or other unpleasantness upon another individual' (Moyer, 1968), and the possibility for aggression exists whenever there is a conflict of interests between two or more individuals. In naturally living species, conflicts arise over the control of resources – principally food, shelter and mates; in most instances a social interaction decides the outcome of a contest, with ritualised displays taking the place of direct physical confrontation. Most contests will be decided quickly, with the 'loser' displaying a submissive posture or gesture, and quickly retreating with little harm done. The term 'agonistic' is normally used to describe all the features of such an encounter, which may or may not include actual physical aggression.

While aggressive behaviour is extremely complex, and there are wide species differences in the execution of such behaviours, studies from diverse species have demonstrated that a common set of limbic and hypothalamic structures are involved in the processing and/or regulation of aggressive behaviours (Goodson, 2005). This then leads to the assumption that there will exist a neuroendocrine basis for such behaviours. However, aggression is extremely complex and is clearly influenced by a host of environmental, genetic, physiological and social factors. For example, agonistic behaviour in animals is sensitive to the environmental context, and several types have been identified. Maternal aggression is displayed when a mother will vigorously defend her offspring and her territory. Fear-induced aggression is displayed when an animal is placed in a life-threatening situation. These types of aggression are relatively rare and are only seen in specific situations, and it has proved difficult to link them to neuroendocrine activity.

A key characteristic of aggressive behaviours throughout the animal kingdom concerns the age and sex of the perpetrator. Young adult males demonstrate a much higher frequency of physical aggression and agonistic interactions with individuals of the same age and sex. This high prevalence of intermale aggression is strongly associated with territoriality, acquisition and protection of valuable resources, and the establishment and maintenance of dominance hierarchies. Most research concerning possible relationships between hormones and aggressive behaviours has thus focussed on intramale aggression, where neuroendocrine–behaviour links appear to be stronger. Indeed, numerous studies across a wide range of species have shown that the androgen testosterone is somehow involved in agonistic behaviours, though the precise physiological neurological mechanisms by which it acts remain to be confirmed; it should be noted that there exist wide species differences (Archer, 1988).

The reduction in aggression seen following castration prior to puberty has been noted in many species historically. In non-castrated males, links between androgen level and aggression have also been observed. For example, Gaines *et al.* (1985) implanted prairie voles with capsules of slow-releasing testosterone or empty capsules, and noted that testosterone-treated males showed higher levels of aggression than the control group. However, not all studies have revealed significant relationships between testosterone and aggressive behaviours. For example, in the dusky-footed wood rat, levels of intermale aggression rise during the breeding season, with a strong relationship being seen between levels of aggression and testosterone. However, if males are castrated as adults they also show a seasonal rise in aggression, and their fighting ability remains unaffected (Caldwell *et al.*, 1984). In golden hamsters, injections of testosterone into a male out of the breeding season do not lead to a rise in aggression (Berndtson and Desjardins, 1974). Most studies reporting no clear relationships between testosterone and aggression have typically relied upon observations of captive males, living in situations far removed from their natural state; as hormone fluctuations are strongly dependent upon appropriate environmental cues (e.g. another male challenging for dominance, or the presence of a fertile female) then it is perhaps not surprising that equivocal relationships have been reported (Wingfield *et al.*, 1990).

## The 'challenge hypothesis'

The principal theoretical explanation for this pattern of aggressive behaviours relates to the Darwinian concept of intersexual selection, where males have to engage in competitive encounters with other males in order first to attract 'choosy' females, and then to monopolise females during the reproductive process in order to ensure their paternity certainty. Wingfield (1985) had noted that in male song sparrows testosterone was most strongly related to aggressive responses when dominance hierarchies were being formed and/or territories were being established at the onset of the breeding season. Once hierarchies/territories had been established and became stable, a decline in testosterone and agonistic behaviours was noted. Individual patterns of alterations in testosterone from a pre-breeding season baseline were found to relate to different reproductive challenges (e.g. establishing a territory, mate-guarding, male challenges, etc.) and so fluctuations in testosterone were assumed to reflect differential reproductive challenges.

The challenge hypothesis was thus proposed by Wingfield *et al.* (1990) in order to explain these observed relationships between testosterone and agonistic behaviours in birds. These authors noted that testosterone showed marked seasonal variations, and rising levels could be reliably associated with changes in secondary sexual characteristics, spermatogenesis, certain territorial/aggressive behaviours, and mating displays (e.g. singing). At the start of the breeding season, levels rise to support reproductive physiology and behaviours associated with reproductive effort and intermale competition. During specific challenges in reproductively relevant contexts, levels of testosterone show a further rise, to enable the individual to meet the challenge successfully. We thus see a corresponding rise in agonistic behaviours, typically in relation to establishing and defending a territory, and mate-guarding.

For example, Wingfield and Wada (1989) simulated territorial intrusions by placing a caged male song sparrow into the centre of another male's territory, and broadcasting a tape of the intruder's territorial song. Resident males responding aggressively to the 'intruder' were captured at either one to four minutes, five to ten minutes, or ten to sixty minutes after the encounter, and blood samples were obtained; levels of testosterone and luteinising hormone were compared with males caught whilst foraging. No hormonal differences were found in males caught one to ten minutes after an aggressive encounter; however, both hormone levels had increased ten minutes after a simulated invasion of territory.

## Evidence for the challenge hypothesis in animals

### Seasonal variations in aggression

In many animal species, reproductive effort is often constrained within a fairly narrow window of opportunity referred to as the 'breeding season'. In such species, aggressive and reproductive behaviours, and secondary sexual characteristics (e.g. plumage, antlers, etc.), are closely associated with changing levels of testosterone. For example, over a two-year period Smith *et al.* (2005) measured testosterone in captured male and female cliff swallows living in colonies of different sizes. Males and females showed a seasonal rise in testosterone when nest ownership was being decided, and a drop in levels when the eggs hatched. Testosterone levels varied significantly with colony size: birds in larger colonies, where competition was more extreme, showed higher levels.

However, numerous other studies have demonstrated that the relationship between testosterone secretion and seasonal aggressive/territorial behaviours may be more complex. For example, in some bird species testosterone is clearly related to singing behaviour, but shows no clear link with aggressive behaviours (Romero *et al.*, 1998). In Japanese quails, Tsutsui and Ishii (1981) noted that the amount of aggressive behaviour following castration and subsequent testosterone supplementation showed no relationship to the differing doses utilised. Wingfield (1994) also observed that aggressive behaviour can persist in male song sparrows even following castration. Finally, some bird species establish and defend a territory outside of the normal breeding season when their testosterone levels are very low (Hau *et al.*, 2000).

Canoine and Gwinner (2002b) suggested that a possible explanation may lie in how testosterone exerts its effects in different situations. The mediation of different behaviours at different times of the year may occur via direct action through androgen receptors, or via conversion to estradiol by aromatase. In their study of male European stonechats, they first established that behavioural responses to a simulated territorial invasion could be observed; indeed such responses were seen in both breeding and non-breeding seasons. In addition, they measured testosterone levels in both seasons, and found that plasma levels were significantly higher in the breeding season. They then compared the male's response to a simulated territorial intrusion before and after simultaneous implantation with an androgen receptor blocker and an aromatase inhibitor, or a placebo, during the breeding and non-breeding seasons. The simulated territorial invasion was then repeated seven days after the implantation, and behavioural responses recorded. During the breeding season all of the placebo-treated males showed the aggressive reaction in response to territorial invasion, but only 25% of the implanted males demonstrated the same response.

In the non-breeding season, the majority of the males responded aggressively to an invasion, with treatment condition having no effect. In this species, then, there are clearly seasonal differences in the hormonal control mechanism underlying territorial aggression. In the breeding season, aggressive behaviours in response to a territorial invasion are mediated by androgens or by their estrogenic metabolites; in the non-breeding season, however, territorial aggression appears to be moderated by a different system. Interestingly, the opposite effect has been noted in western song sparrows, with Soma *et al.* (1999) demonstrating a reduction in aggressive behaviours in response to territorial invasion in the non-breeding season in males implanted with an aromatase inhibitor and an androgen receptor antagonist.

In other mammals, similar relationships have been established. Lincoln *et al.* (1972) studied a population of red deer on the Scottish island of Rhum, in which the males spend much of the year living amicably in large bachelor groups, mostly ignoring the nearby females. In late summer the males move to traditional rutting areas (tracts of rich grassland which can support a large number of females), their antlers lose their soft velvet covering, and they fight vigorously for prime locations within the rutting area for around two months. As dominance rank, and hence mating success, is determined by the ability of a male to acquire and defend a prime spot in the rutting area, the fights are vicious, and around 25% of rutting males become wounded, with some dying (Clutton-Brock *et al.*, 1979). The establishment of such hierarchies is important because the females only come into estrus for a three-week period and will only mate with the males with the highest social rank. After the rutting season finishes, the males shed their antlers and return to a fairly peaceful coexistence with other males in their bachelor herds. Antlers are vitally important to a red deer stag, and the cycle of antler development is dependent upon testosterone. New antlers are covered by soft velvet; high levels of testosterone at the start of the rutting season cause the velvet covering to die off, exposing the hard horn underneath. After rutting, the testes regress, testosterone levels drop and the antlers are cast.

Lincoln *et al.* (1972) found that castration of red deer stags during the winter led to the prompt casting of their antlers and a rapid decline in their social standing. Castrated males provided with continuous infusions of testosterone maintained their antlers, had a higher social rank and were more aggressive. Interestingly they did not show sexual interest any earlier, which suggests that a signal from the females is still required to trigger sexual behaviours in the male. Removing the antlers of gonadally intact males led to similar reductions in dominance, despite the fact that these animals still behaved aggressively (Bouissou, 1983).

In primates, two related mechanisms appear to be important. In a series of studies involving free-living adolescent male rhesus macaques, Higley and colleagues have focussed on relationships between serotonin (as assessed by levels of its metabolite 5HIAA), testosterone and aggressive behaviours. They have reported a negative relationship between serotonin levels and aggression, particularly as regards aggressive behaviours associated with impulsivity and unrestrained aggression: testosterone levels were positively associated with overall aggression, but not with impulsivity (Higley *et al.*, 1992). Higley *et al.* (1996) hypothesised that testosterone and serotonin may thus provide a different contribution to the expression of aggression, testosterone contributing to aggressive drive and motivation, while serotonin may regulate the threshold and frequency of its behavioural expression. They predicted that individuals with above average levels of testosterone but average levels of serotonin might not express violent or unrestrained aggression, though could still display assertive/dominant behaviours. Those with lower levels of serotonin along with higher levels of testosterone would display aggressive motivations coupled with impulsive violent aggression.

In other primates, researchers have just addressed testosterone/aggression links. For example, Muller and Wrangham (2004) took multiple samples of testosterone from the urine of eleven free-living male chimpanzees. When females were in estrus, males showed a significant rise in testosterone and there was a corresponding increase in intermale aggressive competition. Males who had been identified as being more dominant showed higher aggression than low-dominant males, and they produced higher surges of testosterone.

## Artificial manipulation of testosterone levels

A classic study by Allee *et al.* (1939) demonstrated the powerful effects of testosterone on aggressive behaviour. Hens display a clear 'pecking order', with the dominant individuals residing at the top of the hierarchy and claiming all of the benefits associated with their high status. When injected with testosterone propionate, hens observed to be at the bottom of the pecking order showed increased levels of aggression, climbed the status hierarchy, and displayed male-typical secondary sexual characteristics. If the sudden onset of reproductive/agonistic behaviours is associated with a rise in testosterone, then it should be possible to increase testosterone levels artificially during breeding or non-breeding seasons and evaluate the outcomes.

Indeed, Wingfield (1984) implanted testosterone-releasing capsules into monogamous male birds and noted that they became more aggressive, established and maintained larger territories, and displayed polygynous behaviours. Furthermore, increasing testosterone level by using implants just before territories were established led to improvements in territory holding and aggression in several species. However, testosterone provided after such territories have been established did not increase territory size or social dominance (reviewed in Wingfield *et al.*, 1987).

Similarly, Mougeot *et al.* (2005) studied the hormonal regulation of territorial behaviour in the red grouse, a species noted for an aggressive response towards territorial invasions at the onset of the summer breeding season, but also noted for territoriality outside of the breeding season. The authors explained that such behaviours in the non-breeding season are vital, as the establishment of a territory during the autumn and winter months is closely associated with survival rates and the chances of attracting a mate during the subsequent summer breeding season. They first established that testosterone levels rose during the breeding season (they rose two to three times above non-breeding season baselines), and were reflected in an increase in comb size, a secondary sexual ornament signalling to male competitors and potential female partners. They then assessed the effects of testosterone supplementation, or treatment with an aromatase inhibitor in conjunction with an anti-estrogen. During the autumn, 180 male birds were captured and assigned to experimental groups, and aggressive responses to a territorial invasion (the sound of another male's call) were observed. Those participants receiving testosterone supplementation showed a significant increase in their responding to the perceived intruder, while males in the other treatment and placebo groups showed no such effect.

The previously described studies have altered hormone levels within levels typically associated with wild-living animals. A slightly different animal model has focussed on the effects of much higher doses provided by anabolic androgenic steroids (AAS). In such studies the common paradigm is chronically to expose male rodents to AAS and observe changes in their behaviours. These

AAS-treated male rats have been reported to be much more aggressive to other males irrespective of whether they are residents or intruders, and if exposed to mild physical provocation (e.g. a tail pinch) these males respond with greater aggression, suggesting a lowering in the threshold of aggressive responding (e.g. Farrell and McGuiness, 2003; Wesson and McGuinness, 2006).

In hamsters AAS exposure during puberty acts to facilitate aggression during agonistic encounters, by altering the development and activity of vasopressin within the anterior portion of the hypothalamus. Interestingly, aggressive and physiological affects were closely related even after withdrawal from AAS treatment, but only for around twelve days of withdrawal. After this period the behavioural and physical effects were no longer apparent (Grimes et al., 2006). However, other authors have not found this effect in male mice: while testosterone levels rose sharply in response to AAS treatment, aggressive behaviour showed no relationship to this change (Martínez-Sanchis et al., 1998). These authors found that any effects of AAS only appeared in those individuals noted as being more aggressive pre-treatment.

## Puberty

During sexual maturation the testes secrete large amounts of testosterone, raising levels of this hormone from juvenile to adult levels. In numerous animal species males display an increase in aggression towards other males at the onset of puberty, and it is thus not surprising that alterations in aggression have been linked to these dramatic changes in androgens. Indeed, one can view puberty as a particular challenge as the individual enters the breeding market for the first time and is surrounded by a host of other males all eager to establish and defend their social status, and attract potential reproductive partners. Rodent models have shown that intermale aggression seen during sexual maturation is related to changing levels of circulating testosterone (e.g. Albert et al., 1990).

In primates, increased male aggression has been observed at puberty but the evidence is inconsistent, with other studies reporting no clear relationships. For example, Dixson (1980) noted that while testosterone levels rise dramatically in owl monkeys at puberty, agonistic encounters do not increase between juveniles and their parents. Similarly, in squirrel monkeys Coe et al. (1988) suggested that androgen levels during puberty may only play a small role in the behaviours displayed around that time. Instead they argued that androgen secretions during the neonatal period have a long-lasting effect on certain male behaviours such as rough and tumble play and dominance behaviours; behavioural changes at puberty may simply be coincidental, and not be the direct result of androgen secretions.

## Competition and androgen levels in animals

An effect closely related to the challenge hypothesis is the 'winner effect', the observation that an individual with a record of winning agonistic encounters shows an increased probability of winning future encounters (Dugatkin,

1997). An early indication that this effect may reflect a hormonal basis was provided by Rohwer and Rohwer (1978). They observed Harris's sparrows, which form large mixed-sex groups within which individuals compete for limited resources via an established 'pecking order'. As the group is large and changes frequently, the costs involved in constantly having to establish a pecking order would be too large. Natural selection has thus provided a convenient and honest marker of dominance for the males in the form of dark feathers on the head and breast. This colouration is established during the autumn, with individuals having higher testosterone levels exhibiting darker plumage. Birds with darker plumage invariably win agonistic encounters with birds that have lighter plumage. The authors bleached the feathers of some dominant individuals and darkened the plumage of subordinates. Both groups did not fare well: the bleached individuals were faced with constant dominance battles, and the darkened birds failed to live up to their newly acquired high status, being easily ousted by other birds. However, if subordinates were dyed and received testosterone injections, then they a showed dramatic increase in their social standing.

In mammals the situation is slightly more complex as it is very difficult to control for intrinsic fighting abilities, and it is not yet clear whether individuals simply become more skilled at fighting after repeated encounters, or whether winning is indeed associated with alterations in hormone levels, which then influence fighting behaviour. Some studies in mice have shown that even a single aggressive encounter can lead to an increase in future aggression (shorter attack latency, increased frequency of initiated attacks, etc.), despite the fact that a clear 'winner' is not established (e.g. Martinez *et al.*, 1994), but here the role of the neurohormonal system remained unaddressed. An ideal model to assess this effect appears to be the California mouse (*Peromyscus californicus*), as males of this species show territorial aggression all year round, and high levels of aggressive responding when challenged.

Oyegbile and Marler (2005) investigated how winning initial territorial encounters may affect the likelihood of winning a more evenly matched encounter. Fifty males were assigned to be 'residents', forty of whom were randomly assigned to win between zero and three fights against 'intruders' who were not only smaller but also slightly sedated. The remaining ten individuals served as controls. During each encounter the males' behaviours were observed, and the frequency of certain aggressive actions were recorded; a 'winner' was established when at least three attacks occurred by the same individual that resulted in the opponent demonstrating typical submissive/ loser behaviours. The experience of winning did indeed increase the probability of winning the final (unrigged) encounter, but only in the males who had experience of winning all three previous encounters. The only behaviour that appeared to be affected was that of attack latency, which was reduced in experienced males (they attacked more quickly when faced with an intruder);

when faced with these experienced males the intruders also displayed submissive behaviours more rapidly. Males with more experience of winning two or three previous encounters were found to have significantly higher testosterone levels than those winning only one or no previous encounters. Succeeding in the final encounter also led to another rise in testosterone levels, thus confirming the winner effect. Precisely how testosterone exerts these effects remains to be ascertained, but these authors suggested that it could be via interactions with neurochemical systems such as vasopressin, serotonin and dopamine – systems strongly suspected of playing a role in aggressive behaviours (e.g. Ferris and Delville, 1994).

As winners have been seen to experience a rise in testosterone, one would predict that the opposite would occur for those individuals losing a competitive encounter. Indeed the 'loser effect' is well established. For example, Lloyd (1971) reported that male mice losing an aggressive encounter showed reductions in testosterone, this hormone suppression lasting several days. Similarly, Bernstein et al. (1974) found that defeated male rhesus monkeys had reduced levels of testosterone for weeks after a contest, while levels in the winners showed a large increase. Not surprisingly, the outcomes of tied fights do not seem to lead to an alteration in testosterone levels. Oliveira et al. (2005), for example, demonstrated that cichlid fish exposed to their reflection in a mirror displayed considerable aggression towards the apparent intruder, but showed no alteration in testosterone levels. Such alterations are observed when faced with a real opponent. The authors suggested that the androgen response is an adaptive mechanism for controlling an individual's social status after he has assessed the relative fighting ability of a challenger: a rise would only be seen where the individual suspects that he has a good chance of winning. Thus far I am unaware of any studies in mammals that have addressed hormonal responses to tied fights.

## The role of estrogen/aromatase

In animals with a clearly defined breeding season we have already seen that testosterone may exert its behavioural effects via differing mechanisms at different stages of the season. Trainor et al. (2006) reviewed the effects of aromatase in birds and mammals, and how interactions between aromatase and the environment may moderate aggressive behaviours. In birds, estrogen has been seen to increase aggressive behaviours in some species, but not others. Aromatase activity in the preoptic region of the hypothalamus has been associated with aggressive responses in males, as males treated with an aromatase inhibitor show a reduction in aggressive responses (e.g. Schlinger and Callard, 1990).

In mammals, castrated mice treated with estradiol showed more aggressive responses than mice treated with DHT or a placebo; those treated with a non-aromatisable androgen showed more fighting behaviours (Simon and Whalen,

1986). Genetic manipulation studies have been able to create mice in which the aromatase gene remains inactive. These ARKO mice display reduced aggression unless regularly treated with estrogen throughout their development (Toda *et al.*, 2001). Similar studies have been conducted in mice lacking functional estrogen receptors. These ERKO mice lack the estrogen alpha receptor (ERα), and Ogawa *et al.* (1998) confirmed that such males showed a complete suppression of normal offensive attacks; injections of testosterone propionate were ineffective in inducing aggressive responses.

## Human aggression/competition

In animals, aggression is typically defined by objective behavioural acts. In humans the scope and definition is much wider, with a distinction being made between aggression (seen as a biological behaviour) and violence (seen more as a social construction). Archer and Browne (1989) described aggression in terms of three components. The first component relates to the intention to harm another individual, the second relates to the behaviour(s) accompanying that intention, and the third consists of the accompanying emotion(s) (ranging from irritation to rage). Studies of human aggression have tended to focus on these components separately, and have typically utilised self-report assessments, though in a minority of cases observational or experimental techniques have been used.

While defining human aggression has been problematic and is still dogged by controversy, as in other animal species, a key characteristic of aggressive behaviour in humans relates to the age and the sex of the aggressor. However aggressive acts are defined, males engage in them more frequently than do females; for example, in a meta-analysis of numerous studies Hyde (1986) revealed that, while males and females do not differ in terms of 'hostility', males scored much higher on behaviours such as 'aggressive fantasies', 'physical aggression', 'imitative aggression' and 'willingness to shock others'. A casual glance at homicide statistics from various countries will reveal that the proportion of such aggressive crimes committed by males far outweighs those committed by females (Daly and Wilson, 1988). In the majority of cases the perpetrators are young males, with violent crimes showing a peak in the mid-twenties, a phenomenon so robust it has been termed the 'young male syndrome' (Wilson and Daly, 1985).

Many researchers have focussed their attention on discovering clear relationships between hormones and human aggressive behaviour, with the majority of studies addressing testosterone. One major limitation of the majority of studies concerns their ecological validity. In the animal studies described in previous sections, aggressive behaviours were typically viewed within the context of a real-life event, i.e. the animal is responding in a genuine way to an important situation (e.g. repelling an intruder, gaining status to attract a potential mate) that could have significant social/reproductive outcomes for the individual. Ideally, researchers investigating humans would take hormone measures before, during and after equivalent social encounters. Needless to say, because of numerous methodological and ethical considerations, such studies remain rare.

Typically, human investigators assess hormone–aggression relationships within the context of a contrived laboratory setting, often using young male undergraduates (a social group not noted for their violent behaviours) and often making use of subjective self-reported aggressive behaviours or paper-and-pencil measures of aggression, both of which have considerable limitations. Finally, many studies have utilised measures of hormones from blood plasma. Recall that these molecules of hormone are bound and not capable of acting biologically. Not surprisingly then, while some studies have revealed significant associations between testosterone and aggressive behaviours (see review by Harris, 1999), many other studies find no clear relationships, and some authors have questioned the extent to which we will be able to determine simple testosterone–aggression links in humans (Archer, 1991; Archer et al., 1998; Simpson, 2001).

## Can the challenge hypothesis be applied to humans?

Recently, Archer (2006) has evaluated links between testosterone and aggression in humans by considering such relationships in terms of the challenge hypothesis. He points out that the original hypothesis requires some modifications as it is based on species with clear-cut breeding seasons, but notes that the theory could provide a useful predictive model within which to view hormone–behaviour relationships in humans. The caution remains, however, that most human studies thus far conducted have not been specifically designed directly to test this hypothesis. Archer generates a series of predictions from the challenge hypothesis as applied to humans, and some key ones are evaluated as follows:

### Increases in aggression at puberty?

While testosterone at puberty is associated with aggression in rodents, evidence from primates suggests that the pubertal increase is not associated with aggressive behaviours. Archer thus predicts that we will find no significant links between hormone levels at puberty and aggressive behaviours. I am not yet fully convinced by this prediction, as I view puberty as a distinctly challenging social period when human males are clearly competing with other males for social status, and access to an opposite-sex reproductive partner. The young male syndrome, as described previously, reflects this intense competition, which is highest in young males entering the breeding market for the first time, as such males have to gain a higher status to enable them to compete against older males of higher social rank and greater resources.

Wilson and Daly (1985) found that young males are more likely to engage in dangerous confrontations when the reward is a rise in social status. Furthermore, young males are more likely to escalate trivial altercations when there is potential 'loss of face' in front of other competing males, or potential female partners. At adolescence, the killing of males drastically increases, reaching a peak in the early twenties. By this age males are six times more likely to be murdered by other young males!

However, crime surveys only reveal the basic facts and not the reasons behind such behaviours. What about studies investigating testosterone and aggressive behaviours in human adolescents? There is, in fact, conflicting evidence that androgen levels correlate with higher aggression in young males. For example, Olweus et al. (1980) found significant positive correlations between verbal aggression, physical aggression, lack of frustration tolerance and androgen levels in fifty-eight adolescent males. In another study apparently involving exactly the same sample, Olweus et al. (1988) reported that high levels of testosterone were associated with an increased readiness to respond to provocation. However, Udry (1990) found no relationship between testosterone and behaviour in a three-year longitudinal study of adolescent boys. Over the same time period, Halpern et al. (1994) conducted a longitudinal study of one hundred adolescent males undergoing puberty. While testosterone levels rose dramatically during puberty, no change in direct aggression was observed, and there were no correlations between testosterone levels and aggression.

In a review and meta-analysis, Archer (1991) reported a weak positive relationship between testosterone and aggression, a finding echoed a decade later by Book et al. (2001). One study has in fact reported a significant relationship between testosterone and disruptive behaviour in girls, but *not* in boys (Granger et al., 2003). Pajer et al. (2006) also found that adolescent girls with 'conduct disorder' had lower levels of cortisol and higher levels of free testosterone than age-matched girls without such problems. The challenge hypothesis of course relates specifically to males, and so at the moment it is difficult to reconcile the female evidence with any appropriate theory. One could, I suppose, argue that certain reproductive life events are just as challenging for females as for males, and that their neuroendocrine system should also be geared towards coping with such challenges. As yet there is no specific theory addressing female life history, the neuroendocrine system and specific behaviours (such as aggression), though some authors are making headway in this area (e.g. Cashdan, 2003; Taylor et al., 2000). Indeed, Wingfield et al. (2000) did suggest that in species where males and females display joint parental care and demonstrate reduced sexual dimorphism, then testosterone may play an important role in female competitiveness. Clearly this issue remains to be resolved.

Schaal et al. (1996) found that boys with a history of physical aggression between the ages of six and twelve actually had significantly lower levels of testosterone at age thirteen than boys without such a history (though by age sixteen this had reversed). A possible confound here could be physique. Tremblay *et al.* (1998) investigated physical development, social dominance, antisocial behaviour and testosterone levels in fifty-seven boys aged six to thirteen. Testosterone level and body size were predictors of social dominance, such that adolescents with high testosterone levels were more likely to be socially dominant (but not aggressive), especially if they had a large body mass, but those who had a large body mass were more likely to be aggressive irrespective of their testosterone levels.

Another possible confound could relate to the hormonal mechanisms underpinning the behaviours in question. In a study of adolescent males and females considered at risk for later delinquent behaviour, Maras *et al.* (2003) found that plasma levels of testosterone and DHT were significantly higher in males demonstrating behaviours considered to be precursors of aggressive behaviours ('externalising'). In those demonstrating persistent externalising behaviours, DHT showed a closer association. As DHT has a higher affinity for the androgen receptor than testosterone, the authors suggested that future studies could perhaps focus on this androgen rather than on testosterone.

Van Bokhoven *et al.* (2006) pointed out a series of problems with such studies that renders their conclusions equivocal. First, some studies used clinical samples referred for disruptive behavioural problems, whereas others relied upon non-clinical populations. Second, studies differed widely not only in terms of their sample sizes, but also in the number of samples taken from which to analyse testosterone (a single sample being often used rather than the more valid use of multiple samples). Third, a wide array of psychometric tests have been utilised to assess aggressive behaviours; different types of aggression (e.g. disruptive, assertive, violent, physical, etc.) have been measured, and whether such behaviours were reactive or proactive has not always been clearly established. Finally, the studies have a very broad age range of participants, some assessing young children not undergoing puberty, while others have assessed adolescents during puberty or even afterwards. Longitudinal studies assessing children before, during and after puberty are rare.

In their study van Bokhoven *et al.* (2006) assessed relationships between testosterone, aggression, delinquency and dominance, using multiple behavioural measures over a period covering late childhood, through early adolescence and on to adulthood (the age range was six to twenty). An initial sample of over 1000 males were assessed by their teachers at age six; in later years (aged ten, eleven and twelve) teachers assessed physical aggression in 893 of the sample. From age thirteen to fifteen, 203 boys attended laboratory sessions for observational and experimental testing on a yearly basis, testosterone was assayed using multiple samples, and their teachers also provided information concerning their reactive and proactive aggression. A final group of ninety-six was examined when they were twenty-one years old. A key finding was that at age sixteeen, boys with a criminal record had significantly higher testosterone compared to boys lacking a criminal record; this effect remained at age twenty-one, when delinquent males had higher testosterone. In addition, at age sixteen, testosterone was higher in a subgroup of boys scoring higher for pro-active aggression, but overall, throughout puberty, while testosterone levels rose there was no increase in teacher-rated aggression, or self-rated delin-quency. The authors suggested that fluctuating levels of testosterone do not appear to be related to aggressive behaviours. However, this did appear to be related to antisocial behaviours (which sometimes included aggression).

This result echoes an earlier conclusion by Archer *et al.* (1998), who found no relationships between androgen levels and psychometric measures of aggression in 101 male medical students. They suggested that such links may only be found in groups where levels of aggression may already be high. In support, Dabbs and Morris (1990) assessed antisocial behaviour in over 4000 military veterans and found that those classified as being 'high' in testos-terone were more likely to report being in trouble with parents and teachers, and to have broken rules whilst undergoing military service. In another study Dabbs *et al.* (1991) assessed relationships between testosterone and aggres-sive behaviour in 113 late-adolescent male offenders currently undergoing a prison sentence. Those higher in testosterone had committed more violent crimes and violated prison rules more often than those lower in testosterone. Similarly, Dabbs *et al.* (1995b) assessed testosterone levels and criminal behaviour in 692 adult prison inmates. Those who had committed sexual and/or violent offences had significantly higher testosterone levels than those who had committed crimes such as burglary and drug dealing; the inmates with higher levels also committed more rule violations (especially ones involving direct confrontations) whilst in prison.

Perhaps the possible relationships between testosterone and aggression during puberty are too obscured by the potential confounds outlined by van Bokhoven *et al.* (2006). It is also possibly the case that the challenges of puberty remain rather too subjective to be related to hormonal fluctuations. We might expect to find clearer associations in adult males responding to a situation that can be unequivocally designated as challenging.

## Males respond to competition with an increase in testosterone?

In human societies aggression has been ritualised in the form of competition and sport, and several studies have analysed relationships between androgen levels and competitive outcomes. Mazur and Lamb (1980) reported three experiments concerning testosterone and competition. In the first they obtained blood samples from undergraduate tennis players one hour before and one hour after a match in which prize money was at stake. Winners showed a rise in testosterone after the matches, and losers displayed a fall in testosterone. In the second, they measured testosterone levels in male stu-dents as they participated in a cash prize lottery over which they had no control. In this situation, becoming a winner had no influence on testosterone levels, indicating that such changes may only be apparent in situations in which an individual wins through his own efforts. The nature of the competition also does not appear to be limited to sporting contexts, because in their third study they found a rise in testosterone levels shortly after a university graduation ceremony, though whether this reflects a subjective feeling of winning, a rise in social status, or a reduction in the stress-induced inhibition of gonadal steroids remains unclear. In a competitive video game contest, Mazur *et al.* (1997) found that males exhibited a pre-competition rise in testosterone, but after the contest levels did not differ between winners and losers. The authors suggested that the nature of the task was not sufficient to induce a strong feeling of failure or success.

A seemingly important factor relates to the mood of the competitor. Booth *et al.* (1989), for example, measured mood, testosterone and cortisol in six top university tennis players fifteen minutes before and immediately after they took part in singles and doubles matches. Testosterone rose just before most matches, and players with the highest pre-match levels of testosterone also had the most positive improvement in mood before their matches. After the competitions, testosterone rose in winners relative to losers, especially for winners who displayed a positive mood after their victories. This post-match rise in winners and drop in losers carried over to the next match. This could therefore be a factor in winning and losing streaks commonly seen in individuals and in teams in a sporting context. Mazur (1985) had proposed a biosocial theory of status that hypothesised a feedback loop between an individual's testosterone level and his assertiveness in attempting to achieve dominance. As testosterone rises, the theory assumes that the individual becomes increasingly motivated to achieve higher status, and the experience of winning produces a further rise in testosterone, or maintains an already existing high level. The opposite occurs in a loser, and in this way losing and winning streaks are initiated and maintained.

However, other studies have not shown such clear-cut results. Salvador *et al.* (1987) measured testosterone levels in fourteen young male judo competitors ten minutes before and forty-five minutes after a training session and a competitive bout. They found that, in general, testosterone increased after training and decreased after competition, but winning or losing did not change testosterone levels. However, the competitive encounter did not involve any prize or reward and it is perhaps likely that the competitors simply viewed it as an extension of their training programme.

Similarly, Gonzalez-Bono *et al.* (1999) measured testosterone and mood in two teams of professional basketball players playing a single competitive match. While testosterone did rise in the winners and fall in the losers compared to pre-match levels, this remained non-significant, though pre-match levels did not appear to be equitable. However, these authors did find that testosterone correlated positively to 'score/time playing' ratio, a measure of an individual's contribution to the outcome of the result. In addition, testosterone correlated negatively with external attribution in winners, and positively with external attribution in losers.

Other confounding factors may relate to certain social perceptions. Edwards *et al.* (2006) assessed the possible role of status with team-mates and social connectedness, in male and female undergraduate soccer players. In the males, compared to team-mates who did not play in the game, testosterone and cortisol both showed a rise from pre-game to post-game following a winning encounter (comparisons were not conducted before and after a losing game). In the female sample, testosterone and cortisol rose from pre-game to post-game in both the winning and losing games. In males, post-game testosterone was significantly related to scores on the social connectedness and social status questionnaires. Higher ratings of social connectedness, and other players' ratings of an individual player (especially in terms of their communication skills), were associated with higher testosterone during competition. In females, the questionnaires yielded positive associations with before-game testosterone, but not post-game levels.

Another important variable may relate to how an individual perceives the outcome of his or her competitive efforts. Van Anders and Watson (2007b) used a computerised task in which males and females were asked to match a target word to one of five possible words in terms of its meaning. The test was programmed so that those scoring above a certain amount were classed as winners, while those scoring below that amount were classed as losers. At the end of the programme the outcome ('You won!' or 'You lost!') appeared on the screen. Male winners showed a smaller decrease in testosterone levels from pre-game to post-game than did losers; female winners showed no difference from losers. In a second version of the task, participants were assigned to win or lose, irrespective of their actual ability, and no significant changes in testosterone were noted pre- to post-game in either males or females. This suggests then that an earned win may attenuate a decline in testosterone, but note that winning did not lead to an increase in testosterone. Perhaps the nature of the contrived task and/or the solitary nature of the competition played a role here. One would perhaps expect that a genuine competitive encounter with a clearly defined outcome (a change in self-perceived status in front of team-mates and a crowd) might be expected to lead to more clear-cut hormonal events.

Interestingly, testosterone changes may not be limited to competitors but may also be seen in fans. Bernhardt *et al.* (1998) conducted two studies in which sports fans of two opposing teams provided testosterone samples before and after a game. The first sample involved eight basketball fans (four per team), and while their levels did not differ before the match, levels rose in the winners and dropped in the losers. In their second study, twenty-one football fans (twelve and nine per team) watching their teams play in the World

Cup final also provided samples before and after the game. As before, levels rose in the winning-team fans and dropped in the losing-team fans.

### The 'home advantage'

The studies just described did not set out to assess the challenge hypothesis. In fact no human studies have yet explicitly done so. However, we recently conducted some research using a competitive phenomenon that may prove to be a useful human analogue of the challenge hypothesis (Neave and Wolfson, 2003). The home advantage is a robust effect seen in many team sports, in which a team wins more games, and scores more goals/points, when playing at its home ground compared to playing at an away venue. The home advantage in team sports is pervasive, but the potential causes remain under debate. Popular explanations include factors relating to increased crowd support at home, referee bias towards home teams, familiarity with the home venue, and travel and fatigue issues when playing away; there is some support for all of these explanations (reviewed in Neave and Wolfson, 2004).

We reasoned that if testosterone levels are linked with aggression and dominance, and if humans also fight harder to defend their perceived home territory, then there may be a relationship between testosterone levels in sports competitors when playing at home versus playing away. In an initial study, players in a non-league football team provided salivary samples of testosterone, and completed mood ratings before a home match and an away match against the same team (a team at a similar position in the league table). While mood ratings did not differ, testosterone levels before a home game were significantly higher than before the away game. As data were not obtained from a neutral training session, we were unable to tell if this change represented a surge in testosterone before the home game (as anticipated) or simply a decrease before the away game.

In a second study, twenty-five players in a Premiership under-nineteen football team provided salivary samples and completed questionnaires before two home games, two away games and three training sessions. The home and away games were against the same two sides – one described as a 'bitter local rival' and the other as a 'moderate rival'. Again, testosterone levels were significantly higher before the home games; levels before away games and training sessions did not differ. This pre-home surge in testosterone was particularly striking when the team played against a side described as being a 'bitter rival' (Neave and Wolfson, 2003).

This rivalry effect is not surprising, as previous experiences of competing against a variety of opponents of differing abilities are likely to influence subsequent encounters. In support, Wagner et al. (2002) had shown that testosterone surges before competitive encounters against males from an opposing village were higher than before encounters with members of the same village. More recently, Carré et al. (2006) have also reported that testosterone levels in elite hockey players are significantly higher before home than away games, but this was apparently due not to a pre-home surge, but rather to a pre-away decline. Psychological measures also indicated that players were more self-confident when playing at home and more anxious when playing away. Clearly, as only two studies have directly assessed the challenge hypothesis as applied to human sporting situations, and have revealed potentially different mechanisms, additional research is required to confirm and possibly extend the human challenge hypothesis.

### The testosterone response to a challenge increases aggression?

A key aspect of the challenge hypothesis is that a competitive situation should lead to a rise in testosterone, which in turn should influence subsequent aggressive/competitive behaviours. This has not been easy to assess in humans: while the home advantage seen in many sports could be seen to be a reflection of this, it is unlikely that aggression is the key factor in this phenomenon. I am not aware of sporting statistics showing, for example, that teams playing at home commit more 'fouls' or are penalised for overly aggressive behaviours, compared to when playing away, though some studies have indicated that aggression levels are higher in the team playing at home (e.g. Kerr and Vanschaik, 1995; McGuire *et al.*, 1992).

Some studies do suggest that within a sporting context testosterone might be associated with 'aggressive behaviours' during the competition. For example, Suay *et al.* (1996) asked coaches to rate judo competitors during competitive bouts. Increases in testosterone from before the fights were associated with 'looking angry', 'responding to a challenge' and measures of 'offensive play' (study cited in Archer, 2006). In addition, Salvador *et al.* (1999) measured testosterone levels in twenty-eight male judo competitors before and after a competitive bout. The encounters were videotaped and judo specialists evaluated 'fighting', 'domination', 'attack' and 'defensive' behaviours. Testosterone levels before and after a bout were positively associated with the number of threats, fights and attacks made by an individual, with dominating behaviours only being associated with post-bout levels.

Surprisingly, few studies have assessed whether testosterone changes after a win or a loss influence subsequent behaviours. Mehta and Josephs (2006) took saliva samples from sixty-four males just before and fifteen minutes after a rigged competition (the males played against one another, with one being given an easier set of problems to solve). After the contest the players were asked whether or not they would like to compete again. Winners did not show the expected post-competition rise in testosterone; however, pre-test levels of this androgen were associated with subsequent alterations in testosterone fluctuations in the losers. Losers who showed an increase in testosterone were more likely to opt to play again, while losers who showed a decrease in testosterone were more likely to refuse to play again. Winners did not show this relationship, and so the authors speculated that losers who increased in testosterone chose to compete again in order to reclaim their lost status, while losers who showed a drop in testosterone did not want to compete again in order to avoid any further loss of status.

These authors also measured cortisol, and found that those high in baseline cortisol may have been especially vulnerable to the stress of a loss of status. Several studies have also routinely measured cortisol as well as testosterone within the context of competition, and there is evidence that cortisol also shows a pre-match rise (e.g. Bateup *et al.*, 2002; Booth *et al.*, 1989; Wagner *et al.*, 2002) but appears not to be related to other parameters (e.g. Gonzalez-Bono *et al.*, 1999; Salvador *et al.*, 1987). Clearly, future studies may wish to consider the role of this hormone in more detail. One might predict, for example, that individuals experiencing a loss may show a reduction in cortisol.

Other studies have relied upon laboratory paradigms in order to assess relationships between testosterone and aggressive behaviours. For example, Berman *et al.* (1993) measured testosterone in young males and then gave them a competitive reaction time task in which they were required to administer electric shocks to another individual. Initial levels of testosterone were associated with aggression (as measured by the strength of the shocks given), and higher testosterone individuals showed more motivation for the task.

Other studies have simply assessed the effects of testosterone supplementation on subsequent behaviours. While these have not been conducted in order directly to assess the challenge hypothesis, their findings are of some relevance. In a sample of hypogonadal males who were receiving either testosterone supplementation (at different doses) or a placebo over a three-month period, Finkelstein *et al.* (1997) reported that the males receiving testosterone scored significantly higher on physical aggression and aggressive impulses, but there were no effects on verbal aggression. O'Connor *et al.* (2002) assessed dose–response relationships among testosterone levels, behaviour and mood, in eight hypogonadal and thirty eugonadal males over an eight-week period. The hypogonadal males received doses of testosterone sufficient to elevate their levels to a normal baseline, while the eugonadal males received doses to boost their levels to a supraphysiological range. Testosterone administration did not lead to significant changes in a range of aggression and mood measures in the eugonadal males; the hypogonadal males displayed a reduction in negative mood.

In normal males, Kouri *et al.* (1995) gave increasingly high doses of testosterone cypionate over a six-week period (and a placebo), using a double-blind, cross-over design. Participants were tested for aggressive responses using a task in which they were paired with an unseen (fictitious) partner where they could reduce the amount of money given to the partner by pressing a button. They were led to believe that the partner was using this tactic against them, and those receiving higher doses of testosterone were more likely to make punitive responses in reply. As this paradigm could be argued to contain an element of challenge, then this study is nicely in line with the challenge hypothesis.

However, in his review of such studies, Archer (2006) cautions that overall there are few clear, strong positive relationships between testosterone administration and aggressive behaviours. This may be because the studies are highly variable, incorporating different methodologies and using widely different assessments of aggression, particularly measures that were designed to assess trait rather than state aggression.

A final piece of evidence concerns the administration of anabolic steroids. Increasing numbers of athletes, especially those involved in body building, weightlifting or field sports resort to anabolic steroids to increase muscle mass and reduce fatigue (Lamb, 1984), with anecdotal accounts of 'roid rage' being reported by steroid abusers. The dose levels in such instances are extremely high, and Strauss *et al.* (1985) reported that in female steroid abusers increases in libido and aggression were very common. Choi *et al.* (1990) monitored three male anabolic steroid users and three non-users over several months in which assessments were made on-drug and off-drug. Self-rated aggression increased significantly in the steroid users when on-drug, and multiple drug use led to severe hostility and aggression. However, anabolic steroids do not have the same physiological or neurological effects as testosterone, and abusers may well form a biased sample. In mice, recall that high doses of anabolic steroids only led to increases in aggressive behaviour in mice that already showed aggressive tendencies (Martínez-Sanchis *et al.*, 1998). Indeed, in humans, it has been noted that the personality profile of those who use AAS and display aggressive responses had already displayed such aggressive tendencies prior to using AAS (Bond *et al.*, 1995).

## Aggressive dominance is associated with testosterone levels?

Mazur and Booth (1998) pointed out that it is important to distinguish aggressive behaviour from dominance behaviour. They described dominance as 'apparent intent to achieve or maintain high status ... over a conspecific', and while overt physical aggression may form part of dominance, amongst primates (especially humans) direct aggression is rare. Human interpersonal behaviour is subtly concerned with dominance without causing actual physical harm, and they predicted that higher levels of testosterone encourage dominant behaviours that are intended to achieve, and then maintain, a higher social status. There are several lines of evidence in support of this assertion, though exactly what constitutes dominance behaviours, and how such behaviours can be reliably measured, still remains to be confirmed.

In a large sample of more than 1700 males aged thirty-nine to seventy, Gray *et al.* (1991) reported that score on a dominance inventory was significantly positively related to both free and bound testosterone, and to DHEA, but such relationships were small. Some societies exhibit a 'culture of honour', whereby, when challenged by others, males will lose face (and hence social status) if they fail adequately to defend their honour. Cohen *et al.* (1996) compared physio-logical and behavioural outcomes among male students from northern and southern states of the USA following an insult to their honour (a brave volunteer deliberately bumped into them and called them an 'asshole'). The southern students (the South is traditionally noted for its honour culture) showed a larger increase in testosterone and cortisol in response to the insult (the northerners remained relatively unaffected), and questionnaire items relat-ing to willingness to 'challenge' and 'domineer' also increased.

Dabbs *et al.* (2001) suggested that relationships between testosterone and dominance may be stronger in everyday situations when individuals engage in face-to-face social interactions. They argued that individual differences in testosterone may be reflected in expressive behaviours (mainly non-verbal) which may thus then influence the outcome of the situation. In their study, baseline testosterone levels were established in 122 male and 126 female undergraduates. Each was then videotaped as they walked into a room and spoke directly to a camera, met an experimenter, received an interview or talked with a peer. In the camera condition, high testosterone participants focussed more on the camera and displayed less nervousness. In the person condition, high testosterone individuals behaved in a more forward manner, though the authors did not elaborate on this further. In the interview condi-tion, high testosterone individuals walked more quickly to the interview table; in the peer condition the high testosterone participants were rated by judges as being more confident and relaxed, less friendly and less nervous. In both males and females, testosterone was associated with a more focussed and confident manner, expressive behaviours which, when displayed in the early stages of an encounter, lead to impression formation.

Other paradigms have assessed individual responses to facial stimuli. Faces displaying anger are particularly useful in this context as it can be argued that they signal imminent verbal or physical threat, and not surprisingly individ-uals selectively focus their attention on such faces (this makes good adaptive sense). In one study van Honk *et al.* (1999) assessed salivary testosterone in males and females, six hours, four hours and just before they took part in a task assessing selective attention to threat. In this task the participants were shown a series of eighty same-sex faces displaying either a neutral emotion or anger. Salivary testosterone six hours prior to the test was significantly associated with performance on the task – those with higher levels demon-strating greater attention to the angry faces. The relationship between testos-terone and the perception of a potential threat is not surprising, but the time lag is, and if correct surely does not represent an adaptive response. As testos-terone was measured in the morning (when levels show a natural diurnal peak) there could be a potential confound here.

In another study utilising a double-blind, placebo-controlled design, van Honk *et al.* (2001) demonstrated that a single administration of testosterone to women led to an accelerated heart rate, but only when they were exposed to angry faces. The authors suggested that this was due to the encouragement of dominance behaviours and an inclination towards aggression, but the alternative explanation is that the females felt more afraid when faced with such threatening faces.

Utilising controls not incorporated by the previously described studies, Wirth and Schultheiss (2007) assessed the possible relationships between testosterone and responses to angry faces in females and males. In both sexes similar responses were observed: morning levels of testosterone were associated with better processing of angry faces, but only in faces that had been presented too quickly to be consciously processed. The authors suggested that basal testosterone mediates the salience and/or incentive value of certain facial signals, such that high-testosterone individuals are more motivated to approach and engage in a dominance challenge, while low-testosterone individuals would be more likely to avoid such challenging signals. Such processing may be mediated by the amygdala, a structure vital for emotional processing and which contains androgen receptors.

## Additional factors

### Personality

It might be expected that testosterone levels would show some relationships with certain personality characteristics associated with dominance/aggressive behaviours, and associations have been reported between testosterone and various risky behaviours such as drug taking, gambling, seeking multiple sex partners, etc. (e.g. Dabbs and Morris, 1990; Mazur, 1995). One personality trait that has received much attention is that of 'sensation seeking', the extent to which an individual takes risks in order to experience a variety of new sensations. A commonly used test has been the 'Sensation-Seeking Scale-V', which consists of four subscales: Thrill and Adventure Seeking: AS; Disinhibition: DIS; Experience Seeking: ES; and Boredom Susceptibility: BS (Zuckerman, 1979).

Daitzman and Zuckerman (1980) had reported that males with higher testosterone levels scored higher on disinhibition (described in relation to the display of uninhibited behaviours, and a disregard of social constraint) than those with lower levels. Testosterone also correlated positively with extraversion, dominance, activity levels and sexual experiences, and correlated negatively with socialisation, self-control, introversion and depression. Rosenblitt et al. (2001) measured testosterone and cortisol in sixty-eight males and seventy-five females and asked them to complete the SSS-V. Males scored significantly higher on the total score, as well as on three of the subscales (TAS, ES and BS), but there were no significant associations between testosterone level and scores on the test, though lower levels of cortisol were associated with total score and all subscales except for TAS.

## Organisational effects

A key feature of the challenge hypothesis concerns the role of testosterone in activating certain dominance/aggressive behaviours within an appropriate social context. However, recall that the organisational/activational hypothesis (see chapter 3) states that certain behaviours are first organised (prenatally or shortly after birth) before being activated in adulthood. Is there thus any evidence that aggressive/dominance behaviours can be related to prenatal hormone exposure?

While such evidence is as yet limited, of interest are reports concerning relationships between prenatal hormone levels and certain personality traits assessed in adulthood. Resnick *et al.* (1993) reasoned that female members of opposite-sex fraternal twins might show masculinised behaviour patterns as they have shared a womb with a male foetus and thus perhaps have received greater exposure to testosterone as a result. While this remains speculative in humans, in mice it has been demonstrated that female foetuses located in-between two males do display higher levels of testosterone, and subsequently display increased aggressive behaviours (Vom Saal and Bronson, 1978; 1980). In their study, 422 pairs of twins completed the SSS-V form and results were as predicted, i.e. the female co-twins who shared a womb with a male displayed significantly higher scores on the DIS and ES subscales (performance on the other subscales was in the expected direction but was non-significant). Of course, as female co-twins were also reared closely alongside their brothers, a psychosocial influence cannot be ruled out.

Another line of enquiry relates to the 2D:4D ratio. Myself and colleagues measured 2D:4D in a sample of forty-eight males. We then showed facial photographs of these males to females, and asked the females to rate the males on how dominant they looked. While circulating testosterone was not related to dominance, 2D:4D ratio was significantly related, with a low ratio (higher prenatal testosterone exposure) being associated with higher ratings of dominance. We suggested that prenatal testosterone organises male facial features that are subsequently activated at puberty to reflect dominance characteristics (Neave *et al.*, 2003). Our findings are in accord with Campbell *et al.* (1998), who suggested that human dominance behaviours may reflect organisational rather than activational processes.

Bailey and Hurd (2005) measured 2D:4D in 298 male and female undergraduates and also asked them to complete an aggression questionnaire. As expected, males scored significantly higher in relation to 'physical aggression', 'verbal aggression' and 'hostility'; males with lower finger length ratios scored significantly higher on physical aggression only, and there were no relationships seen in the female sample. Fink *et al.* (2006) assessed 2D:4D and sensation seeking (using the SSS-V) in 278 German and UK undergraduates. In the male sample only, they reported a negative correlation between digit ratio and the total sensation-seeking score, and on the boredom susceptibility subscale. Finally, Mcintyre *et al.* (2007) looked at 2D:4D in relation to behaviours during a simulated war game in which players could opt to negotiate or attack the opponent. Males showed a greater propensity to engage in unprovoked attacks and, amongst males only, those who adopted such aggressive tactics were found to have a lower 2D:4D ratio.

## Conclusions

Previous conceptualisations of relationships between testosterone and aggressive/dominance behaviours have not really been viewed within a coherent theoretical context. Thus, researchers have simply spoken about unidirectional relationships in which it is assumed that increasing levels of testosterone lead to an increase in aggressive behaviours. Some animal models have conformed to this conception, but it soon became clear that such a simple way of viewing the relationship was missing the point somewhat. The challenge hypothesis was derived from a strong evolutionary position in viewing aggressive/dominance behaviours from an adaptive and life-history perspective. Thus, to have high levels of testosterone on a permanent basis would lead to negative physiological and health consequences, because androgens are known to impair the functioning of the immune system. Instead, if androgens can be maintained at a relatively low level, and then surge when the appropriate occasion demands, then this will be of greater benefit to the individual.

In his review, Archer (2006) concludes that the challenge hypothesis provides a fairly good 'fit' to the evidence as regards human aggressive/dominance behaviours and hormone levels, but notes that we remain a long way from completely understanding the possible adaptive basis of human aggression/dominance, and their neurohormonal underpinnings. There are, of course, other kinds of human aggressive behaviours that may not fit neatly into such conceptualisations, and it remains to be seen whether such behaviours can be linked to any hormonal processes. The roles played by testosterone and its metabolites, and by hormones such as estradiol and cortisol, remain to be fully ascertained. In addition, the mechanism(s) by which these hormones may work in relation to their receptors, their interactions with other neurotransmitters, and their effects within the central nervous system to trigger or maintain aggressive behaviours, remains to be determined.

# 11  Sex steroids and cognition

Previous chapters have identified the key role played by the endocrine system (especially the sex steroids) in sexual determination and differentiation, these effects stemming from both organisational and activational factors. The resulting effects on physiology and morphology are large, and are usually referred to in terms of being sexually dimorphic.[1] Chapter 7 also discussed the possible influence of hormones on neural differentiation, and, while contentious, the evidence appears to suggest that hormones (specifically the sex steroids), acting during prenatal and pubertal periods, sculpt certain brain regions into more masculine or feminine forms. If this is indeed the case, then we might expect that such neurological dimorphisms would be reflected in sexually dimorphic processing capabilities, especially ones related to the different hemispheres (e.g. verbal versus spatial processing). While this initially appears to be simple, there are several key issues that render the interpretation of available evidence difficult:

### What do we mean by cognitive processing?

A glance through any general cognitive psychology textbook (they all contain approximately the same information) will reveal a wide range of cognitive processes that we could consider. They normally include perception, attention, memory (long-term, short-term and working memory), visuospatial processes, executive processes, decision-making, problem-solving, reasoning and language. These processes can be assessed by a wide variety of tests utilising various methods of presentation and data capture. It is beyond the scope of this text to describe all such processes and how they are measured, but specific examples will be described in relation to supposed associations with the neuroendocrine system. A major problem is that while some tests are certainly more 'popular' than others, researchers often use widely different tests, and are often in disagreement as to precisely what each test might be measuring. Thus, tests may be described as 'spatial' but it soon becomes obvious that a spatial test might also be tapping into

---

[1] The word 'dimorphism' stems from the Greek for 'two forms'.

working memory, executive memory, reference memory, attention, etc., and may be measured in terms of accuracy, reaction times, errors made, etc. It is thus quite difficult to compare between different studies and draw definitive conclusions; exactly the same problem arises for verbal tests. Should one test show a relationship to the neuroendocrine system, then it is not easy to judge exactly which type of processing is supposedly being affected by hormones – if a spatial task contains various cognitive components then is it one and not another process being affected, or are all components similarly affected? While there is strong evidence that hormones do have an impact upon cognition, exactly what is being affected and how remains rather mysterious.

## Do the sexes differ in cognitive processing?

Deciding if there is a genuine difference between males and females in their performance of various cognitive tasks remains a highly controversial topic. Sex differences have been consistently reported for certain cognitive tasks, with the basic difference seeming to reflect better performance by males on certain spatial tasks, and better performance by females on certain verbal, memory and perceptual speed tasks. So, for instance, males have been found to excel at visuospatial, spatiotemporal and spatial-motor tasks, while females have been found to excel at verbal fluency, synonym generation, immediate processing, spelling and episodic memory (Halpern, 2000; Kimura, 2002). However, other studies report few consistent differences between the sexes on verbal and spatial processing (e.g. Caplan *et al.*, 1985; Hyde and Linn, 1988), and the dichotomy between verbal and spatial ability is by no means clear-cut, as females have been found to outperform males on certain spatial tasks, while males have been shown to outperform females on certain verbal tasks. In addition, there are several factors that undoubtedly have to be considered. These include age (cognitive performance changes over time, and males and females mature at slightly different rates) and other factors such as practice effects and sociocultural influences. These issues will be raised as appropriate when the evidence for the effects of hormones on such tasks are considered. There are numerous lines of evidence suggesting that sex steroids are related to certain aspects of cognition. These are as follows:

### Animal studies

Once more, rodent models have formed the backbone of evidence addressing hormone–behaviour relationships. Many studies have demonstrated that certain aspects of rodent cognitive performance differ between the sexes. For example, males outperform females on certain tests of spatial memory. This ability relates to the processing of non-verbal spatial information that is used to assist the individual when navigating around the environment, and remembering the location of certain important objects (i.e. food). Standard testing paradigms have utilised various types of maze. For example, the radial-arm maze was devised by Olton and Samuelson (1976) to measure spatial learning and memory in rats. The apparatus consists of eight equidistantly spaced arms, radiating out from a circular central platform. At the end of each arm there is a small depression where food rewards can be hidden out of sight of the hungry rodent. In a standard test session, the animal is placed in the central area and left free to roam around the maze collecting the food rewards. The walls of the arms are normally made of plexiglass so that the animal can use environmental features (e.g. posters on the walls of the laboratory) to help it to navigate successfully. As arms are sequentially visited then the food supplies disappear. By returning to an arm visited previously (now bereft of food), the animal is regarded as having made an error. As there are eight arms (some radial mazes contain as many as forty-eight arms), then perfect performance would be eight out of eight, and this presumably reflects superior working (i.e. short-term) memory for spatial information. Rats demonstrate excellent performance in this procedure as they only tend to make about a single error (they enter one previously visited arm), and thus have a success rate of around 88 (Olton and Samuelson, 1976).

Another commonly used task has been the Morris[2] water maze. This is not a maze as such, but rather a large tub of water with a small platform hidden beneath the surface (the water is made opaque so that the animal cannot see the platform). On the walls of the tub are visual cues, such as coloured shapes, which act as navigational reference points. When placed into the water the rat will swim around until it locates the platform. It climbs out and wet fur can be groomed. Various performance parameters can be recorded, such as the time spent in each quadrant of the pool, the total distance swum, but the most useful is perhaps the time taken (latency) to find the platform when the rat is replaced in the water (the platform does not move). It is assumed that a shorter latency reflects a better spatial memory for the platform's location. After sufficient practice, a rat will swim directly to the platform from any release point within the tub (Morris, 1984). It is assumed that the standard version of this task does not utilise spatial working memory, but rather reference memory (other types of memory can, however, be assessed).

Successful performance on such tasks appears to rely strongly upon the hippocampus, a complex structure in the telencephalon that plays a key role in learning and memory (especially that of a spatial nature). Recall that in chapter 4 I discussed the morphological effects of gonadal steroids within this structure, and provided the example of steroidal effects on dendritic spines. Both androgen and estrogen receptors are expressed in this structure (particularly on cholinergic terminals), so testosterone, or its aromatised metabolite estradiol, can act in a direct fashion, probably by influencing

[2] Named after its inventor Richard Morris.

dendritic spine density (Wooley *et al.*, 1997). In addition, the basal forebrain sends cholinergic and GABAergic projections to the hippocampal formation. If these pathways are severed then testosterone-induced increases in dendritic spine density are prevented (Kovacs *et al.*, 2003). The cholinergic neurons within the basal forebrain are also rich in estrogen receptors, and in females estradiol has been shown to have a direct influence on these neurons by increasing levels of choline acetyltransferase (ChAT), an important enzyme that is involved in creating molecules of the neurotransmitter acetylcholine (Gibbs, 1996).

As male rodents have been observed routinely to outperform females on the spatial tasks previously described (note, however, that not all researchers report a strong sex difference), studies began to focus on possible hormonal effects of this differential performance. Several reports showed that female rats exposed to testosterone during gestation or shortly after birth showed a pattern of male-typical performance in such tasks; male rats castrated before puberty displayed a more female-typical pattern of performance (e.g. Dawson *et al.*, 1975; Joseph *et al.*, 1978). Williams *et al.* (1990) attempted to discover if such differences in spatial ability were related to the organisational effects of gonadal steroids. In their study, four groups of rats were utilised: normal males; males castrated shortly after birth; females treated with estradiol benzoate for the first ten days postnatally; and normal females. To remove the potentially confounding effects of increased steroid activity at puberty, all animals were gonadectomised at around this time. Individuals were required to learn an eight-arm radial maze task, and then perform the test again under a variety of different conditions. The normal males and the females treated with estradiol performed significantly better than the castrated males and normal females. In an additional experiment the authors established that animals exposed to steroid hormones solved the task by relying upon a single environmental cue to assist with their navigation; in contrast, unexposed individuals appeared to use several different cues. The authors suggested that one possible action of gonadal steroids was thus to cause a perceptual bias such that the animal will selectively attend to a single environmental cue, rather than multiple ones, and thus acquire the task more quickly.

Using the Morris water maze, Roof and Havens (1992) assessed the effects of testosterone injections (or a control substance) during postnatal days 3–5 on spatial ability and hippocampal morphology, in male and female rats. When ninety days old, all animals were tested on this task, with latency to find the hidden platform on each trial being recorded. As often reported, normal males outperformed normal females, but the females who received testosterone performed as well as the control males. In terms of the morphology of the hippocampus, in the right hemisphere a region called the dentate gyrus was found to contain a thicker layer of granule cells in normal males compared to normal females. In the females receiving testosterone, these cells showed the same hemispheric asymmetry, being thicker in their right hemisphere. A strong correlation was observed between thickness of these cells and performance in the task, suggesting that testosterone actively changes this cell layer during the organisational period (remember that this period extends into the first few weeks of postnatal life in rats) and these alterations were reflected in enhanced spatial processing.

Using the same task but a different species (the meadow vole) Galea *et al.* (1995) focused on activational effects of gonadal steroids and spatial learning in males and females. Females were split into those that were paired with males (they were in constant behavioural estrus and displayed high levels of estrogens), and those that were not (they were not in estrus and displayed low levels of estrogens), and males were separated into low and high testosterone groups. Females exhibiting high levels of estradiol took significantly longer to reach the hidden platform than both of the male groups, and the female group with low levels of estradiol. In fact, females with low levels of estradiol performed no differently from the male animals. Testosterone levels did not appear to be related to spatial ability within males, as those with higher circulating levels performed no differently from those with low circulating levels. Other studies have noted that ovariectomised female rats subsequently treated with estradiol and progesterone showed impaired acquisition of the water maze task, compared to ovariectomised females treated with an inert substance (e.g. Chesler and Juraska, 2000).

Gibbs (2005) set out to assess the possible differential effects of testosterone and estradiol on cognitive performance in male rats. In this study male rats were first castrated and then implanted with slow-releasing capsules of either testosterone propionate, estradiol or a placebo substance. The animals were then trained on a delayed matching-to-position task (DMP) using another type of maze called a T-maze.[3] All of the rats were able to learn this task, with castration and testosterone supplementation in males having no effect upon task acquisition. Treatment with estradiol, however, did appear to enhance the rate at which this group learnt the task. When the task had been learnt to a criterion the group treated with testosterone were less affected by an increase in the delay (thirty, sixty and ninety second delays were used) between first and second choices. Thus, it appears that the effects of hormone treatment were task specific, estradiol enhancing task acquisition and testosterone enhancing working memory. In female rats ovariectomised and subsequently treated with estradiol, the same effect on the acquisition of a DMP task has also been noted (Gibbs, 2002).

---

[3] This is T-shaped. The animal is housed at the base of the T and allowed to explore the alleyway. At the end of the two arms is a small well hiding the bait. The animal is allowed free choice to enter a single arm and eat the food. It is then replaced at the base of the alley. On its next choice it is rewarded for entering the same arm that it entered previously (the well has been re-baited). The delay between first and second choice can of course be increased to make the task more difficult, and again this is assumed to be a test of spatial working memory.

These hormonal manipulations appear to be having a significant effect on dendritic spine density within the hippocampus, effects that appear to underlie the kinds of performance deficits seen. For example, Sandstrom and Williams (2001) ovariectomised female rats and then provided replacement therapy in the form of estradiol and progesterone prior to testing on a working memory task using the Morris water maze. Successful performance was observed in the replacement group, and the best performance was found to correlate closely with high spine density; poorer performance was associated with lower spine density. Estradiol does not, however, influence spine density in castrated male rats; density is reduced following castration and is restored by testosterone or dihydrotestosterone replacement (Leranth *et al.*, 2003).

Sandstrom *et al.* (2006) pointed out some inconsistencies in the evidence concerning the effects of sex steroids on spatial ability in rats. They observed that performance on reference memory tasks (as measured by the Morris water maze) seems to be impaired by the presence of estradiol and progesterone, while performance on spatial working memory tasks (radial arm, DMP) seems to be enhanced. Similarly, castration may have little effect on reference memory, but seems to have a consistently negative effect on performance in working memory tasks. To test this hypothesis they assessed the effects of castration on acquisition of a reference memory task (Morris maze) and a working memory task (DMP) using the same apparatus. Castration did not affect reference memory, but working memory was severely impaired, the implantation of testosterone-releasing capsules restoring the performance of the castrated males in the DMP task to that of the normal males. It is thus very important not to view all tasks containing elements of spatial processing as tapping into a generic 'spatial' ability. It is clear that different tests are tapping into slightly different aspects of visuospatial processing, and such processing may be differentially affected by the gonadal steroids.

## Organisational effects in humans

As previous chapters have highlighted the permanent organisational effects of the sex steroid hormones on certain brain regions, it is not surprising that investigators have attempted to establish possible relationships between hormonal exposure before birth and subsequent cognitive performance. Needless to say, establishing such relationships is less than simple, as of course we have no simple way in which to determine levels of hormones during this time.

### Evidence from 2D:4D

The previously discussed ratio between the second and fourth fingers (2D:4D) provides such a possible window (albeit a narrow one) into prenatal hormone events. Manning and Taylor (2001) established that a lower ratio (higher testosterone exposure) in males was associated with better performance on a standard test of visuospatial processing called the Mental Rotation Task (MRT).[4] It has since been established that performance on this task is sexually dimorphic, as males outperform females. Indeed out of all of the tests of spatial performance it yields the largest and most consistent sex difference (Voyer *et al.*, 1995). However, Coolican and Peters (2003) replicated this experiment but also included a sample of females. While they found the expected sex difference in digit ratio, and males performed significantly better than females on the MRT, there was no relationship between 2D:4D and performance on the task split by sex. Similarly, using just a sample of females, van Anders and Hampson (2005) failed to find a relationship between digit ratio and performance on three spatial tests (one was the MRT), and Rahman *et al.* (2004) also failed to find a relationship between 2D:4D and MRT performance in heterosexual and homosexual participants.

Using a different version of the MRT and another test involving the recall of object locations (a spatial task in which it has been reported that females excel), Poulin *et al.* (2004) found no relationships between 2D:4D and cognitive performance in the male sample, but did find significant positive relationships in the female sample. The higher the ratio (high estrogenylow testosterone) then the better the performance. However, utilising another version of the MRT, Kempel *et al.* (2005) reported that females with a more male-typical pattern of finger length ratios performed significantly better on such tasks compared to females possessing a more feminised finger length ratio, though the small sample in this study (twenty-three females as opposed to 132 in the Poulin *et al.*, experiment) renders their results speculative.

Burton *et al.* (2005) were able to replicate the finding reported by Poulin and colleagues; in their sample of ninety-three females a significant negative relationship between 2D:4D and performance on the MRT (and on a test of verbal fluency) was established. Thus, females with the more male-typical pattern performed the best. Interestingly, they also found that in their male sample, those with a more female-typical finger length ratio performed better on the MRT and on the verbal task. The authors suggested that this evidence is best interpreted within the concept of a curvilinear relationship between prenatal testosterone and subsequent cognition. In participants possessing a 'normal' hormonal profile before birth, there may be an optimal level of sex steroids around the centre of the male–female continuum, such that higher testosterone in females but lower testosterone in males may predispose towards optimal cognitive performance. This idea of a curvilinear relationship is not unprecedented. In support the authors point out that both

---

[4] The participant is usually shown a pair of three-dimensional objects (geometric shapes) and asked to decide whether they represent the same image or not (they are rotated differently). Shepard and Metzler (1971) established that the time taken for individuals to decide whether the shapes were the same or different was determined by the angle of rotation; the greater the angle of rotation then the longer the time to decide.

Geschwind and Galaburda (1987) and Nyborg (1983) have suggested similar mechanisms (testosterone for the former and estradiol for the latter). This issue will be further discussed in a subsequent section.

The evidence concerning 2D:4D and spatial ability is thus somewhat contradictory. Even if we focus on the most commonly utilised spatial test (MRT), some studies find no significant associations, others a relationship in males, and others a relationship in females. The direction of these relationships also demonstrates some variability. It is thus hard to know what to conclude: perhaps 2D:4D provides only a limited window into the development of this facet of spatial ability with its neurological substrate possibly being organised during different developmental time periods, and not necessarily the same in males and females (Putz *et al.*, 2004). Another issue to consider relates to the fact that performance on these paper-and-pencil spatial tasks may be strongly influenced by differential learning experiences, practice or sociocultural influences. It is also possible that individuals solve such problems using different strategies. Indeed there is some evidence that males rely on a more spatial strategy while females rely upon verbal strategies (Allen, 1974). The previously described studies have not really taken such considerations into account.

Relationships between prenatal hormone exposure and cognitive ability might be expected to be stronger in simple tasks assessing very basic fundamental cognitive processes that are perhaps less influenced by sociocultural factors, practice, differential strategies, etc. Surprisingly, little headway has been made here, though some authors have now begun to focus on certain numerical processing tasks. The rationale here is that while general mathematical ability is likely to be based upon learned skills partly derived from verbal reasoning and spatial aptitude abilities, evidence now strongly suggests that core aspects of numerical processing may be based around a primitive capacity to represent numerical quantity, this in itself being a category-specific, hard-wired process (Dehaene, 1997). Some preliminary evidence does suggest that numerical skills are better in individuals with more masculinised digit ratios (Luxen and Buunk, 2005), and that in boys specifically, lower digit ratio is associated with better performance on number knowledge, counting and visual numerical representations (Fink *et al.*, 2006).

Numerical processing is argued to consist of two core systems, the first being an exact system for representing small quantities, and the second being an approximate system for representing or comparing large magnitudes. This second system is characterised as being analogous to a mental number line. Evidence for this comes from a study in which participants were asked to judge whether two numbers were of the same or different magnitude. Individuals were found to respond faster to lower magnitude numbers with their left hand, but faster to higher magnitude numbers with their right hand. This link between the magnitude of number and their spatial position (left to right in individuals from cultures where reading is left to right) has been called the 'Spatial Numerical Association of Response Codes', or SNARC (Dehaene *et al.*, 1993).

Bull and Benson (2006) measured 2D:4D in thirty-seven males and thirty-eight females and asked them to complete a number judgement task from which they could calculate the SNARC effect. Irrespective of sex, individuals with a more masculine digit ratio showed a stronger SNARC effect. The authors suggested that this effect may represent the influence of prenatal testosterone on the automatic transcoding between the visual number code and the core magnitude representation of a mental representation of magnitude along a number line. However, as they did not include a control task they could not be certain of this relationship. Perhaps prenatal testosterone is simply related to any kind of (non-numerical) judgement related to the organisation of material in an ordinal sequence (e.g. days of the week).

More recently Brookes *et al.* (2007) assessed 2D:4D in relation to subitising, the rapid labelling of simultaneously presented small quantities. In this study, eighty participants made reaction time judgements to the number of dots in a random pattern presented very quickly. In females, lower 2D:4D was associated with higher response–hand difference scores (the difference between left and right hand response times), while this was lower in females with higher 2D:4D. No relationships were found in males. This may reflect the effects of prenatal testosterone on the degree of cerebral lateralisation for subitising, though of course hand difference may not be a truly accurate reflection of cerebral lateralisation. These latter studies do seem to suggest, though, that prenatal testosterone exposure might be better associated with basic elements of cognitive processing, elements that occur early in processing and perhaps tap into fundamental neurological processes. Further research on similar unconscious aspects of cognition, such as reaction time and perceptual processing, would clearly be of benefit here.

### Evidence from foetal hormone samples

A second line of organisational evidence concerns relationships between hormone levels measured directly in the womb, and subsequent cognitive performance. For example, Jacklin *et al.* (1988) took blood samples from the umbilical cord at birth in ninety-six infants, and then when the children were aged six and a half, their performance in reading, number, listening and spatial tests was assessed. While no sex differences were found in performance on these tasks, higher levels of perinatal testosterone and androstenedione were associated with poorer spatial performance in the girls. No relationships were found for the boys. However, the authors admit that hormone levels obtained at birth from the umbilical cord may not be representative of hormonal levels experienced during early stages of gestation when neural systems are being organised.

To address this methodological problem Finegan *et al.* (1992) therefore measured testosterone levels from amniotic fluid taken between weeks 14 and 20 of gestation in thirty males and thirty females. Four years later the children were asked to perform a range of cognitive tasks including language ability, puzzle solving, block building, form copying, counting, number knowledge and verbal memory. In the girls, a significant quadratic relationship was found between testosterone and language comprehension and conceptual grouping, such that low and high levels predicted poorer performance in these tasks; in addition an inverse linear relationship was found between testosterone and mathematical performance. No associations were found in males, and the authors suggested that the time of sampling may not have reflected a period of testosterone activity and subsequent neural differentiation. In addition, hormones obtained from the amniotic fluid are of course reflecting levels derived from the mother's adrenal glands; testosterone from the male's own testes may be more critical but of course this was impossible to measure. For the females, of course, exposure to the mother's testosterone is their prime source of this hormone, and thus one might expect to see some relationships between amniotic samples and subsequent cognitive ability.

Grimshaw *et al.* (1995b) performed a similar experiment. They took measures of testosterone from amniotic fluid between weeks 14 and 20 of gestation in twenty-nine girls and thirty-one boys. When the children were seven years old they performed a mental rotation task involving the judgement of whether a rotated teddy bear had the same or different arm raised. The authors controlled for spatial play experiences and made a note of the kinds of strategy used by the children to solve this tricky task. They found that prenatal testosterone was positively correlated with female performance on the rotation task; in those using a spatial strategy, higher testosterone levels were associated with faster response times and quicker rates of rotation. Once more no such relationships were found in boys.

Finally, Lutchmaya *et al.* (2002b) obtained samples of amniotic fluid from eighty-seven pregnant women and assessed levels of testosterone and estradiol. Their infants were tested at age eighteen months and twenty-four months on the size of their vocabulary.[5] At both testing stages the girls had a significantly larger vocabulary than the boys; within the sexes there was no association between vocabulary size and prenatal testosterone. However, when the sample was treated as a whole then testosterone was a significant predictor of vocabulary size, lower levels being associated with a larger vocabulary.

## Studies in hormonally abnormal groups

Various clinical conditions have been described in chapter 6 that involve atypical hormone exposure during the prenatal period, and these provide

---

[5] Parents simply ticked off the words they could say from a large standardised list.

investigators with another technique by which possibly to assess the organisational effects of hormonal exposure on subsequent cognition.

Females with congenital adrenal hyperplasia (CAH) have been exposed to high levels of adrenal androgens, resulting in physical masculinisation; as young children they also display masculinised toy preferences, tomboyism and more male-typical interests. One might perhaps expect that such females would display more male-typical cognitive skills, i.e. better spatial performance but reduced verbal performance. Indeed, Resnick *et al.* (1986) gave a battery of cognitive tests and a measure of early childhood activities to seventeen female and eight male children with CAH, and matched controls. While the CAH patients did not differ in terms of general intellectual functioning, compared to unaffected females the CAH girls showed significantly better spatial performance (on three out of the five spatial tests used). Other studies have not, however, demonstrated that CAH girls show enhanced spatial ability (e.g. McGuire *et al.*, 1975; Perlman, 1973), though it has been suggested that these studies did not use tests that demonstrate a sex difference between normal males and females (Collaer and Hines, 1995).

With regard to verbal skills, Resnick *et al.* (1986) found no differences between their female samples on a test of verbal fluency (in which females are thought to excel and CAH females might be expected to be correspondingly poorer). In support, other studies have reported that CAH girls show no evidence of impairments in verbal processing (McGuire *et al.*, 1975; Sinforiani *et al.*, 1994), but Nass and Baker (1991) reported that CAH girls had a significantly lower verbal IQ score compared to their unaffected sisters. In addition, Plante *et al.* (1996) reported that individuals with CAH had a higher prevalence of language disorders suggestive of a specific impairment in left-hemisphere processing; when MRI scans were conducted on these individuals it was confirmed that they showed an atypical pattern of cortical asymmetry, with the left hemisphere being reduced in relation to the right. More recently, Kelso *et al.* (2000) administered a battery of cognitive tests to seventeen CAH patients and seventeen normal controls. They also assessed handedness and cerebral lateralisation using a dichotic listening task. While a higher incidence of left-handedness was found in the CAH group (suggesting atypical hemispheric dominance), they did not display atypical cerebral lateralisation. The CAH group did however show a higher spatial IQ than verbal IQ.

In her review, Berenbaum (2001) criticised the majority of the studies cited above on methodological grounds, especially as regards the nature of the tests used supposedly to identify verbal or spatial impairments, though she did suggest that the evidence for an improvement in spatial ability was stronger than evidence suggesting a deficit in verbal ability. Berenbaum also pointed out that the majority of studies have focussed on the possible effects of high adrenal androgen levels, but there is a dearth of knowledge concerning the possible cognitive effects of the other hormonal problems associated with this group – e.g. high levels of ACTH.

Individuals with androgen insensitivity syndrome (AIS) are genetic and gonadal males who are insensitive to circulating levels of androgens before birth. Those with the complete form of AIS have a typical female phenotype, and are feminine in gender and behaviour. Imperato-McGinley *et al.* (1991) compared cognitive performance in ten AIS individuals with that of normal males and females. On a measure of perceptual organisation and various subtests of spatial ability, the AIS group performed significantly worse than the male group, and interestingly they also performed significantly worse than normal females on these same tests. The authors argued that this exaggerated female pattern of performance suggests that some androgen exposure in essential for normal females to show some spatial ability.

Another example concerns girls born with Turner syndrome, a variable condition but which typically involves pathological alterations to one of the X chromosomes (deletion, translocation or total absence). An additional feature is gonadal dysgenesis, such that affected females are unable to produce sex steroid hormones; while such females display a female phenotype (though with various physical abnormalities) they remain sexually immature unless provided with hormone replacement therapy at puberty. Early studies suggested that such individuals displayed mental retardation, but subsequent studies showed that Turner girls had normal intelligence, but showed a dissociation between verbal and spatial IQ, in that performance on verbal tasks was higher than performance on spatial tasks (e.g. Silbert *et al.*, 1977). Other authors failed to find a specific deficit in spatial ability per se, but instead suggested that the deficits observed were indicative of impairments in parietal lobe and frontal lobe functioning. Thus, Waber (1979) noted that Turner patients had specific difficulties with visual memory and motor coordination, deficits that may then be reflected in seemingly poorer spatial ability; visuospatial tasks not relying upon such basic processes appeared to remain unaffected. Waber suggested that the lack of exposure to prenatal estrogens does not have a specific effect on a certain type of cognitive ability, but rather a general effect on various brain regions.

Support for this came from Rovet and Netley (1982), who assessed performance by thirty-one Turner syndrome girls and the same number of matched controls on the mental rotation test. The Turner group performed significantly worse than the control girls on this task, implying a specific spatial deficit. However, analysis of their performance revealed that they were significantly slower to solve the task, and they differed in the slope component of the linear function relating reaction times to angular disparity (recall that as the angle of rotation between items increases, then reaction times to decide if they are same or different increases in a linear fashion – this is the slope function). The authors suggested that this then reflects a deficit in reaction times rather than in spatial ability. In turn this may reflect a general encoding problem. In a second experiment they compared performance on a verbal task (a test of sentence verification) and the groups did not differ in terms of performance, but analysis of reaction times showed once more that the Turner girls were significantly slower to make their judgement. Other studies have also found that Turner individuals display a specific deficit in long-term memory, further evidence that this condition reflects global gener-alised impairments rather than specific ones affecting primarily spatial processing (Pennington *et al.*, 1985).

Following initial suggestions by Money (1973), that were later echoed by Waber (1979), McCauley *et al.* (1987) hypothesised that the pattern of deficits observed in Turner syndrome might reflect specific functional impair-ments in right-hemispheric processing. They noted that damage to certain regions of the right hemisphere is also associated with deficits in facial and emotional processing; as Turner girls have also been reported to have psy-chosocial problems, especially in relation to poor peer relationships, a deficit in their ability to process facial and affective information may underlie this. McCauley and colleagues thus tested seventeen Turner girls and matched controls on several cognitive tests, an assessment of social competence and a measure of affective discrimination. Several cognitive impairments were found (especially in tests assessing spatial and attentional processing). In addition, the Turner girls were less accurate at discriminating between faces displaying various emotions, and were rated as being less socially competent. However, a study utilising measurements of regional cerebral glucose utilisa-tion in Turner girls revealed decreases in activation in both left *and* right parietal hemispheres, thus providing evidence against selective right parietal hemisphere deficits (Clark *et al.*, 1990).

A possible explanation for these discordant findings comes from work by Skuse *et al.* (1997). Turner's individuals inherit two X chromosomes – one from their mother and one from their father. One of these remains normal while the other is affected to some degree or other. Previous studies have not differentiated between which of the chromosomes has been affected, and have thus tended to describe Turner girls in homogenous terms – perhaps focussing on the extent of the damage to an X chromosome, but not reveal-ing which chromosome has been affected. In their study, Skuse *et al.* (1997) compared social cognition, and verbal and spatial skills in eighty Turner females, in whom fifty-five received their unaffected X chromosome from their mother, while the remainder received a normal X chromosome from their father. Those carrying a single maternally derived X chromosome performed significantly worse on all cognitive tasks than those whose X was paternally derived. They were also more likely to demonstrate social behav-ioural problems at school. Future studies should thus take this crucial factor into account.

A final example concerns evidence from children exposed to very high levels of synthetic estrogens during prenatal development, via diethylstilbestrol (DES) prescribed to their mothers to reduce the likelihood of miscarriage. DES has been shown to masculinise and defeminise the foetus (see chapter 7) and thus one would perhaps predict that such individuals might display enhanced male-typical cognitive skills. However, studies have failed to demonstrate that DES-exposed females perform in a male-typical manner on various cognitive tests, though they may display a more male-typical pattern of language lateralisation (studies reviewed in Collaer and Hines, 1995).

Evidence from individuals exposed to an abnormal hormonal environment before birth is thus somewhat difficult to conceptualise. While some evidence suggests that individuals exposed to higher levels of androgens perform more like males on certain spatial tasks, the evidence is contradictory. This may partly stem from the fact that a variety of different spatial tests are used, though whether these tests tap into genuine spatial processing, or perhaps other domains of cognitive processing, remains to be determined.

## Circulating hormone levels and cognitive performance

It is known that key aspects of physiology and behaviour are organised before, and shortly after, birth, and then perhaps again at puberty. After this time it is assumed that the behaviours that have been organised are then activated by fluctuating hormone levels. We might thus expect to see relationships between levels of certain hormones and cognitive ability, especially perhaps in those domains that have shown a reliable sex difference. The evidence for this simple idea will be addressed in males and females separately.

### Relationships between testosterone and cognition in males

Before hormone assays were routinely available, researchers used physical markers to 'guess' hormone status. Thus, males characterised as having a 'masculine' body build were assumed to have higher levels of testosterone than males with a more androgynous build (e.g. Petersen, 1976). More recently, Beech (2001) pointed out that male pattern baldness is mainly caused by increases in dihydrotestosterone, which attacks the hair cells.[6] Beech examined variations in male pattern baldness and performance on the MRT, and found a curvilinear relationship in that mild/moderate hair loss was related to better performance. Needless to say, such relationships (while based on good reasoning) may be rather variable, and the results from these kinds of studies should be treated with caution. By the beginning of the 1980s, hormone assays were routinely available, and researchers were able to rely upon more quantitative assessments of hormone status.

Shute *et al.* (1983) noted that sex differences in spatial ability seem to emerge at around the ages of eight to ten when males begin to produce high levels of testosterone, and become maximal during puberty when the sexes are very different in terms of their hormonal profiles. In their study they investigated the relationship between androgen levels from blood plasma

---

[6] The drug Finasteride inhibits 5-alpha reductase and thereby reduces DHT expressed in the scalp and is an effective hair loss therapy in some males.

(their radioimmunoassay appears not to have been that selective) and performance on four standard spatial ability tests in males and females aged sixteen to forty-one. They reported the expected sex differences in performance on these spatial tasks, with males outperforming females, and not surprisingly males also displayed significantly higher levels of androgens. In terms of the relationship between androgens and spatial ability, a curvilinear relationship was found: in females, those with the highest levels performed the best, but in males, those with low/median levels performed better.

In a second experiment, males and females were split into those having high or low levels of androgens, and the authors confirmed that females with high levels and males with low levels performed better than females with low levels and males with high levels. Similarly, Gordon and Lee (1986) focussed on levels of follicle stimulating hormone (FSH) and luteinising hormone (LH), gonadotropins that stimulate the gonads to produce the sex steroids. In males, higher concentrations of FSH were related to poorer performance in four spatial tests. In females, higher levels were associated with poorer performance on one spatial task, but better performance in two verbal tasks. Testosterone levels were only significantly related (positively) to performance on one spatial task.

Christiansen and Knussmann (1987) carried out a similar experiment, taking serum and salivary assays of testosterone and dihydrotestosterone in 117 males, along with measures of performance on five spatial and six verbal tests. They, however, found a linear relationship, with levels of both hormones correlating negatively with verbal performance, but positively with spatial performance. Using the same two hormones, McKeever and Deyo (1990) assessed their relationship to performance on two spatial tests in fifty-eight males. Neither showed any significant relationship to task performance. However, the ratio between dihydrotestosterone and testosterone was associated with performance on one of the tasks; those participants whose values deviated most from the group means (higher testosterone being implicated) performed significantly better on the tests.

Gouchie and Kimura (1991) took salivary measures of testosterone from forty-two males and forty-six females and grouped the participants in terms of them having high or low testosterone levels. The volunteers then performed a battery of cognitive tasks incorporating assessments of spatial ability, mathematical ability, perceptual speed, verbal articulation and vocabulary. Low-testosterone males were found to outperform high-testosterone males and low-testosterone females on the paper folding task, with high-testosterone women outperforming the low-testosterone women. The same pattern of performance was revealed on the mathematical aptitude tasks, but on mental rotation ability only low-testosterone males performed better than low-testosterone females. In tests favouring females, there was no clear relationship between testosterone and cognition.

Using a sample of 114 !Kung San bushmen from Namibia, Christiansen (1993) assessed relationships between a range of hormones derived from both serum and saliva samples and cognitive performance. While estradiol levels showed no significant relationships, testosterone (from both blood and saliva) showed significant positive associations with performance on tests of spatial ability, but a negative association with verbal fluency.

Thus far we are seeing a complex pattern emerging, with some studies reporting linear relationships, others reporting curvilinear relationships (seemingly different between the sexes), and some finding no significant relationships at all. One possible explanation for these discordant findings comes from a study by Moffat and Hampson (1996), who assessed relationships between salivary testosterone and performance on two spatial and two verbal tasks in forty males and females. A key difference between their study and the preceding experiments was that they made a note of the hand preference of their participants. One must assume, though, that previous studies have used predominantly right-handed individuals. In right-handed individuals only, they found a non-linear relationship between testosterone and spatial performance (a composite measure from scores on both tasks), with moderate levels of testosterone being associated with better spatial ability. They thus suggested that a curvilinear relationship might only be found in right-handed individuals. However, this only applied to the data as a whole (i.e. including males and females); in the male sample alone, they actually found a negative linear relationship. It is perhaps not surprising that if we take a sexually dimorphic task such as mental rotations and a sexually dimorphic pattern of hormone levels (as normally seen between males and females) and look at them in conjunction, what emerges is a curvilinear relationship.

Thus, myself and colleagues found a curvilinear relationship between circulating testosterone and mental rotation performance when data from males and females were included together (Neave et al., 1999). Silverman et al. (1999), however, suggested that possible relationships between hormones and cognitive performance should be assessed within and not between sexes. In their study, fifty-nine males provided salivary samples at 8 a.m. and 10 p.m. and performed the mental rotation test and two control tasks at the same times. Testosterone was significantly higher in the morning session, as was performance on the mental rotation task. Here then a significant positive relationship was found between testosterone levels and mental rotation ability.

One issue relates to the mechanism by which androgens produce their effects. In animals it has been shown that testosterone exerts its physiological effects after being converted into estradiol or dihydrotestosterone. The studies just described provide no indication of whether testosterone is indeed the critical hormone or whether its metabolites are more important. Indeed it has been suggested that in humans estrogen may be the crucial hormone, with a curvilinear relationship being expected between levels of this hormone and cognition (Nyborg, 1983). That would fit neatly with those studies reporting curvilinear associations between testosterone and certain cognitive abilities. Clearly studies need to take a range of hormone parameters in order to begin to address this issue.

Another problem with these studies that have supposedly assessed the activational effects of steroid hormones concerns the issue that adult hormone levels may reflect to a greater or lesser extent prenatal sex steroid exposure. As such, studies only typically take a snapshot of hormone levels and cognitive performance, and thereby might not be expected to display consistent relationships (e.g. Halari *et al.*, 2005). Of potentially greater interest is seeing if alterations in hormone levels lead to differential performance on certain tests. In males this could be done by assessing performance at different times of the day (testosterone levels are higher in the morning than in the evening). Indeed, Furnham and Rawles (1988) observed that a group of males tested at 9.30 a.m. performed better than groups tested at 1.30 p.m. and 5.30 p.m., on a mental rotation task. This suggests that higher testosterone led to better performance but the authors did not directly assess hormone levels, nor indeed consider their variability in their study. Moffat and Hampson (1996) did conduct hormone assays and found that males tested later on in the day (11.45 a.m.) outperformed those tested earlier on (8.15 a.m.), despite the fact that there was only a few hours separating the groups.

Another problem relates to the fact that different studies have relied upon different cognitive tests. Even studies using the most common test of spatial ability have used slightly different versions that have the same general principle, but differ in terms of presentation, timing and scoring. It is also the case that studies typically relate hormone levels to the overall score obtained and describe that score as reflecting 'mental rotation performance' while not explicitly defining precisely what aspects of performance may have been influenced. Hooven *et al.* (2004) pointed out that studies have not distinguished between the various processes involved, namely encoding the stimuli, transforming the objects in mental imagery, comparing between different objects and producing a response. In their study they made some attempt to address this by focussing specifically on response times (reaction times) and error rates that enabled them to compute the slope (the effect of rotating the object in terms of time or accuracy) and the intercept (the contribution of non-rotational processes). In a sample of twenty-eight males, higher levels of salivary testosterone were associated with faster responding and reduced error rates. In addition, testosterone showed no relationship to the slope function, but did with the intercepts.

This suggests that testosterone is not specifically influencing the spatial component of the task (the rotational aspect) but rather non-spatial elements such as processing speed. Support for this notion comes from a study by Müller (1994) in which it was demonstrated that higher levels of testosterone in males were associated with faster reaction times. However, Falter *et al.* (2006) were unable to find a relationship between testosterone and either slope function or

the intercepts. They pointed out that Hooven *et al.* (2004) had shown participants a video prior to assessing cognitive performance. One such video contained sexually arousing material which did not directly influence testosterone
levels, but could have influenced arousal, something that the intercept values
are apparently sensitive to. More confusingly, a recent study by Yang *et al.*
(2007) reported that in a sample of ninety-two Chinese males (the largest
sample thus far reported in studies of this kind), testosterone was significantly
associated with the slope function, but not the intercept – the opposite finding
to that reported by Hooven and colleagues! To clarify, as the task became
more difficult when the angular disparity increased, high testosterone males
did not slow down as much as low testosterone males. Clearly, further studies
are required here to solve this conundrum.

Recently, an additional issue has been raised. Newman *et al.* (2005)
pointed out that the main assumption has been that testosterone influences
cognitive performance by initially shaping brain structures and then activating the same structures during and after puberty. In an interesting side-step
they note that in terms of the challenge hypothesis (see previous chapter) a
key assumption is that testosterone should only influence behaviour when
there is a perceived threat to one's social status. They hypothesised that individuals with higher circulating levels of testosterone may have a greater need
for status than those lower in testosterone, and this need may be activated
when their status is challenged. They thus predicted that the cognitive performance of high-testosterone individuals will reflect their perceived status in
the testing situation: when their perceived status is high they should perform
well, but when they perceive that their status is lower they will activate behaviours to redress the balance and their performance will be negatively affected.
In order to test this, males and females performed two cognitive tasks (mental
rotation and verbal fluency) in two conditions (high status and low status).
Perceived status was manipulated by telling the volunteers that they were
taking part in a group task in which they were either a leader or a follower.
As predicted, on both tasks high-testosterone individuals performed worse
when in the low-status condition, and better when in the high-status condition. In a neutral condition where status was not manipulated task performance did not differ. This study then suggests that cognitive performance may
be influenced not only by hormonal events but also by the social environment, in this case perceived social status.

*Fluctuations in cognitive performance across the menstrual
cycle in females*

Most women between the ages of fifteen and fifty are regularly affected by the
endocrinological and physiological changes that are associated with the cyclical process of ovulation and menstruation (see chapter 2). For the sake of
clarity I have grouped the evidence for these relationships in terms of specific
cognitive domains.

**General intellectual ability**     A characteristic feature of the phase of the cycle immediately before and after the onset of menstruation (paramenstruum) is the subjective perception of reduced intellectual efficiency. If such impairments are genuine, then this could have a major impact upon academic achievement in the many thousands of females currently in the education system. While Wickham (1958) reported no effect of menstrual cycle phase on academic test performance, considerable shockwaves were felt when Dalton (1960) reported that schoolgirls aged eleven to seventeen showed clear decrements in academic performance during their premenstrual and menstrual phases. The conclusions of this influential study were criticised on statistical and methodological grounds, but it had a major impact on stimulating research in this controversial topic. For example, Sommer (1972) assessed critical thinking and coursework examination performance in females during different phases of the cycle, and also incorporated a group of contraceptive pill users. There was no effect of cycle phase on performance, but Sommer did admit that the test of critical thinking utilised was not designed specifically to assess fluctuations over time. Walsh *et al.* (1981) looked at examination performance over an academic year in 244 female medical students. Performance on exams taken during the menstrual phase showed no impairment compared to those taken at other stages of the cycle. A similar finding was reported by Asso (1986), who found no significant effects of cycle phase on exam performance in female psychology students. Richardson (1989) conducted a survey of 277 female students and found that each reported on average around thirteen negative symptoms during their premenstrual phase (mood swings, weight gain, lethargy, irritability, etc.) and clearly felt subjectively that their performance did vary according to their cycle. Objective assessments of this, however, revealed no major impact.

**Basic cognitive processing**     An initial element of cognitive processing of course relates to the actual perception of the stimulus, and thus some researchers have attempted to see if there are cyclical differences in visual perceptual processing. Thus, it has been reported that visual sensitivity alters as a function of the menstrual cycle, with acuity being lower during ovulation compared to menstruation (Scher *et al.*, 1985). However, other studies have shown that scotopic visual sensitivity (night vision) is increased during ovulation (Barris *et al.*, 1980). In terms of psychophysical processes, Dye (1992) reviewed the effects of visual information processing during the cycle, focussing on her own studies using critical flicker fusion (CFF).[7] In a sample of thirty-four women, the CFF threshold was found to vary significantly as

---

[7] This task requires the participant to discriminate between flicker and fusion in a set of lights that are rapidly lit in an ascending or descending sequence, and is assumed to reflect CNS activation.

a function of the menstrual cycle, with a higher threshold (reflecting better performance) being found during the premenstrual phase.

If visual processing is affected, then this might have knock-on effects for later stages of cognitive processing. Indeed, researchers have also assessed possible effects of cycle phase upon reaction time performance. Results have, however, been equivocal. For example, Zimmerman and Parlee (1973) reported no changes in simple and choice reaction time performance, Hutt *et al.* (1980) found no influence of phase on choice reaction time speed, while Gimerale *et al.* (1975) reported a significant impairment in choice reaction time during menses, and Ho *et al.* (1986) found faster choice reaction time performance during ovulation. Hunter *et al.* (1979) assessed performance on three reaction time tests, each varying in complexity, over the course of two menstrual cycles in thirty-six females, half of whom were taking the contraceptive pill. Estrogen concentration was established by radioimmunoassay. For simple and complex reaction times, no effects of the cycle were seen. However, choice reaction time performance did show an effect of phase as performance was significantly slower during the premenstrual phase only in those females not using the contraceptive pill, suggesting that some aspects of rapid decision-making are being influenced by the phase of the cycle.

**Memory**   Hartley *et al.* (1987) assessed performance on several memory tasks in thirty females who were asked to monitor their body temperature on a daily basis in order to identify the well-documented rise in temperature that accompanies ovulation. When ovulation occurred, and again during menstruation, the volunteers completed a test of logical reasoning, the recall of acoustically or semantically similar words, and the immediate and delayed recall of prose. At ovulation, performance on the logical reasoning task was impaired, as was performance on the recall of semantically similar words. Recall of acoustically similar words was correspondingly better during menstruation. While this study was more concerned with establishing relationships between hormone fluctuations and circadian performance changes, it did suggest that semantic processing may be affected by higher levels of estradiol associated with ovulation.

Phillips and Sherwin (1992) assessed visual memory performance in twenty-five females during their menstrual and luteal phases, with hormone concentrations being established by radioimmunoassay. Performance on a delayed recall element of a visual reproduction test was significantly worse during menses. In addition, levels of estradiol were positively correlated with paired-associate recall during the luteal phase. This decrease in visual memory appeared to be particularly apparent in some of the women and was associated with levels of progesterone during the luteal phase. However, this subsample reported more dysphoric mood changes during the menstrual phase and thus a key variable could relate to the well-documented affective symptoms associated with the paramenstruum. Most women experience a variety of physical, psychological and behavioural changes during this phase, these symptoms were originally described by Frank in the 1930s, who also coined the term 'Premenstrual Tension' or PMT (now called 'Premenstrual Syndrome' or PMS) to describe their negative effects.

The general pattern of symptoms associated with this phase has been thought to equate with the theoretical construct of state anxiety, defined by Spielberger (1972) as 'subjective, consciously perceived feelings of tension and apprehension, and activation of the autonomic nervous system'. If one assumes that the physiological processes that occur during menstruation, or indeed the anticipation of the occurrence of such symptoms, constitute an internal source of stress and anxiety, and as anxiety is known to interfere with cognition, then we may expect that premenstrual symptoms would disrupt cognition. In general, it is agreed that anxiety and stress interfere with working memory more so than consolidation or retrieval, so it could be predicted that tests of short-term retention (i.e. immediate recall) would be most affected during the premenstruum. Richardson (1991) tested this hypothesis in pill-users and non-pill-users, and a control group of males. Each group was assessed on the immediate serial recall of sequences of phonemically similar and phonemically distinct words at two fortnightly sessions. The results demonstrated that there was no overall difference between male and female performance, there were no differences between females tested during menstruation or during the intermenstruum, and while females taking oral contraceptives produced higher scores, this did not reach significance. So, the menstrual phase per se did not appear to be associated with academic impairment, or with deficits in specific cognitive domains.

In her review of previous studies, however, Sommer (1992) noted some issues had typically not been addressed. First, it is understood that the menstrual cycle is both a physical and a psychological process, and it is rare then, for example, for hormone levels to be ascertained along with individual perceptions concerning the effects of the physical changes to be measured, within the same study. Second, studies vary markedly in how the phases of the cycle have been delineated. For example, major problems exist when researchers assume particular levels of certain hormones based upon counting the days from the onset of menstruation. Indeed, Gordon et al. (1986) took blood samples from twenty-four volunteers over the course of their cycle and found that almost half of the women were not in their 'expected' phase as regards counting off the days, when precise hormone levels were established. Thirdly, many studies have not used the more powerful repeated-measures design and have not included adequate control groups. Finally, cognitive assessments have been utilised that have not been all that specific, or perhaps sensitive enough in order to detect perhaps what are likely to be subtle changes.

If there are robust effects on memory caused by fluctuations in hormone levels then it would help if researchers could pinpoint which regions of the brain are being affected. In light of the critical role played by the hippocampus in certain aspects of mnemonic processing, and the evidence concerning alterations in dendritic spine density via hormonal fluctuations in rodents (chapter 4), it is not surprising that researchers have focussed on this structure in humans. However, thus far there is little direct evidence to associate changes in the hippocampus with hormonal fluctuations and performance on memory tasks. Keenan *et al.* (2001) suggested that searching for such relationships might well prove to be fruitless, as brain regions beyond the hippocampus also play a vital role in encoding, storing and retrieving certain kinds of information. They suggest that attention should be directed towards the frontal lobes, because learning and memory are under the direction of frontally mediated processes referred to as executive functioning, a generic term that covers aspects such as attention, working memory, response inhibition, set switching, behavioural monitoring and dual task processing. Evidence for the effects of estrogens on prefrontal cortex has been assessed using hormone replacement paradigms, usually in postmenopausal females, and as such will be briefly reviewed later in this chapter.

**Tasks sensitive to sex differences**    Other researchers have tried to focus on specific aspects of cognition that may be more sensitive to hormonal fluctuations, and have also attempted to provide neurological explanations for their predictions/findings. Thus, Komnenich *et al.* (1978) utilised more sensitive tests to address this issue, and took blood samples from which to measure gonadal steroids at four different menstrual phases in pill-using and non-pill-using females. Performance on automatic tasks (these require simple repetitive responses) was enhanced around ovulation when estrogen levels were high, but performance on tasks requiring the inhibition of attention was impaired during this phase. To explain these findings, Broverman *et al.* (1981) noted that performance on automatic tasks is improved by adrenergic stimulants such as caffeine, while performance on perceptual-restructuring tasks is impaired by such stimulants. They suggested that estrogen may act as an adrenergic stimulant by prolonging the action of norepinephrine by suppressing the concentration of monoamine oxidase (MAO), and so argued that performance on automatic tasks may improve when estrogen levels are high (pre-ovulation) but drop when levels are low (menstruation). They assessed this notion in eighty-seven female students (not using oral contraceptives) who performed the two types of task at days 10 and 20 of the cycle. Results indicated that the predicted changes in performance on the two tasks over the cycle did indeed occur, but recent advances in the understanding of neuropharmacology have indicated that the hormone-neurotransmitter mechanism described by Broverman *et al.* may not be strictly correct.

Hampson and Kimura (1988) instead proposed that high levels of estrogen and progesterone (seen after ovulation) would lead to better performance on tasks in which females typically excel, whilst low levels of these hormones (at menses) would be detrimental. The opposite would be true for tasks on which females typically perform badly. In their study, thirty-four non-pill-using women were tested during menstruation and the midluteal phases on a perceptual task normally favouring males, and several tests of speeded tests of manual coordination normally favouring females. The expected dissociation was found, in that performance on the spatial task was better during menstruation and worse during the midluteal phase; in contrast, performance on the tasks in which females normally excel was enhanced during the midluteal phase compared to the menstrual phase.

In a subsequent set of studies, Hampson used a wider set of tests to assess performance at varying phases of the cycle, confirming that performance on tasks favouring females was enhanced during the luteal phase, relative to the menstrual phase (Hampson, 1990a). In another study Hampson (1990b) noted that assessing cognitive performance during the midluteal phase may be inappropriate, as both progesterone and estradiol are high at this time. Assessing performance during the late follicular phase (just prior to ovulation) might provide a clearer picture as only estradiol levels are high during this phase. So, female performance was assessed on a battery of cognitive and motor tasks during these phases and, as predicted, performance on articulatory and fine motor skills was improved in the preovulatory phase compared to menses, while performance on spatial tests showed the opposite pattern. In addition, levels of estradiol were taken from blood samples, and a non-linear relationship between estradiol levels and performance on one spatial test was found, such that medium levels predicted better performance. This then was in accord with Nyborg's (1983) prediction that estradiol levels and cognitive performance should show a curvilinear relationship.

Utilising the test that typically reveals a robust sex difference (mental rotations), Silverman and Phillips (1993) compared males, pill-using females and non-pill-using females on MRT performance during menstruation and the luteal phase. In an initial experiment they reported the usual male advantage on this test, and that the pill-using females were more accurate. At menstruation, female performance was significantly better than at post-ovulation, and again the pill-users performed better. Other tasks (digit symbol, space relations and anagram solving) did not show any of these features. Several years later Phillips and Silverman (1997) focused on possible changes in spatial performance between menstrual and midluteal phases in sixty non-pill-using females. As in previous studies, spatial ability during the midluteal phase was decreased relative to the menstrual phase; this was especially so for tests involving three-dimensional processing. As both of these studies tested females in the luteal phase (they did not use hormone assays to verify this though), it is impossible to say whether the change in performance reflected the impact of estradiol, progesterone or both.

Halpern and Tan (2001) assessed immediate processing and mental rotation ability in females over the course of their menstrual cycle. A small enhancement on immediate processing performance was observed during the preovulatory phase (estrogen levels are rising), but in addition they found that performance on the mental rotation task also showed two peaks, corresponding to early follicular and midluteal phases, when levels of estrogen are high (in the former) and estrogen and progesterone are high (in the latter). Rosenberg and Park (2002) tested eight women at four different times during their cycle on a modified version of the mental rotation test, and a test of verbal working memory. A group of ten women currently using the contraceptive pill served as controls. While spatial ability showed no fluctuation over the four test phases (only eight trials were conducted each time though), verbal working memory did show a curvilinear relationship with cycle phase, with higher levels of estrogen being associated with improved memory span. This fluctuation was not seen in the pill-users.

Epting and Overman (1998) criticised previous studies for not utilising direct hormonal assessments and instead relying upon other indirect means to determine hormone levels (e.g. by simply counting the days from menses). In their review of some sixty-two studies thus far that had assessed cognition during the menstrual cycle, only 17 has used direct hormone measures, and they suggested that this could be a reason for the equivocal results obtained. In their study, upon determining ovulation by an ovulation-detection kit, they compared performance during menstruation and midluteal phases (a sample of males was also included). While they found sex differences in performance in the predicted direction on four out of the six tests used, they found no effect of menstrual cycle phase on female cognitive performance. However, using a more detailed method of assessing hormone levels, Hausmann *et al.* (2000) collected blood samples in three-day intervals over six weeks from twelve women, and correlated levels of testosterone, estradiol, progesterone, LH and FSH with performance on three spatial tests during menses and midluteal phases. Performance on the mental rotation task altered significantly over the cycle, with performance being better at menses; this was related positively to testosterone level, but negatively to estradiol level.

One theory that may explain fluctuations in cognitive performance over the cycle relates to how the brain processes visually presented information. Studies have established that the left hemisphere is faster and more accurate at processing language-related information, while the right hemisphere is better at processing spatial/facial information (see chapter 7). Kimura and Hampson (1993) proposed that fluctuations in hormone levels (specifically estrogen) may alter hemispheric processing, such that high estrogen levels may facilitate visual processing in the left hemisphere relative to the right hemisphere. In a test of this theory, Rode *et al.* (1995) measured levels of estrogen and progesterone throughout the cycle, and correlated fluctuations in these hormones with female performance on a lexical decision task (shown to yield a left-hemisphere advantage) and a figure comprehensions test (yields a right-hemisphere advantage). The volunteers were tested at menses and the luteal phase, and while the lexical decision task showed no effect of menstrual cycle, performance on the figural comparison task showed an alteration in hemispheric asymmetry over the cycle. Thus, during the luteal phase (high estrogen and progesterone) lateralisation showed a reduction, in that performance was equivalent in both hemispheres; during menses, on the other hand, the right hemisphere performed significantly faster than the left hemisphere. However, this degree in the change of lateralisation was not related to fluctuations in estrogen or progesterone.

According to Compton and Levine (1997), a possible confound here is mood, a factor that is known to vary markedly throughout the cycle, and has been found to have a negative influence on response times and errors, specifically in the left visual field (e.g. Banich *et al.*, 1992). In studies assessing possible fluctuations in cerebral lateralisation over the cycle, mood has often not been adequately controlled for. Thus, Compton and Levine asked thirty-three women to perform several visual laterality reaction time tasks during menses and the follicular and luteal phases, and at each session asked them to complete a mood questionnaire. No effects of menstrual cycle phase were found for perceptual asymmetry performance (they did not, however, directly measure hormone levels); but negative mood was associated with a reversal in the typically reported right-hemisphere advantage on a face perception test.

## Hormonal supplementation and cognitive performance

### Hypogonadal men

Males suffering from idiopathic hypogonadotropic hypogonadism (IHH) have a normal 46,XY karotype, show normal masculinisation during prenatal development and show normal development until puberty, when pubescence fails to occur owing to a failure of gonadotropin-releasing factor. As they have experienced no other developmental disorders, or hormonal deficiencies, they therefore form a unique group in which to investigate the role played by pubertal androgens on cognitive performance. Hier and Crowley (1982) compared nineteen IHH males with the same number of control males, and five other males who had developed IHH after puberty (acquired IHH), on a range of psychometric tests. On tests of verbal ability the three groups showed no differences. However, on three tests of spatial processing the IHH males performed significantly worse then the other two groups. Within this sample, there was a significant positive relationship between testicular size (testicular mass provides an indirect measure of gonadotropins, gonadotropins-releasing factor and testosterone levels) and performance on two out of the three spatial tests. In six of these males, the effects of androgen replacement therapy for a three-month period was then investigated. After this time, the males were asked to perform the same spatial tests but no significant improvements were found. The authors suggested that the lack of androgens during puberty leads to a permanent effect on spatial ability. If such a deficit is experienced after puberty then spatial ability will not be affected (the acquired IHH group showed no problems). This adds credence to the notion that puberty is a key time when certain neurological process are being organised and not simply activated (see chapter 3).

In a similar study, O'Carroll (1984) assessed spatial ability in eight hypogonadal males and sixteeen males suffering from sexual dysfunction (who were described as being eugonadal). The hypogonadal males were currently receiving testosterone replacement therapy, but the treatment was halted for two months, at the end of which they were retested. Following that, they resumed their androgen therapy for a further five months and were retested again. The eugonadal males were also receiving replacement therapy and they were tested after six weeks of therapy or following six weeks of a placebo. The two groups did not differ on spatial ability, and the hypogonadal males showed no change in performance following androgen therapy, thereby confirming the results by Hier and Crowley (1982), though the spatial test used (Minnesota Paper Form Board Test) may not have been sufficiently sensitive to detect any changes.

Alexander *et al.* (1998) recruited a larger sample of thirty-three hypogonadal males, and compared their performance on a battery of tests shown to be sensitive to sex differences (visuospatial ability, verbal ability and perceptual speed) with twenty-nine eugonadal males. The hypogonadal males were all assessed before and after they received testosterone replacement therapy; a subsample of the control males were also tested before and after they received testosterone enanthate (they were undergoing clinical trials for a possible male contraceptive), and the remainder of the eugonadal males received nothing. Group differences in testosterone levels were not associated with differential cognitive performance, though the hypogonadal males were impaired at verbal fluency, and performance on this task improved to match that of the eugonadal males following testosterone therapy. This study seemed to suggest, then, that testosterone may enhance verbal fluency (in androgen-deficient males) but did not utilise a placebo-controlled design.

O'Connor *et al.* (2001) replicated this study by comparing the effects of supraphysiological doses of testosterone in fifteen normal males (fifteen others received a placebo) and replacement doses of testosterone in seven hypogonadal males, on verbal and spatial cognitive performance. All groups performed a battery of neuropsychological tests before treatment commenced, and then again after four and eight weeks of treatment. The hypogonadal group performed at a lower level compared to the eugonadal groups, but testosterone therapy had no effect on their cognitive performance. In the normal males, a reduction in performance on one spatial task (block design subtest of the Weschler Adult Intelligence Test – Revised: WAIS – R), but an improvement in performance on verbal fluency, was seen after four weeks of treatment. The authors argued that this reflects the possibility that circulating testosterone influences different cognitive processes in opposite ways – an inverted U-shape for certain aspects of spatial ability, but a U-shape for certain types of verbal ability.

## Transsexuals

This group of individuals appear to have experienced no abnormalities in sexual differentiation (either physiological, genetic or hormonal) yet undergo drastic surgery in order to change physically into the sex that they feel they are (see chapter 6). As part of this treatment the individuals are routinely administered cross-sex hormones, and they thus provide a potentially valuable group within which to assess the effects of exposure to gonadal steroids in various aspects of behaviour (including cognition). Thus, van Goozen *et al.* (1994) conducted the first study assessing the effects of testosterone administration in twenty-two female-to-male transsexuals. Androgen administration (to a level equivalent to that seen in normal males) led to a significant improvement on performance of the visuospatial task, but verbal ability was significantly reduced. This finding is in accord with the differential curvilinear hypothesis proposed by O'Connor *et al.* (2001), in that low–normal testosterone seems to enhance spatial ability, but impairs verbal ability. A problem is, of course, that a placebo group was not included, but such a group would be difficult to recruit because of the ethical problems. Normal females exposed to testosterone in this manner would display alterations in their physical characteristics that could be permanent.

In a subsequent study, van Goozen *et al.* (1995) replicated their previous findings by showing that three months of testosterone administration to female-to-male transsexuals was associated with the same pattern of results, namely an enhancement of spatial ability and an impairment of verbal ability. In this study, though, they were also able to incorporate a group of fifteen male-to-female transsexuals who received both anti-androgen treatment and estrogen therapy. In this latter group, the opposite pattern of performance was found (spatial impairment but verbal improvement) following hormone therapy, though whether this was due to the effects of the anti-androgen, the estrogen or synergistic effects of both is difficult to determine. Importantly, the authors noted that these effects did not come about via changes in self-perceived masculinity/femininity, and thus concluded that these reflected genuine hormonal effects.

Miles *et al.* (1998) compared performance on a range of cognitive tasks shown to reveal sex differences in a normal population, in twenty-nine male–female transsexuals currently receiving estrogen treatment (this ranged from three to seventy-two months), and thirty who were awaiting treatment. While group performance on the mental rotation task, controlled associations test or an assessment of vocabulary did not differ, those receiving estrogen performed significantly better on paired-associate learning, a verbal memory task often performed better by females. Here, then, estrogen therapy did not lead to an impairment in spatial ability (as reported by van Goozen and colleagues), but note that in the Miles *et al.*, study most individuals only received estrogen and not antiandrogens as well.

Other studies have yielded more conflicting results. For example, Slabbekoorn *et al.* (1999) reported an enhancement of spatial performance in female-to-male transsexuals following long-tern androgen therapy, but did not find that the same treatment had a negative effect on verbal performance. In male-to-female transsexuals the provision of an antiandrogen combined with estrogen supplementation did not lead to an impairment of spatial ability and an improvement in verbal ability. More recently, using a more robust design, Miles *et al.* (2006) assessed performance on a range of cognitive tasks incorporating memory, verbal skills and spatial ability, in 103 male-to-female transsexuals. Participants were either tested before treatment began and then again following three to twelve months of treatment, or tested during current estrogen therapy (at least two years of treatment) and again after the therapy was discontinued as a prerequisite for sex-reassignment surgery. After controlling for a range of possible confounds, the authors found no evidence that estrogen treatment influenced memory or cognition and raised several possible methodological reasons as to why previous studies may have found such effects.

## Hormone replacement therapy in the elderly

### Females

In females, from around the age of forty-three the mass of the ovaries begins to decline, and it becomes no longer possible to initiate and maintain a viable corpus luteum. The ovaries then produce less and less progesterone, and the pituitary initiates a corresponding rise in FSH to compensate, and thus estrogen levels rise accordingly. This is the period of the 'perimenopause', the time following the last menstrual period when initial alterations in endocrinology, physiology and perhaps behaviour signal the onset of the menopause proper (Cutler and Genovese-Stone, 2000). The menopause itself occurs at around the age of fifty, and is characterised by a marked decline in production of both estradiol and progesterone from the ovaries. This dramatic alteration in hormone production thus renders menopausal females a fascinating group in which to assess the effects of hormonal withdrawal on various aspects of physiology and cognition. They also form a group in which it is possible first to observe the effects of hormone removal, and then observe what might happen if those same hormones are reinstated.

In chapter 2 I described organotherapy, the 'science' pioneered by Charles Brown-Séquard, with the idea being that injections of various hormone extracts could rejuvenate the ailing human being, and perhaps act as a cure for certain physical conditions. As humans in many societies are now living longer than before, they are experiencing physical, emotional and psychological changes that perhaps rarely troubled their ancestors. It is thus not surprising that we are witnessing a more scientific rebirth of organotherapy in the form of hormone replacement therapy (HRT), as aging individuals attempt to delay the inevitable, and achieve a better quality of life. As we have seen in previous chapters, and in earlier sections of this chapter, the sex steroids play an important role in the central nervous system, not just in subserving certain sexual behaviours, but also in terms of their effect on areas of the brain that underlie certain aspects of cognitive processing. Many elderly individuals display characteristic impairments in learning and memory, and often such impairments are degenerative (e.g. Alzheimer's disease) and appear to involve pathological alterations to the same brain regions (McEwen and Alves, 1999). The possible protective and preventative actions of HRT thus make it a potentially major weapon in the war against age-related physical and mental decline.

Early studies assessing the effects of HRT indicated that estrogen supplementation could indeed have beneficial effects on cognition. For example, Caldwell and Watson (1952) injected either estrogen or a control substance into twenty-eight elderly women once per week for a year. The women who had received estrogen showed a significant increase in their verbal intelligence, while performance on the same tasks showed a decline in the control group. A year after both treatments had been withdrawn, scores in both groups decreased relative to baseline. Thus, initial studies provided a very positive outlook: simply restoring estrogen could ameliorate the decline in intellectual performance, a decline often reported subjectively by women during their menopause. However, these early studies were criticised by Sherwin (1988), who noted that they used very different hormone replacements (viable comparisons could thus not be made), did not actually measure levels of circulating hormones, and used many different tests (again rendering comparisons difficult).

Sherwin argued that studies assessing the effects of HRT should use more the rigorous repeated-measures, placebo-controlled, cross-over designs, i.e. testing cognitive function in premenopausal women, and again post-menopausally after receiving HRT therapy. As this could be tricky in terms of waiting for the menopause to occur naturally, many studies elected to focus on those women undergoing surgical menopause. In one such study, Sherwin and Phillips (1990) evaluated groups before and after surgical menopause on paired-associate learning and paragraph recall. By the second month following surgery the performance of the HRT group on the retention of paired-associates learned previously remained at the preoperative baseline, while the performance of the placebo group declined significantly. On the paragraph recall, performance of the HRT group increased significantly compared to the preoperative baseline, while the performance of the placebo group was maintained at baseline level.

However, such effects may only be limited to a small number of cognitive domains. Kampen and Sherwin (1994) found that estrogen users performed significantly better than non-estrogen users on paragraph recall, but there were no group differences on other verbal or spatial tests. Duff and Hampson (2000) argued that the explanation for the mixed findings was that the tests apparently sensitive to estrogen are those which tap into working memory processes governed by the prefrontal cortex. In their study, the performance of thirty-five post-menopausal women not taking HRT was compared with sixty-one postmenopausal women taking HRT, on a verbal and spatial working memory test. The HRT group performed significantly better on both working memory tasks, whilst performance on verbal and spatial non-working memory tasks did not differ. In support of this notion, Keenan *et al.* (2001) proposed that menopausal cognitive decline may be due to executive dysfunction in prefrontal cortex caused by loss of estrogen receptors. They compared performance on a battery of cognitive tests assessing memory and executive functioning in postmenopausal women taking and not taking HRT. Those not receiving HRT showed poorer performance on a range of working memory tasks, and had difficulty inhibiting inappropriate responses (a classic problem associated with frontal cortex impairment). However, Duka *et al.* (2000) had assessed the effects of three weeks of estradiol supplementation in nineteen healthy elderly females; a further group of eighteen individuals were provided with a placebo. Assessments of memory, frontal lobe function and mental rotation ability were taken before and after treatment. Performance on the mental rotation test and memory tasks showed a significant improvement in the estrogen-treated group, though frontal cortex functions showed no changes. Many other studies, however, did not report significant benefits of HRT (e.g. O'Hara *et al.*, 2005), and it may be the case that HRT can only provide some benefit if provided early enough following the menopause.

In an in-depth meta-analytic review of studies conducted thus far, Hogervorst *et al.* (2000) provided some insight into the important methodological issues surrounding this type of research. A key area of concern is that women who agree to take part in clinical trials where they may receive HRT after their menopause are typically healthier before they enter menopause; those who do use HRT are also likely to be younger, to be better educated and to be from a higher social class. Studies that have followed such groups of women before and during their HRT may thus be drawing their conclusions from a biased sample. Indeed, in support of this notion, epidemiological studies routinely report positive outcomes of HRT, whereas experimental studies (which carefully control for age, education and health) do not.

Another major factor relates to the type of HRT given. There are many different forms of HRT, differing on dose, type of compound administered and the duration over which the therapy has been provided. Brain estrogen receptors are more sensitive to estradiol, but the most commonly used therapy provides estrone rather than estradiol, and this could be why many studies have consistently failed to find positive effects. Other studies have assessed therapies that contained a mixture of estrogens and progestins (combination therapy) and it has been suggested that the progestins may actually have an adverse effect on cognition. A final problem relates to the fact that it is very difficult to maintain double-blind conditions, as women receiving estrogen quickly observe the characteristic alterations in their physical condition that accompany the therapy (e.g. reduction in hot flushes and night sweats). This then creates an 'expectancy effect' in that knowledge that one is receiving therapy may then bias one's perceptions and performance.

Hogervorst *et al.* (2000) concluded that the effects of HRT in healthy elderly women are small and inconsistent, but note that there is a dearth of longitudinal studies assessing the effects of HRT in older females. If there is little effect in healthy women, what about those suffering from pathological cognitive problems, i.e. those with dementia? Alzheimer's disease is characterised by progressive memory dysfunction, and women appear to have a higher risk of suffering from this condition than males (studies cited in Hogervorst *et al.*, 2000). Interestingly, one study (Doraiswamy, 1997) has shown that women with Alzheimer's who were not receiving HRT scored significantly worse on a dementia checklist than males with Alzheimer's. Another study has demonstrated that females with Alzheimer's who were receiving HRT performed significantly better on a semantic memory task than females matched for dementia severity but not currently receiving HRT (Henderson *et al.*, 1996). If providing HRT after diagnosis of dementia can ameliorate the severity of some of the cognitive deficits, then can HRT act as a protective agent against Alzheimer's disease? In their review Hogervorst *et al.* (2000) identified fourteen studies that had set out to test whether HRT could indeed act as a protector against the development of dementia. Some support for this notion was indeed found, as the relative risk of dementia was reduced in those women receiving HRT. However, it remains unclear how this might work, as studies have reported contradictory information as to the optimal dose or duration of therapy. Several experimental studies have in fact indicated that a longer duration of therapy (defined as being twelve months or more) may result in even more cognitive problems as compared to those receiving a placebo (Mulnard *et al.*, 2000)!

The reviewers point out that the evidence concerning the beneficial effects of estrogen on neural structures is derived from short-term studies in animals; longer-term effects might be very different, perhaps as a result of the reduction in estrogen binding and the down regulation of estrogen receptors following long-term exposure. As premenopausal females do not experience a continual steady state of estrogen exposure (estradiol shows a cyclical pattern) then perhaps therapies could be managed to achieve a more natural rhythm. Some evidence for this comes from Krug *et al.* (2006), who provided fourteen healthy postmenopausal females with either a single boost of estrogen over three days to mimic the midcycle rise, or a placebo. Performance was assessed on tests sensitive to hippocampal function (immediate and delayed verbal memory) or prefrontal function (ordering of events, and susceptibility to interference). A beneficial effect of estrogen was found primarily on the tasks thought most sensitive to frontal lobe functioning, though immediate recall was also enhanced; the authors suggested that hormone replacement therapies may have more consistent and positive effects if they utilise shorter temporary increases, rather than continuous long-term infusions.

## Males

While the effects of hormonal depletion and subsequent restoration have been extensively studied in elderly females, there is a paucity of research concerning possible links between hormonal decline/restoration and cognition in elderly males. An earlier section of this chapter suggested that testosterone replacement therapy may alleviate certain cognitive deficits in hormonally abnormal males. Elderly males have been found to experience an age-related decline in serum testosterone levels, with particular decrements in bioavailable testosterone, and many of the clinical features of this so-called 'andropause' resemble those seen in hypogonadal males (Kaufman *et al.*, 2004). One might thus expect that as levels of androgen fall then one could see corresponding reductions in the performance of certain cognitive tasks.

However, the picture is likely to be complicated by the fact that if testosterone is related to certain aspects of cognition in a curvilinear fashion (as seems likely from evidence previously discussed), then elderly males with lower levels of testosterone might actually show an improvement in certain abilities. Barrett-Connor *et al.* (1999) assessed cognitive performance in a sample of 547 elderly males and found that those with lower estradiol combined with higher testosterone performed better on several cognitive tests, though a limitation of this study is that the samples from which hormones were analysed were taken several years before the cognitive tests were conducted. Wolf and Kirschbaum (2002) measured estradiol, testosterone and cognitive performance in elderly males and females. While higher levels of estradiol and testosterone were associated with various aspects of cognition in females, the only significant association in males was a negative relationship between testosterone and verbal fluency. In a larger study incorporating over 900 males, Fonda *et al.* (2005) found that older age was clearly associated with cognitive decline but were unable clearly to associate such decline with circulating hormone levels. However, in a more recent longitudinal study of more than a thousand males and females aged thirty-five to ninety, Thilers *et al.* (2006) found that in males higher levels of testosterone were associated with better performance on visuospatial, semantic and episodic memory tasks. This effect became stronger in the older males.

As regards supplementation, Janowsky *et al.* (1994) randomly assigned fifty-six healthy males aged sixty to seventy-five to testosterone treatment or to a placebo for a three-month period. Using a battery of neuropsychological tests, the authors demonstrated that testosterone supplementation significantly enhanced performance on a spatial test (block design). Using similar methodology, Cherrier *et al.* (2001) gave twenty-five males aged fifty to eighty injections of either testosterone or a placebo for a six-week period, cognitive evaluations being conducted before treatment, and again at weeks three and six. They reported significant improvements in both spatial memory (recall of a route taken, and block construction) and verbal recall of a short story. More recently, Cherrier *et al.* (2007) conducted a similar study with fifty-seven males aged fifty to eighty-five. Three different doses of testosterone were utilised, and an additional test session six weeks after the treatment had finished was incorporated. On this occasion they found significant non-linear relationships between testosterone and verbal and spatial memory, such that better performance was associated with moderate increases in serum testosterone (levels approximated high to high normal levels in younger males). These studies thus suggest some relationships between testosterone and cognition in older males but they are unable to determine whether this represents a specific effect of testosterone, or that of its metabolite estradiol (both are typically increased at a similar rate in those receiving supplementation).

**Food additives**

HRT appears to have some benefits for postmenopausal females, but such therapies have been associated with various medical complications, including an increased risk of breast cancer and cardiovascular disease. In light of such health scares, there has been renewed interest in natural products that may boost estrogen activity. Certain foodstuffs and dietary supplements that are derived from the soya bean contain isoflavones. These are weak non-steroidal estrogens and are referred to as 'phytoestrogens', two important ones being genistein and daidzein. Genistein is structurally similar to 17β estradiol and therefore is thought to act as a partial agonist as it binds principally to the estrogen receptors ERβ, though with less affinity than estradiol. Genistein has also been found to alter expression of progesterone, androgen and oxytocin receptors (Fitzpatrick, 2003). It has been shown that consumption of soya-enriched foods leads to high plasma concentrations of phytoestrogens (Rowland *et al.*, 2000) and so it is likely that these compounds can reach the brain in sufficient quantities to activate the various receptors. In young healthy males and females, File *et al.* (2001) showed that a soya diet containing high levels of phytoestrogens led to a significant enhancement of verbal and non-verbal memory, and a measure of mental flexibility (a measure of frontal lobe function) after a ten-week period.

If isoflavones influence memory in young participants, then it was widely expected that they may have even greater positive effects in postmenopausal females. Duffy *et al.* (2003) assessed the effects of soy isoflavones on a battery of cognitive tests in thirty-three postmenopausal women not using conventional HRT. In a double-blind trial the volunteers received either 60 mg of isoflavones per day or a placebo, for a twelve-week period. During that time they completed a battery of cognitive tests and provided ratings of their mood and menopausal symptoms. Those receiving isoflavones showed a significant improvement in delayed picture recall, sustained attention, learning rule reversals and planning. However, in a study utilising 175 healthy postmenopausal females, Kreijkamp-Kaspers *et al.* (2004) examined the effects of soy protein on cognition and bone mineral density. The participants were randomly assigned to receive soy isoflavones or a placebo, and performed cognitive assessments at baseline and then again after one year of treatment. On the tests of memory the soy group did show some improvements, but the effects were not significant. The authors suggested, though, that as the women in their sample were on average eighteen years into their menopause, the intervention may have come too late to have any clear effect.

Another source of dietary isoflavones (especially in Western cultures) is lignans, formed by the action of intestinal bacteria on lignan precursors found in food such as berries, legumes, vegetables (especially broccoli and alfalfa) and flaxseeds. Franco *et al.* (2005) evaluated long-term dietary intake of lignans from around 400 women who were split into two groups in relation to how long they had been in a menopausal state: a long time (twenty to thirty years) or a shorter time (eight to twelve years). A higher intake of lignans was associated with a higher probability of intact cognitive function, but this was only apparent in the group who had experienced menopause for longer.

There are numerous possible confounds with human studies, but some recent evidence from an experimental animal study demonstrates that such compounds may enhance particular aspects of cognition and have direct effects on certain brain regions. Luine *et al.* (2006) ovariectomised seventeen female rats and then fed eight of them on a diet rich in phytoestrogens, while the remainder received a diet containinig minimal amounts of phytoestrogens. After seven weeks all animals were tested on a spatial task and the phytoestrogen group performed significantly better (performance on tests not requiring spatial ability showed no group differences). After nine weeks of the diet, dendritic spine density in the hippocampus and prefrontal cortex was also significantly greater in the phytoestrogen group.

### Effects of hormonal reductions

It is rare that hormone levels are artificially reduced. This of course occurs in transsexual patients undergoing sex reversals, but is normally done in combination with the provision of opposite-sex hormones. One group of patients provides a unique window into the possible effects of specific androgen deprivation. Males being treated for prostrate cancer undergo androgen deprivation therapy (ADT) such that circulating levels of androgens are reduced to levels typically seen in castrated males. Normally, the effects of such therapy are viewed within the context of so-called 'quality of life' but now several researchers are beginning to focus on possible effects on cognition. For example, Salminen *et al.* (2003) assessed cognitive performance in twenty-five males at baseline (before treatment) and then after they received ADT for six and twelve months. Significant improvements in the immediate and delayed recall of objects and in semantic memory were observed. Using the same methodology, Salminen *et al.* (2004) assessed the effects of ADT in twenty-three males suffering from prostate cancer. This time, along with an improvement in episodic memory, testosterone decline was associated with impairments in speeded performance in a digit symbol test, an increase in errors on a choice reaction time test, and an impaired hit rate in a vigilance task. These effects were particularly evident at twelve months, suggesting that the magnitude of change in performance was perhaps related to the rate of testosterone decline. Thus, testosterone appears to have differential effects on cognition, but as only a few studies have been specifically conducted using this methodology, these results remain preliminary. As more and more males each year are diagnosed with this condition, and receive ADT, then further clarification is likely.

## Conclusion

The overall picture remains complex. At a broad level there appears to be strong evidence for relationships between sex steroids and cognition. While evidence from experimental animals shows that hormonal manipulation is related to cognitive performance, and specific morphological changes in the brain, obtaining similar evidence from humans is difficult. In addition, while the animal studies require individuals to navigate their way around the environment in a goal-directed fashion (i.e. to search for food or to escape from drowning) comparative situations are completely lacking in human studies, which typically involve a sheet of paper and a pencil. While studies of humans with specific hormonal deficiencies provide slightly clearer evidence than correlational studies conducted in 'normal' individuals, there remain a host of confounding factors that render any conclusions tentative. It would be surprising indeed if hormones were not related to human cognitive processing, but determining which hormones are involved in which processes involving which areas of the brain remains to be demonstrated.

# References

Abitbol, J., Abitbol, P., and Abitbol, B. (1999). Sex hormones and the female voice. *Journal of Voice* 13: 424–46.

Aboitiz, F., Scheibel, A.B., and Zaidel, E. (1992). Morphometry of the Sylvian fissure and the corpus callosum, with emphasis on sex differences. *Brain* 115: 1521–41.

Adams, D.B., Gold, A.R., and Burt, A.D. (1978). Rise in female-initiated sexual activity at ovulation and its suppression by oral contraceptives. *New England Journal of Medicine* 299: 1145–50.

Adkins-Regan, E. (1981). Hormone specificity, androgen metabolism, and social behaviour. *American Zoologist* 21: 257–71.

Aggleton, J.P. (1993). The contribution of the amygdala to normal and abnormal emotional states. *Trends in Neurosciences* 16: 328–33.

Aggleton, J.P., Kentridge, R.W., and Good, J.M.M. (1994). Handedness and musical ability: a study of professional orchestral players, composers, and choir members. *Psychology of Music* 22: 148–56.

Agid, O., Kohn, Y., and Lerer, B. (2000). Environmental stress and psychiatric illness. *Biomedicine and Pharmacotherapy* 54: 135–41.

Ågmo, A. (1997). Male rat sexual behaviour. *Brain Research Protocols* 1: 203–9.

(1999). Sexual motivation: an enquiry into events determining the occurrence of sexual behavior. *Behavioral Brain Research* 105: 129–50.

(2003). Uncondition sexual incentive motivation in the male Norway rat (*Rattus norvegicus*). *Journal of Comparative Psychology* 117: 3–14.

Ågmo, A., and Ellingsen, E. (2003). Relevance of non-human animal studies to the understanding of human sexuality. *Scandinavian Journal of Psychology* 44: 293–301.

Akcam, T., Bolu, E., Merati, A.L., Durmus, C., Gerek, M., and Ozkaptan, Y. (2004). Voice changes after androgen therapy for hypogonadotrophic hypogonadism. *The Laryngoscope* 114: 1587–91.

Al-Ayadhi, L.Y. (2005). Altered oxytocin and vasopressin levels in autistic children in central Saudi Arabia. *Neurosciences* 10: 47–50.

Albert, D.J., Jonik, R.H., Watson, N.V., Gorzalka, B.B., and Walsh, M.L. (1990). Hormone-dependent aggression in male rats is proportional to serum testosterone concentration but sexual behaviour is not. *Physiology and Behavior* 48: 409–16.

Alexander, G.M. (2006). Associations among gender-linked toy preferences, spatial ability, and digit ratio: evidence from eye-tracking analysis. *Archives of Sexual Behavior* 35: 699–709.

Alexander, G.M., and Hines, M. (1994). Gender labels and play styles: their relative contribution to children's selection of playmates. *Child Development* 65: 869–79.

Alexander, G.M., and Sherwin, B.B. (1993). Sex steroids, sexual behaviour, and selection attention for erotic stimuli in women using oral contraceptives. *Psychoneuroendocrinology* 18: 91–102.

Alexander, G.M., Sherwin, B.B., Bancroft, J., and Davidson, D.W. (1990). Testosterone and sexual behaviour in oral contraceptive users and nonusers: a prospective study. *Hormones and Behavior* 24: 388–402.

Alexander, G.M., Swerdloff, R.S., Wang, C., Davidson, T., McDonald, V., Steiner, B., and Hines, M. (1997). Androgen–behavior correlations in hypogonadal men and eugonadal men. I. Mood and response to auditory sexual stimuli. *Hormones and Behavior* 31: 110–19.

(1998). Androgen–behavior correlations in hypogonadal men and eugonadal men. II. Cognitive abilities. *Hormones and Behavior* 33: 85–94.

Alford, F.P., Baker, H.W.G., Patel, Y.C., Rennie, G.C., Youatt, G., Burger, H.G., and Hudson, B. (1973). Temporal patterns of circulating hormones as assessed by continuous blood sampling. *Journal of Clinical Endocrinology* 36: 108–16.

Allee, W., Collias, N., and Lutherman, C. (1939). Modification of the social order in flocks of hens by the injection of testosterone propionate. *Physiological Zoology* 12: 412–40.

Allen, E., and Doisy, E.A. (1923). An ovarian hormone: preliminary report of its localization, extraction and partial purification, and action in test animals. *Journal of the American Medical Association* 81: 819–21.

Allen, L.S., and Gorski, R.A. (1990). Sex difference in the bed nucleus of the stria terminalis of the human brain. *Journal of Comparative Neurology* 302: 697–706.

Allen, L.S., Hines, M., Shryne, J.E., and Gorski, R.A. (1989). Two sexually dimorphic cell groups in the human brain. *Journal of Neuroscience* 9: 497–506.

Allen, M.J. (1974). Sex differences in spatial problem solving style. *Perceptual and Motor Skills* 85: 249–77.

Allen, R.S., Richey, M.F., Chai, Y.M., and Gorski, R.A. (1991). Sex differences in the corpus callosum of the living human being. *Journal of Neuroscience* 11: 933–42.

Alliende, M.E. (2002). Mean versus individual hormonal profiles in the menstrual cycle. *Fertility and Sterility* 78: 90–5.

Anderson, R.A., Bancroft, J., and Wu, F.C.W. (1992). The effects of exogenous testosterone on sexuality and mood of normal men. *Journal of Clinical Endocrinology and Metabolism* 75: 1503–7.

Anderson-Hunt, M., and Dennerstein, L. (1994). Increased female sexual response after oxytocin. *British Medical Journal* 309: 929.

Angelopoulou, R., Lavranos, G., and Manolakou, P. (2006). Establishing sexual dimorphism in humans. *Collegicum Antropologicum* 30: 653–8.

Anonymous (1972). Effects of sexual activity on beard growth in man. *Nature* 226: 869–70.

Archer, J. (1988). *The Behavioural Biology of Aggression*. Cambridge: Cambridge University Press.

(1991). The influence of testosterone on human aggression. *British Journal of Psychology* 82: 1–28.

(2006). Testosterone and human aggression: an evaluation of the challenge hypothesis. *Neuroscience and Biobehavioral Reviews* 30: 319–45.

Archer, J., Birring, S.S., and Wu, F.C.W. (1998). The association between testosterone and aggression among young men: empirical findings and a meta analysis. *Aggressive Behaviour* 24: 411–20.

Archer, J., and Browne, K. (1989). Concepts and approaches to the study of aggression. In J. Archer and K. Browne (eds.), *Human Aggression: Naturalistic Approaches*. London: Routeledge, pp. 4–24.

Argiolas, A., and Gessa, G.L. (1991). Central functions of oxytocin. *Neuroscience and Biobehavioral Reviews* 15: 217–31.

Arletti, R., Bazzani, C., Castelli, M., and Bertolini, A. (1985). Oxytocin improves male copulatory performance in rats. *Hormones and Behavior* 19: 14–20.

Arletti, R., and Bertolini, A. (1985). Oxytocin stimulates lordosis behaviour in female rats. *Neuropeptides* 6: 247–53.

Arnold, A.P. (1980). Effects of androgens on volumes of sexually dimorphic brain regions in the zebra finch. *Brain Research* 185: 441–4.

(1996). Genetically triggered sexual differentiation of brain and behaviour. *Hormones and Behavior* 30: 495–505.

Arnold, A.P., and Breedlove, S.M. (1985). Organizational and activational effects of sex steroids on brain and behaviour: a re-analysis. *Hormones and Behavior* 19: 469–98.

Arnold, A.P., and Schlinger, B.A. (1993). Sexual differentiation of the brain and behaviour: the zebra finch is not just a flying rat. *Brain Behavior and Evolution* 42: 231–41.

Aron, D.C., Findling, J.W., and Tyrell, J.B. (1997). Hypothalamus and pituitary. In F.S. Greenspan and G.J. Strewler (eds.), *Basic and Clinical Endocrinology*. Stamford: Appleton and Lange, 5th edition, pp. 95–156.

Asso, D. (1986). Psychology degree examinations and the premenstrual phase of the menstrual cycle. *Women and Health* 10: 91–104.

Babler, W.J. (1987). Development of dermatoglyphic patterns: associations with epidermal ridge, volar pad, and bone morphology. *Collegium Antropologicum* 11: 297–304.

Bagatell, C.J., Heiman, J.R., Rivier, J.E., and Bremner, W.J. (1994). Effects of endogenous testosterone and estradiol on sexual behavior in normal young men. *Journal of Clinical Endocrinology and Metabolism* 78: 711–16.

Bagemihl, B. (1999). *Biological Exuberance: Animal Homosexuality and Natural Diversity*. New York: St Martin's Press.

Bahr, N.I., Martin, R.D., and Pryce, C.R. (2001). Peripartum sex steroid profiles and endocrine correlates of postpartum maternal behavior in captive gorillas (*Gorilla gorilla*). *Hormones and Behavior* 40: 533–41.

Bailey, A.A., and Hurd, P.L. (2005). Finger length ratio (2D:4D) correlates with physical aggression in men but not in women. *Biological Psychology* 68: 215–22.

Bailey, J.M., and Pillard, R.C. (1991). A genetic study of male sexual orientation. *Archives of General Psychiatry* 48: 1089–96.

Bailey, J.M., Pillard, R.C., Dawood, K., Miller, M.B., Farrer, L.A., Trivedi, S., and Murphy, R.L. (1999). A family history study of male sexual orientation using three independent samples. *Behavior Genetics* 29: 79–86.

Bailey, J.M., Pillard, R.C., Neale, M.C., and Agyei, Y. (1993). Heritable factors influence sexual orientation in women. *Archives of General Psychiatry* 50: 217–23.

Bailey, J.M., Willerman, L., and Parks, C. (1991). A test of the maternal stress theory of human male homosexuality. *Archives of Sexual Behavior* 20: 277–93.

Baker, F. (1888). Anthropological notes on the human hand. *American Anthropologist* 1: 51–76.

Ball, G.F., and Balthazart, J. (2006). Androgen metabolism and the activation of male sexual behaviour: it's more complicated than you think! *Hormones and Behavior* 49: 1–3.

Ball, J. (1937). Sex activity of castrated male rats increased by estrin administration. *Journal of Comparative Psychology* 24: 135–44.

Balthazart, J., and Ball, G.F. (1995). Sexual differentiation of brain and behaviour in birds. *Trends in Endocrinology and Metabolism* 6: 21–9.

(1998). New insights into the regulation and function of brain estrogen synthase (aromatase). *Trends in Neurosciences* 21: 243–9.

Bancroft, J. (2005). The endocrinology of sexual arousal. *Journal of Endocrinology* 186: 411–27.

Bancroft, J., Davidson, D.W., Warner, P., and Tyrer, G. (1980). Androgens and sexual behavior in women using oral contraceptives. *Clinical Endocrinology* 12: 327–40.

Bancroft, J., Sherwin, B.B., Alexander, G.M., Davidson, D.W., and Walker, A. (1991). Oral contraceptives, androgens, and the sexuality of young women: II. The role of androgens. *Archives of Sexual Behaviour* 20: 121–35.

Banich, M.T., Stolar, N., Heller, W., and Goldman, R.B. (1992). A deficit in right hemisphere performance after induction of a depressed mood. *Neuropsychiatry, Neuropsychology, and Behavioral Neurology* 5: 20–7.

Bardi, M., French, J.A., Ramirez, S.M., and Brent, L. (2004). The role of the endocrine system in baboon maternal behavior. *Biological Psychiatry* 55: 724–32.

Baron-Cohen, S. (2002). The extreme male brain theory of autism. *Trends in Cognitive Sciences* 6: 248–54.

Barrenetxe, J., Delagrange, P., and Martinez, J.A. (2004). Physiological and metabolic functions of melatonin. *Journal of Physiology and Biochemistry* 60: 61–72.

Barretti-Connor, E., Goodman-Gruen, D., and Patay, B. (1999). Endogenous sex hormones and cognitive function in older men. *Journal of Clinical Endocrinology and Metabolism* 84: 3681–5.

Barris, M.C., Dawson, W.W., and Theiss, C.L. (1980). The visual sensitivity of women during the menstrual cycle. *Documenta Opthalmologia* 42: 293–301.

Bartels, A., and Zeki, S. (2000). The neural basis of romantic love. *Neuroreport* 11: 3829–34.

Bass, A.H., and Zakon, H.H. (2005). Sonic and electric fish: at the crossroads of neuroethology and behavioral neuroendocrinology. *Hormones and Behavior* 48: 360–72.

Bateup, H.S., Booth, A., Shirtcliff, E.A., and Granger, D.A. (2002). Testosterone, cortisol, and women's competition. *Evolution and Human Behavior* 23: 181–92.

Baulieu, E.E. (1998). Neurosteroids: a novel function of the brain. *Psychoneuroendocrinology* 23: 963–87.

Baumeister, R.F. (2000). Gender differences in erotic plasticity: the female sex drive as socially flexible and responsive. *Psychological Bulletin* 126: 347–74.

Baxter, J.D. (1997). Introduction to endocrinology. In F.S. Greenspan and G.J. Strewler (eds.), *Basic and Clinical Endocrinology*. Stamford: Appleton and Lange, 5th edition, pp. 1–38.

Bayliss, W.M., and Starling, E.H. (1902). The mechanism of pancreatic secretion. *Journal of Physiology* 28: 325–53.

Beach, F.A. (1956). Characteristics of masculine 'sex drive'. *Nebraska Symposium in Motivation* 4: 1–32.

  (1975). Behavioural endocrinology: an emerging discipline. *American Scientist* 63: 178–87.

  (1976). Sexual attractivity, proceptivity, and receptivity in female mammals. *Hormones and Behavior* 7: 105–38.

  (1981). Historical origins of modern research on hormones and behavior. *Hormones and Behavior* 15: 325–76.

Bean, R.B. (1906). Some racial peculiarities of the negro brain. *American Journal of Anatomy* 5: 353–415.

Beato, M., and Sánchez-Pacheco, A. (1996). Interaction of steroid hormone receptors with the transcription initiation complex. *Endocrinology Review* 17: 587–609.

Beckford, N.S., Schaid, D., Rood, S.R., and Schanbacher, B. (1985). Androgen stimulation and laryngeal development. *Annals of Otology, Rhinology and Laryngology* 94: 634–40.

Beech, J.R. (2001). A curvilinear relationship between hair loss and mental rotation and neuroticism: a possible influence of sustained dihydrotestosterone production. *Personality and Individual Differences* 31: 185–92.

Benbow, C.P. (1988). Sex differences in mathematical reasoning ability in intellectually talented preadolescents: their nature, effects and possible causes. *Behavioral and Brain Sciences* 11: 169–232.

Benedek, T. (1970). Motherhood and nurturing. In E.J. Anthony and T. Benedek (eds.), *Parenthood: Its Psychology and Psychopathology*. Boston, MA: Little Brown, pp. 153–66.

Benelli, A., Bertolini, A., Poggioli, R., Menozzi, B., Basaglia, R., and Arletti, R. (1995). Polymodal dose-response curve for oxytocin in the social recognition test. *Neuropeptides* 28: 251–5.

Benes, F.M., Turtle, M., Khan, Y., and Farol, P. (1994). Myelination of a key relay zone in the hippocampal formation occurs in the human brain during childhood, adolescence, and adulthood. *Archives of General Psychiatry* 51: 477–84.

Berenbaum, S.A. (2001). Cognitive function in congenital adrenal hyperplasia. *Endocrinology and Metabolism Clinics of North America* 30: 173–92.

Berenbaum, S.A., and Hines, M. (1992). Early androgens are related to childhood sex-typed toy preferences. *Psychological Science* 3: 203–6.

Berg, S.J., and Wynne-Edwards, K.E. (2001). Changes in testosterone, cortisol, and estradiol in men becoming fathers. *Mayo Clinic Proceedings* 76: 582–92.

Berman, M., Gladue, B., and Taylor, S. (1993). The effects of hormones, type A behaviour pattern, and provocation on aggression in men. *Motivation and Emotion* 17: 125–38.

Bernal, J., and Nunez, J. (1995). Thyroid hormones and brain development. *European Journal of Endocrinology* 133: 390–8.

Berndtson, W.E., and Desjardins, C. (1974). Circulating LH and FSH levels and testicular function in hamsters during light deprivation and subsequent photoperiodic stimulation. *Endocrinology* 95: 195–205.

Bernhardt, P.C., Dabbs, J.M. Jr., Fielden, J.A., and Lutter, C.D. (1998). Testosterone changes during vicarious experiences of winning and losing among fans at sporting events. *Physiology and Behaviour* 65: 59–62.

Bernstein, I.S., Rose, R.M., and Gordon, T.P. (1974). Behavioural and environmental events influencing primate testosterone levels. *Journal of Human Evolution* 3: 517–25.

Beyer, C., Morali, G., Naftolin, F., Larsson, K., and Pérez-Palacios, G. (1976). Effects of some antiestrogens and aromatase inhibitors on androgen induced sexual behaviour in castrated male rats. *Hormones and Behavior* 7: 353–63.

Bhasin, S., Woodhouse, L., Casaburi, R., Singh, A.B., Bhasin, D., Berman, N., Chen, X., Yarasheski, K.E., Magliano, L., Dzekov, C., Djekov, J., Bross, R., Phillips, J., Sinha-Hikim, I., Shen, R., and Storer, T.W. (2001). Testosterone dose-response relationships in healthy young men. *American Journal of Physiology, Endocrinology and Metabolism* 281: E1172–81.

Bibawi, D., Cherry, B., and Hellige, J.B. (1995). Fluctuations of perceptual asymmetry across time in women and men: effects related to the menstrual cycle. *Neuropsychologia* 33: 131–8.

Bishop, D.V.M. (1990). *Handedness and Developmental Disorder*. Oxford: Blackwell.

Bishop, K.M., and Wahlsten, D. (1997). Sex differences in the human corpus callosum: myth or reality? *Neuroscience and Biobehavioral Reviews* 21: 581–601.

Blaicher, W., Gruber, D., Bieglmayer, C., Blaicher, A.M., Knogler, W., and Huber, J.C. (1999). The role of oxytocin in relation to female sexual arousal. *Gynecologic and Obstetric Investigation* 47: 125–6.

Blanchard, R. (2001). Fraternal birth order and the maternal immune hypothesis of male homosexuality. *Hormones and Behavior* 40: 105–14.

Blanchard, R., and Bogaert, A.F. (1996). Homosexuality in men and number of older brothers. *American Journal of Psychiatry* 153: 27–31.

Blanchard, R., and Ellis, L. (2001). Birth weight, sexual orientation and the sex of preceding siblings. *Journal of Biosocial Science* 33: 451–67.

Blanchard, R., and Klassen, P. (1997). H-Y antigen and homosexuality in men. *Journal of Theoretical Biology* 185: 373–8.

Blanchard, R., Zucker, K.J., Cavacas, A., Allin, S., Bradley, S.J., and Schachter, D.C. (2002). Fraternal birth order and birth weight in probably prehomosexual feminine boys. *Hormones and Behavior* 41: 321–7.

Bloch, G.J., and Gorski, R.A. (1988). Estrogen/progesterone treatment in adulthood affects the size of several components of the medial preoptic area in the male rat. *Journal of Comparative Neurology* 275: 613–22.

Bobrow, N.A., Money, J., and Lewis, V.G. (1971). Delayed puberty, eroticism and sense of smell: a psychological study of hypogonadotropinism, osmatic and anosmatic (Kallmann's syndrome). *Archives of Sexual Behavior* 1: 329–44.

Boccia, M.L., Razzoli, M., Prasad Vadlamudi, S., Trumbull, W., Caleffie, C., and Pedersen, C.A. (2007). Repeated long separations from pups produce depression-like behaviour in rat mothers. *Psychoneuroendocrinology* 32: 65–71.

Bond, A., Choi, P.Y.L., and Pope, H.G. (1995). Assessment of attentional bias and mood in users and non-users of anabolic-androgenic steroids. *Drug and Alcohol Dependence* 37: 241–5.

Bonsall, R.W., Rees, H.D., and Michael, R.P. (1983). Characterization by high-performance liquid chromatography of nuclear metabolites of testosterone in the brains of male rhesus monkeys. *Life Sciences* 33: 655–63.

Bonsall, R.W., Zumpe, D., and Michael, R.P. (1978). Menstrual cycle influences on operant behaviour of female rhesus monkeys. *Journal of Comparative and Physiological Psychology* 92: 846–55.

Book, A.S., Starzyk, K.B., and Quinsey, V.L. (2001). The relationship between testosterone and aggression: a meta-analysis. *Aggression and Violent Behavior* 6: 579–99.

Booth, A., and Dabbs, J.M. Jr. (1993). Testosterone and men's marriages. *Social Forces* 72: 463–77.

Booth, A., Shelley, G., Mazur, A., Tharp, G., and Kittok, R. (1989). Testosterone, and winning and losing in human competition. *Hormones and Behaviour* 23: 556–71.

Booth, J.E. (1977). Sexual behavior of neonatally castrated rats injected during infancy with oestrogen and dihydrotestosterone. *Journal of Endocrinology* 72: 135–42.

Borell, M. (1978). Setting the standards for a new science: Edward Schäfer and endocrinology. *Medical History* 22: 282–90.

Bosinski, H.A.G., Peter, M., Bonatz, G., Arndt, R., Heidenreich, M., Sippell, W.G., and Wille, R. (1997). A higher rate of hyperandrogenic disorders in female-to-male transsexuals. *Psychoneuroendocrinology* 22: 361–80.

Bouissou, M.F. (1983). Androgens, aggressive behaviour and social relationships in higher primates. *Hormones Research* 18: 43–61.

Bowlby, J. (1982). *Attachment and Love*, vol. 1: *Attachment*. New York: Basic Books, 2nd edition.

Bradley, S.J., Oliver, G.D., Chernick, A.B., and Zucker, K.J. (1998). Experiment of nurture: ablatio penis at 2 months, sex reassignment at 7 months, and a psychosexual follow-up in young adulthood. *Pediatrics* 102: e9.

Braunstein, G.D. (1997). Testes. In F.S. Greenspan and G.J. Strewler (eds.), *Basic and Clinical Endocrinology*. Stamford: Appleton and Lange, 5th edition, pp. 403–33.

Breedlove, S.M. (1994). Sexual differentiation of the human nervous system. *Annual Review of Psychology* 45: 389–418.

Broad, K.D., Curley, J.P., and Keverne, E.B. (2006). Mother–infant bonding and the evolution of mammalian social relationships. *Philosophical Transactions of the Royal Society, B* 361: 2199–2214.

Bröder, A., and Hohmann, N. (2003). Variations in risk taking behaviour over the menstrual cycle. An improved replication. *Evolution and Human Behavior* 24: 391–8.

Brody, S., and Krüger, T.H.C. (2006). The post-orgasmic prolactin increase following intercourse is greater than following masturbation and suggests greater satiety. *Biological Psychology* 71: 312–15.

Broks, P., Young, A.W., Maratos, E.J., Coffey, P.J., Calder, A.J., Isaac, C.L., Mayes, A.R., Hodges, J.R., Montaldi, D., Cezayirli, E., Roberts, N., and Hadley, D. (1998). Face processing impairments after encephalitis: amygdala damage and recognition of fear. *Neuropsychologia* 36: 59–70.

Bronson, F., and Desjardins, C. (1982). Endocrine responses to sexual arousal in male mice. *Endocrinology* 111: 1286–91.

Brookes, H., Neave, N., Hamilton, C., and Fink, B. (2007). Digit ratio (2D:4D) and lateralization for basic numerical quantification. *Journal of Individual Differences* 28: 55–63.

Broverman, D.M., Vogel, W., Klaiber, E.L., Majcher, D., Shea, D., and Paul, V. (1981). Changes in cognitive task performance across the menstrual cycle. *Journal of Comparative and Physiological Psychology* 95: 646–54.

Brown, R.E. (1994). *An Introduction to Neuroendocrinology*. Cambridge: Cambridge University Press.

Brown, R.E., and McFarland, D.J. (1979). Interaction of hunger and sexual motivation in the male rat: a time sharing approach. *Animal Behaviour* 27: 887–96.

Brown, R.E., and Moger, W.H. (1983). Hormonal correlates of parental behaviour in male rats. *Hormones and Behavior* 17: 356–65.

Brown, W.M., Finn, C.J., Cooke, B.M., and Breedlove, S.M. (2002a). Differences in finger length ratios between self-identified 'butch' and 'femme' lesbians. *Archives of Sexual Behavior* 31: 123–7.

Brown, W.M., Hines, M., Fane, B.A., and Breedlove, S.M. (2002b). Masculinised finger length patterns in human males and females with congenital adrenal hyperplasia. *Hormones and Behavior* 42: 380–6.

Brown-Séquard, C.E. (1893). New therapeutic method consisting in the use of organic liquids extracted from glands and other organs. *British Medical Journal* 2: 1145–7; 1212–14.

Bruckert, L., Liénard, J.-S., Lacroix, A., Kreutzer, M., and Leboucher, G. (2006). Women use voice parameters to assess men's characteristics. *Proceedings of the Royal Society of London, B* 273: 83–9.

Bryden, M.P., McManus, I.C., and Bulman-Fleming, M.B. (1994). Evaluating the empirical support for the Geschwind-Behan-Galaburda Model of cerebral lateralization. *Brain and Cognition* 26: 103–67.

Buck, J.J., Williams, R.M., Hughes, I.A., and Acerini, C.L. (2003). In-utero androgen exposure and 2nd to 4th digit ratio length ratio – comparisons between healthy controls and females with classical congenital adrenal hyperplasia. *Human Reproduction* 18: 976–9.

Bull, R., and Benson, P.J. (2006). Digit ratio (2D:4D) and the spatial representation of magnitude. *Hormones and Behavior* 50: 194–9.

Burley, N. (1979). The evolution of concealed ovulation. *American Naturalist* 114: 835–58.

Burnham, T.C., Chapman, J.F., Gray, P.B., McIntyre, M.H., Lipson, S.F., and

Ellison, P.T. (2003). Men in committed romantic relationships have lower testosterone. *Hormones and Behavior* 44: 119–22.

Burton, L.A., Henninger, D., and Hafetz, J. (2005). Gender differences in relations of mental rotation, verbal fluency, and SAT scores to finger length ratios as hormonal influences. *Developmental Neuropsychology* 28: 493–505.

Byne, W., Tobet, S., Mattiace, L.A., Lasco, M.S., Kemether, E., Edgar, M.A., Morgello, S., Buchsbaum, M.S., and Jones, L.B. (2001). The interstitial nucleus of the human anterior hypothalamus: an investigation of variation with sex, sexual orientation, and HIV status. *Hormones and Behavior* 40: 86–92.

Caldwell, B.M., and Watson, R.I. (1952). An evaluation of psychologic effects of sex hormone administration in aged women: results of therapy after six months. *Journal of Gerontology* 7: 228–44.

Caldwell, G.S., Glickman, S.E., and Smith, E.R. (1984). Seasonal aggression is independent of seasonal testosterone in wood rats. *Proceedings of the National Academy of Science, USA* 81: 5255–7.

Caldwell, J.D., Johns, J., Faggin, B.M., Senger, M.A., and Pedersen, C.A. (1994). Infusion of an oxytocin antagonist into the medial preoptic area prior to progesterone inhibits sexual receptivity and increases rejection in female rats. *Hormones and Behavior* 28: 445–53.

Callard, G.V., Petro, Z., and Ryan, K.J. (1978). Phylogenetic distribution of aromatase and other androgen-converting enzymes in the central nervous system. *Endocrinology* 103: 2283–90.

Campbell, A., Muncer, S., and Odber, J. (1998). Primacy of organising effects of testosterone. *Behavioral and Brain Sciences* 21: 365.

Campbell, B., and Pedersen, W.E. (1953). Milk let down and the orgasm in the human female. *Human Biology* 25: 165–8.

Canoine, V., and Gwinner, E. (2002a). Seasonality in androgenic control of aggressive behavior in captive European stonechats (*Saxicola torquata*). *Hormones and Behavior* 41: 446.

(2002b). Seasonal differences in the hormonal control of territorial aggression in free-living European stonechats. *Hormones and Behavior* 41:1–8.

Caplan, P.J., MacPherson, G.M., and Tobin, P. (1985). Do sex-related differences in spatial abilities exist? A multilevel critique with new data. *American Psychologist* 40: 786–99.

Carani, C., Granata, A.R.M., Bancroft, J., and Marrama, P. (1995). The effects of testosterone replacement on nocturnal penile tumescence and rigidity and erectile response to visual erotic stimuli in hypogonadal men. *Psychoneuroendocrinology* 20: 743–53.

Carlson, N.R. (2004). *Physiology of Behavior*. London: Allyn and Bacon, 8th edition.

Carmichael, M.S., Humbert, R., Dixen, J., Palmisano, G., Greenleaf, W., and Davidson, J.M. (1987). Plasma oxytocin increases in the human sexual response. *Journal of Clinical Endocrinology and Metabolism* 64: 27–31.

Carré, J., Muir, C., Belanger, J., and Putnam, S.K. (2006). Pre-competition hormonal and psychological levels of elite hockey players: relationship to the 'home advantage'. *Physiology and Behavior* 89: 392–8.

Carter C.S. (1992). Oxytocin and sexual behaviour. *Neuroscience and Biobehavioral Reviews* 16: 131–44.

(1998). Neuroendocrine perspectives on social attachment and love. *Psychoneuro-endocrinology* 23: 779–818.

Carter, C.S., and Altemus, M. (1997). Integrative functions of lactational hormones in social behaviour and stress management. *Annals of the New York Academy of Science* 807: 164–74.

Carter, C.S., DeVries, A.C., and Getz, L.L. (1995). Physiological substrates of mammalian monogamy: the prairie vole model. *Neuroscience and Biobehavioral Reviews* 19: 303–14.

Carter, C.S., and Getz, L.L. (1993). Monogamy and the prairie vole. *Scientific American* June: 70–6.

Caruso, S., Maiolino, L., Rugulo, S., Intelisano, G., Farina, M., Cocuzza, S., and Serra, A. (2003). Auditory brainstem responses in premenopausal women taking oral contraceptives. *Human Reproduction* 18: 85–9.

Cashdan, E. (1995). Hormones, sex, and status in women. *Hormones and Behavior* 29: 354–66.

(2003). Hormones and competitive aggression in women. *Aggressive Behaviour* 29: 107–15.

Chae, S.W., Choi, G., Kang, H.J., Choi, J.O., and Jin, S.M. (2001). Clinical analysis of voice change as a parameter of premenstrual syndrome. *Journal of Voice* 15: 278–83.

Chambers, K.C., Thornton, J.E., and Roselli, C.E. (1991). Age-related deficits in brain androgen metabolism, testosterone, and sexual behaviour of male rats. *Neurobiology of Aging* 12: 123–30.

Chavanne, T.J., and Gallup, G.G. (1998). Variation in risk taking behaviour among female college students as a function of the menstrual cycle. *Evolution and Human Behavior* 19: 27–32.

Cheng, M.-F., and Burke, W.H. (1983). Serum prolactin levels and crop-sac development in ring doves during a breeding cycle. *Hormones and Behavior* 17: 54–65.

Cherrier, M.M., Asthana, S., Plymate, S., Baker, L., Matsumoto, A.M., Peskind, E., Raskind, M.A., Brodkin, K., Bremner, W., Petrova, A., LaTendresse, S., and Craft, S. (2001). Testosterone supplementation improves spatial and verbal memory in healthy older men. *Neurology* 57: 80–8.

Cherrier, M.M., Matsumoto, A.M., Amory, J.K., Johnson, M., Craft, S., Peskind, E.R., and Raskind, M.A. (2007). Characterization of verbal and spatial memory changes from moderate to supraphysiological increases in serum testosterone in healthy older men. *Psychoneuroendocrinology* 32: 72–9.

Chesler, E.J., and Juraska, J.M. (2000). Acute administration of estrogen and progesterone impairs the acquisition of the spatial Morris water maze in ovariectomised rats. *Hormones and Behavior* 38: 234–42.

Chiarello, C., McMahon, M.A., and Schaefer, K. (1989). Visual cerebral lateralization over phases of the menstrual cycle: a preliminary investigation. *Brain and Cognition* 11: 18–36.

Cho, M.M., DeVries, C.A., Williams, J.R., and Carter, C.S. (1999). The effects of oxytocin and vasopressin on partner preferences in male and female prairie voles (*Microtus ochrogaster*). *Behavioral Neuroscience* 113: 1071–9.

Choi, P.Y.L., Parrott, A.C., and Cowan, D. (1990). High-dose anabolic steroids in strength athletes: effects upon hostility and aggression. *Human Psychopharmacology* 5: 349–56.

Chopra, I.J., and Sabatino, L. (2000). Nature and sources of circulating thyroid hormones. In L.E. Braverman and R.D. Utiger (eds.), *Werner and Ingbar's the
Thyroid: A Fundamental and Clinical Text*. New York: Lippincott, Williams
and Wilkins, 8th edition, pp. 121–35.

Chopra, I.J., Solomon, D.H., and Chua Teco, G.N. (1973). Thyroxine: just a prohormone or a hormone too? *Journal of Clinical Endocrinology and Metabolism*
36: 1050–7.

Christiansen, K. (1993). Sex hormone-related variations of cognitive performance
in !Kung San hunter-gatherers of Namibia. *Neuropsychobiology* 27:
97–107.

Christiansen, K., and Knussmann, R. (1987). Sex hormones and cognitive functioning in men. *Neuropsychobiology* 18: 27–36.

Clark, A.S., Davis, L.A., and Roy, E.J. (1985). A possible physiological basis for the
dud-stud phenomenon. *Hormones and Behavior* 19: 227–30.

Clark, C., Klonoff, H., and Hayden, M. (1990). Regional cerebral glucose metabolism in Turner's syndrome. *The Canadian Journal of Neurological Sciences*
17: 140–4.

Clutton-Brock, T.H., Albon, S.D., Gibson, R.J., and Guiness, F.E. (1979). The logical
stag: adaptive aspects of fighting in red deer (*Cervus elaphus*). *Animal
Behaviour* 27: 211–25.

Coe, C.L., Hayashi, K.T., and Levine, S. (1988). Hormones and behaviour at puberty:
activation or concatenation? In M.R. Gunnar and W.A. Collins (eds.),
*Development during the Transition to Adolescence*. Hillsdale, NJ: Erlbaum,
pp. 17–41.

Cohen, D., Nisbett, R.E., Bowdle, B.F., and Schwarz, N. (1996). Insult, aggression,
and the Southern culture of honor: an 'experimental' ethnology. *Journal of
Personality and Social Psychology* 70: 945–60.

Cohen-Bendahan, C.C.C., Buielaar, J.K., van Goozen, S.H.M., and Cohen-Kettenis,
P.T. (2004). Prenatal exposure to testosterone and functional cerebral
lateralization: a study of same-sex and opposite-sex twin girls.
*Psychoneuroendocrinology* 29: 911–16.

Cohen-Kettenis, P.T. (2005). Gender change in 46,XY persons with 5α-reductase-2
deficiency and 17β-hydroxysteroid dehydrogenase-3 deficiency. *Archives of
Sexual Behavior* 34: 399–410.

Cohen-Kettenis, P.T., van Goozen, S.H.M., Doorn, C.D., and Gooren, L.J.G.
(1998). Cognitive ability and cerebral lateralisation in transsexuals.
*Psychoneuroendocrinology* 23: 631–41.

Cohen-Kettenis, P., and Pfäfflin, F. (2003). *Transgenderism and Intersexuality in
Childhood. Developmental Clinical Psychology and Psychiatry*, vol. 46.
London: Sage.

Colapinto, J. (2000). *As Nature Made Him: The Boy Who Was Raised as a Girl*.
London: Quartet Books.

Collaer, M.L., and Hines, M. (1995). Human behavioral sex differences: a role for
gonadal hormones during early development? *Psychological Bulletin* 118:
55–107.

Commins, D., and Yahr, P. (1984). Adult testosterone levels influence the morphology of a sexually dimorphic area in the Mongolian gerbil brain. *The Journal
of Comparative Neurology* 224: 132–40.

(1985). Autoradiographic localization of estrogen and androgen receptors in the sexually dimorphic area and other regions of the gerbil brain. *Journal of Comparative Neurology* 231: 473–89.

Compton, R.J., and Levine, S.C. (1997). Menstrual cycle phase and mood effects on perceptual asymmetry. *Brain and Cognition* 35: 168–83.

Connolly, P.B., Handa, R.J., and Resko, J.A. (1988). Progesterone modulation of androgen receptors in the brain and pituitary of male guinea pigs. *Endocrinology* 122: 2547–53.

Connolly, P.B., and Resko, J.A. (1989). Progestins affect reproductive behaviour and androgen receptor dynamics in male guinea pigs. *Brain Research* 305: 312–16.

Constantini, R.M., Park, J.H., Beery, A.K., Paul, M.J., Ko, J.J., and Zucker, I. (2007). Post-castration retention of reproductive behaviour and olfactory preferences in male Siberian hamsters: role of prior experience. *Hormones and Behavior* 51: 149–55.

Conte, F.A., and Grumbach, M.M. (1997). Abnormalities of sexual determination and differentiation. In F.S. Greenspan and G.J. Strewler (eds.), *Basic and Clinical Endocrinology*. Stamford: Appleton and Lange, 5th edition, pp. 487–520.

Contempré, B., Juaniaux, E., Jurkovic, D., Campbell, S., and Morreale de Escobar, G. (1993). Detection of thyroid hormone in human embryonic cavities during the first trimester of pregnancy. *Journal of Clinical Endocrinology and Metabolism* 77: 1719–22.

Coolican, J., and Peters, M. (2003). Sexual dimorphism in the 2D:4D ratio and its relation to mental rotation performance. *Evolution and Human Behavior* 24: 179–83.

Cooper, A.J. (1986). Progestogens in the treatment of male sex offenders: a review. *Canadian Journal of Psychiatry* 31: 73–9.

Cordoba, O.A., and Chapel, J.L. (1983). Medroxyprogesterone acetate antiandrogen treatment of hypersexuality in a pedophiliac sex offender. *American Journal of Psychiatry* 140: 1036–9.

Coren, S. (1992). *Left Hander*. London: John Murray.

Corter, C., and Fleming, A.S. (1995). Psychobiology of maternal behaviour in human beings. In M. Bonstein (eds.), *Handbook of Parenting*. Hillsdale, NJ: Erlbaum, pp. 87–116.

Cowan, W.M. (1979). The development of the brain. *Scientific American* September: 107–17.

Crews, D. (1994). Temperature, steroids, and sex determination. *Journal of Endocrinology* 142: 1–8.

(1998). The evolutionary antecedents to love. *Psychoneuroendocrinology* 23: 751–64.

Crews, D., and Moore, M.C. (2005). Historical contributions of research on reptiles to behavioral neuroendocrinology. *Hormones and Behavior* 48: 384–94.

Csakvari, E., Hoyk, Z., Gyenes, A., Garcia-Ovejero, D., Garcia-Segura, L.M., and Párducz, Á. (2007). Fluctuation of synapse density in the arcuate nucleus during the estrous cycle. *Neuroscience* 144: 1288–92.

Csathó, A., Osváth, A., Bicsák, E., Karádi, K., Manning, J., and Kállai, J. (2003). Sex role identity related to the ratio of the second to fourth digit length in women. *Biological Psychology* 62: 147–56.

Cunha, G.R., Place, N.J., Cao, M., Baskin, L., Conley, A., Cunha, T.J., and Glickman, S.E. (2005). The ontogeny of the urogenital system of the spotted hyena (*Crocuta crocuta Erxleben*). *Biology of Reproduction* 73: 554–64.

Cutler, W.B., and Genovese-Stone, E. (2000). Wellness is women after 40 years of age: the role of sex hormones and pheromones (part I). *Current Problems in Obstetrics, Gynecology and Fertility* 23: 1–32.

Dabbs, J.M. Jr. (1990a). Age and seasonal variations in serum testosterone concentration among men. *Chronobiology International* 7: 245–9.

(1990b). Salivary testosterone measurements: reliability across hours, days, and weeks. *Physiology and Behavior* 48: 83–6.

(1993). Salivary testosterone measurements in behavioral studies. *Annals of the New York Academy of Science* 694: 177–83.

(1997). Testosterone, smiling and facial appearance. *Journal of Nonverbal Behaviour* 21: 45–55.

(2000). *Heroes, Rogues and Lovers: Testosterone and Behavior*. New York: McGraw-Hill.

Dabbs, J.M. Jr., Bernieri, F.J., Strong, R.K., Campo, R., and Milun, R. (2001). Going on stage: testosterone in greetings and meetings. *Journal of Research in Personality* 35: 27–40.

Dabbs, J.M. Jr., Campbell, B.C., Gladue, B.A., Midgley, A.R., Navarro, M.A., Read, G.F., Susman, E.J., Swinkels, L.M.J.W., and Wothman, C.M. (1995a). Reliability of salivary testosterone measurements: a multicenter evaluation. *Clinical Chemistry* 41: 1581–4.

Dabbs, J.M. Jr., Carr, T.S., Frady, R.L., and Riad, J.K. (1995b). Testosterone, crime, and misbehaviour among 692 male prison inmates. *Personality and Individual Differences* 18: 627–33.

Dabbs, J.M. Jr., Hargrove, M.F., and Heusel, C. (1996). Testosterone differences among college fraternities: well-behaved vs. rambunctious. *Personality and Individual Differences* 20: 157–61.

Dabbs, J.M. Jr., Jurkovic, G.J., and Frady, R.L. (1991). Salivary testosterone and cortisol among late adolescent male offenders. *Journal of Abnormal Child Psychology* 19: 469–78.

Dabbs, J.M. Jr., and Mallinger, A. (1999). High testosterone levels predict low voice pitch among men. *Personality and Individual Differences* 27: 801–4.

Dabbs, J.M. Jr., and Mohammed, S. (1992). Male and female salivary testosterone concentrations before and after sexual activity. *Physiology and Behavior* 52: 195–7.

Dabbs, J.M. Jr., and Morris, R. (1990). Testosterone, social class, and antisocial behavior in a sample of 4,462 men. *Psychological Science* 1: 209–11.

Daitzman, R.J., and Zuckerman, M. (1980). Disinhibitory sensation seeking, personality and gonadal hormones. *Journal of Biosocial Science* 10: 401–8.

Dalton, K. (1960). Effect of menstruation on schoolgirls' weekly work. *British Medical Journal* 1: 326–8.

Daly, M., and Wilson, M. (1988). *Homicide*. New York: Aldine.

Damasio, A.R., and Van Hoesen, G.W. (1983). Emotional disturbances associated with focal lesions of the limbic frontal lobe. In K.M. Heilman and P. Satz (eds.), *Neuropsychology of Human Emotion*. New York: Guildford Press, pp. 85–110.

Damassa, D.A., Davidson, J.M., and Smith, E.R. (1977). The relationship between circulating testosterone levels and male sexual behaviour in rats. *Hormones and Behavior* 8: 275–86.

Dancey, C.P. (1990). Sexual orientation in women: an investigation of hormonal and personality variables. *Biological Psychology* 30: 251–64.

Dawson, J.L.M., Cheung, Y.M., and Lau, R.T.S. (1975). Developmental effects of neonatal sex hormones on spatial and activity skills in the white rat. *Biological Psychology* 3: 213–29.

Davidson, J.M., Camargo, C.A., and Smith, E.R. (1979). Effects of androgen on sexual behaviour in hypogonadal men. *Journal of Clinical Endocrinology and Metabolism* 48: 955–8.

De Courten-Myers, G. (1999). The human cerebral cortex: gender differences in structure and function. *Journal of Neuropathology and Experimental Neurology* 58: 217–26.

de Lacoste, M.C., Kirkpatrick, J.B., and Ross, E.D. (1986). Topography of the human corpus callosum. *Journal of Neuropathology and Experimental Neurology* 44: 578–91.

de Lacoste-Utamsing, C., and Holloway, R.L. (1982). Sexual dimorphism in the human corpus callosum. *Science* 216: 1431–2.

De Voogd, T.J., and Nottebohm, F. (1981). Gonadal hormones induce dendritic growth in the adult avian brain. *Science* 214: 202–4.

De Vries, G.J., and Simerly, R.B. (2002). Anatomy, development, and function of the sexually dimorphic circuits in the mammalian brain. In D.W. Pfaff, A.P. Arnold, A.M. Etgen, S.E. Fahrbach, and R.T. Rubin (eds.), *Hormones, Brain and Behavior*, vol. 4. San Diego, CA: Academic Press, pp. 137–54.

De Wied, D., Diamant, M., and Fodor, M. (1993). Central nervous system effects of neurohypophyseal hormones and related peptides. *Frontiers in Neuroendocrinology* 14: 251–302.

Dehaene, S. (1997). *The Number Sense: How the Mind Creates Mathematics*. Oxford: Oxford University Press.

Dehaene, S., Bossini, S., and Giraux, P. (1993). The mental representation of parity and number magnitude. *Journal of Experimental Psychology (General)* 122: 371–96.

Dekaban, A.S., and Sadowsky, D.S. (1978). Changes in brain weights during the span of human life: relation of brain weights to body heights and body weights. *Annals of Neurology* 4: 345–56.

del Abril, A., Segovia, S., and Guillamon, A. (1987). The bed nucleus of the stria terminalis in the rat: regional sex differences controlled by gonadal steroids early after birth. *Brain Research* 429: 295–300.

Delahunty, K.M., McKay, D.W., Noseworthy, D.E., and Storey, A.E. (2007). Prolactin responses to infant cues in men and women: effects of parental experience and recent infant contact. *Hormones and Behavior* 51: 213–20.

Dempsey, E.W., Hertz, R., and Young, W.C. (1936). The experimental induction of oestrus (sexual receptivity) in the normal and ovariectomised guinea pig. *American Journal of Physiology* 116: 201–9.

Dennerstein, L., Dudley, E., Hopper, J.L., and Burger, H. (1997). Sexuality, hormones and the menopausal transition. *Maturitas* 26: 83–93.

Dennerstein, L., Randolph, J., Taffe, J., Dudley, E., and Burger, H. (2002). Hormones, mood, sexuality, and the menopausal transition. *Fertility and Sterility* 77 (Suppl. 4): S42–8.

DeRidder, C.M., Bruning, P.F., Zonderland, M.L., Thijssen, J.H.H., Bonfrer, J.M.G., Blankenstein, M.A., Husveld, L.A., and Erich, W.B.M. (1990). Body fat mass, body fat distribution, and plasma hormones in early puberty in females. *Journal of Clinical Endocrinology and Metabolism* 70: 888–93.

Dessens, A.B., Slijper, F.M.E., and Drop, S.L.S. (2003). Gender dysphoria and gender change in chromosomal females with congenital adrenal hyperplasia. *Archives of Sexual Behavior* 34: 389–97.

Diamond, L.M. (2004). Emerging perspectives on distinctions between romantic love and sexual desire. *Current Directions in Psychological Science* 13: 116–19.

Diamond, M. (1966). Progestagen inhibition of normal sexual behaviour in the male guinea pig. *Nature* 209: 1322–4.

Diamond, M., Diamond, A.L., and Mast, M. (1972). Visual sensitivity and sexual arousal levels during the menstrual cycle. *Journal of Nervous and Mental Diseases* 155: 170–6.

Diamond, M.C., Dowling, G.A., and Johnson, R.E. (1981). Morphologic cerebral cortical asymmetry in male and female rats. *Experimental Neurology* 71: 261–8.

Diamond, M.C., Johnson, R.E., and Ehlert, J. (1979). A comparison of cortical thickness in male and female rats – normal and gonadectomised young and adult. *Neural Biology* 26: 485–91.

Diamond, M.C., Johnson, R.E., and Ingham, C.A. (1975). Morphological changes in the young, adult and aging rat cerebral cortex, hippocampus and diencephalon. *Behavioral Biology* 14: 163–74.

Diamond, M.C., Llacuna, A., and Wong, C.L. (1973). Sex behaviour after neonatal progesterone, testosterone, estrogen or anti-androgens. *Hormonal Behavior* 4: 73.

Diamond, M., and Sigmundson H.K. (1997). Sex reassignment at birth. Long-term review and clinical implications. *Archives of Pediatric and Adolescent Medicine* 151: 298–304.

Dittman, R.W., Kappes, M.H., Kappes, M.E., Borger, D., Stegner, H., Willig, R.H., and Wallis, H. (1990). Congenital adrenal hyperplasia I: gender-related behavior and attitudes in female patients and sisters. *Psychoneuroendocrinology* 15: 401–20.

Dixson, A.F. (1980). Androgens and aggressive behaviour in primates: a review. *Aggressive Behaviour* 6: 37–67.

Dixson, A.F., Everitt, G.J., Herbert, J., Rugman, S.M., and Scruton, D.M. (1973). Hormonal and other determinants of sexual attractiveness and receptivity in rhesus and talapoin monkeys. *Symposia of the IVth International Congress of Primatology*, vol. 2: *Primate Reproductive Behavior*. Basel: Karger, pp. 36–63.

Döhler, K.D., Hancke, J.L., Srivastava, S.S., Hofman, C., Shryne, J.E., and Gorski, R.A. (1984a). Participation of estrogens in female sexual differentiation of the brain: neuroanatomical, neuroendocrine and behavioural evidence. In G.J. De Vries., J.P.C. De Bruin, H.B.M. Uylings, and M.A. Corner (eds.), *Progress in Brain Research*, vol. 61. Amsterdam: Elsevier, pp. 99–117.

Döhler, K.D., Hines, M., Coquelin, A., Davis, F., Shryne, J.E., and Gorski, R.A. (1984b). Pre- and postnatal influence of testosterone propionate and diethylstilbestrol on differentiation of the sexually dimorphic nucleus of the preoptic area in male and female rats. *Brain Research* 302: 291–5.

Döhler, K.D., Srivastava, S.S., Shryne, J.E., Jarzab, B., Sipos, A., and Gorski, R.A. (1984c). Differentiation of the sexually dimorphic nucleus in the preoptic area of the rat brain is inhibited by postnatal treatment with an estrogen antagonist. *Neuroendocrinology* 38: 297–301.

Don, B.R., Biglieri, E.G., and Schamelan, M. (1997). Endocrine hypertension. In F.S. Greenspan and G.J. Strewler (eds.), *Basic and Clinical Endocrinology*. Stamford: Appleton and Lange, 5th edition, pp. 359–80.

Doraiswamy, P.M. (1997). Gender, concurrent estrogen use and cognition in AD. *International Journal of Geriatric Psychopharmacology* 1: 34–7.

Dörner, G. (1976). *Hormones and Brain Sexual Differentiation*. Amsterdam: Elsevier Scientific.

(1979). Psychoneuroendocrine aspects of brain development and reproduction. In L. Zichella and E. Pancheri (eds.), *Psychoneuroendocrinology and Reproduction: Interdisciplinity Approach*. Amsterdam: Elsevier.

Dörner, G., Geier, T., and Ahrens, L. (1980). Prenatal stress as a possible aetiological factor of homosexuality in human males. *Endokrinologie* 75: 365–8.

Dörner, G., Poppe, I., Stahl, F., Kölzsch,, J., and Uebelhack, R. (1991). Gene- and environment-dependent neuroendocrine etiogenesis of homosexuality and transsexualism. *Experimental and Clinical Endocrinology* 98: 141–50.

Dörner, G., Rhode, W., Stahl, F., Krell, L., and Masius, W.G. (1975). A neuroendocrine predisposition for homosexuality in man. *Archives of Sexual Behavior* 4: 1–8.

Dörner, G., Schenck, B., Schmiedel, B., and Ahrens, L. (1983). Stressful events in prenatal life of bi- and homosexual men. *Experimental and Clinical Endocrinology* 81: 83–7.

Doughty, C., Booth, J.E., McDonald, P.G., and Parrot, R.F. (1975). Effects of estradiol benzoate and synthetic estrogen RU-2858 on sexual differentiation in the neonatal rat. *Journal of Endocrinology* 67: 419–24.

Downey, J., Ehrhardt, A.A., Schiffman, M., Dyrenfurth, I., and Becker, J. (1987). Sex hormones in lesbian and heterosexual women. *Hormones and Behavior* 21: 347–57.

Dratman, M.B., Futaesaku, Y., Crutchfield, F.L., Berman, N., Payne, B., Sar, M., and Stumpf, W.E. (1982). Iodine-125-labelled triiodothyronine in rat brain: evidence for localization in discrete neural systems. *Science* 215: 309–12.

Drea, C.M., Weldele, M.L., Forger, N.G., Coscia, E.M., Frank, L.G., Licht, P., and Glickman, S.E. (1998). Androgens and masculinisation of the genitalia in the spotted hyaena (*Crocuta crocuta*). 2. Effects of prenatal anti-androgens. *Journal of Reproduction and Fertility* 113: 118–28.

Duff, S.J., and Hampson, E. (2000). A beneficial effect of estrogen on working memory in postmenopausal women taking hormone replacement therapy. *Hormones and Behavior* 38: 262–76.

Duffy, R., Wiseman, H., and File, S.E. (2003). Improved cognitive function in postmenopausal women after 12 weeks of consumption of a soya extract containing isoflavones. *Pharmacology, Biochemistry and Behavior* 75: 721–9.

Dugatkin, L.A. (1997). Winner and loser effects and the structures of dominance hierarchies. *Behavioral Ecology* 8: 583–7.

Duka, T., Tasker, R., and McGowan, J.F. (2000). The effects of 3-week estrogen hormone replacement on cognition in elderly healthy females. *Psychopharmacology* 149: 129–39.

Dye, L. (1992). Visual information processing and the menstrual cycle. In J.T.E. Richardson (eds.), *Cognition and the Menstrual Cycle*. London: Springer-Verlag, pp. 67–97.

Eaton, G.G., and Resko, J.A. (1974). Ovarian hormones and sexual behaviour in *Macaca nemestrina*. *Journal of Comparative and Physiological Psychology* 86: 919–25.

Edwards, D.A., Wetzel, K., and Wyner, D.R. (2006). Intercollegiate soccer: saliva cortisol and testosterone are elevated during competition, and testosterone is related to status and social connectedness with teammates. *Physiology and Behavior* 87: 135–43.

Ehrhardt, A.A., Epstein, R., and Money, J. (1968). Fetal androgens and female gender identity in the early-treated androgenital syndrome. *Johns Hopkins Medical Journal* 122: 165–7.

Ehrhardt, A.A., and Meyer-Bahlburg, H.F.L. (1981). Effects of prenatal sex hormones on gender-related behaviour. *Science* 211: 1312–18.

Elkadi, S., Nicholls, M.E.R., and Clode, D. (1999). Handedness in opposite and same-sex dizygotic twins: testing the testosterone hypothesis. *NeuroReport* 10: 333–6.

Ellis, H. (1915). *Studies in the Psychology of Sex*, vol. 2: *Sexual Inversion*. Philadelphia, PA: Davis.

Ellis, L. (2006). Gender differences in smiling: an evolutionary neuroandrogenic theory. *Physiology and Behavior* 88: 303–8.

Ellis, L., and Ames, M.A. (1987). Neurohormonal functioning and sexual orientation: a theory of homosexuality–heterosexuality. *Psychological Bulletin* 101: 233–58.

Ellis, L., Ames, M.A., Peckham, W., and Burke, D. (1988). Sexual orientation of human offspring may be altered by severe maternal stress during pregnancy. *Journal of Sex Research* 25: 152–7.

Ellison, P.T. (1988). Human salivary steroids: methodological considerations and applications in physical anthropology. *Yearbook of Physical Anthropology* 31: 115–42.

Elwood, R.W., and Mason, C. (1994). The couvades and the onset of paternal care: a biological perspective. *Ethology and Sociobiology* 15: 145–56.

Enlow, D.H. (1996). Growth of the mandible. In D.H. Enlow and M.G. Hans (eds.), *Essentials of Facial Growth*. Philadelphia: Saunders, pp. 57–78.

Epting, L.K., and Overman, W.H. (1998). Sex-sensitive tasks in men and women: a search for performance fluctuations across the menstrual cycle. *Behavioural Neuroscience* 112: 1304–17.

Erpino, M.J. (1973). Temporary inhibition by progesterone of sexual behaviour in intact male mice. *Hormones and Behavior* 4: 335–9.

Etgen, A.M., Ungar, S., and Petitti, N. (1992). Estradiol and progesterone modulation of norepinephrine neurotransmission: implications for the regulation of female reproductive behaviour. *Journal of Neuroendocrinology* 58: 352–8.

Evans, R.M. (1988). The steroid and thyroid hormone receptor superfamily. *Science* 240: 889–95.

Evans, R.M., and Arriza, J.L. (1989). A molecular framework for the actions of glucocorticoid hormones in the nervous system. *Neuron* 2: 1105–12.

Fadem, B.H., Barfield, R.J., and Whalen, R.E. (1979). Dose-response and time-response relationships between progesterone and the display of patterns of receptive and proceptive behaviour in the female rat. *Hormones and Behavior* 13: 40–8.

Fagot, B.I. (1978). The influence of sex of child on parental reactions to toddler children. *Child Development* 49: 459–65.

Fagot, B.I., and Leinbach, M.D. (1993). Gender-role development in young children: from discrimination to labelling. *Developmental Review* 13: 205–24.

Fahrbach, S.E., and Mesce, K.A. (2005). 'Neuroethoendocrinology': integration of field and laboratory studies in insect neuroendocrinology. *Hormones and Behavior* 48: 352–9.

Fahrbach, S.E., Morrell, J.I., and Pfaff, D.W. (1985). Possible role for endogenous oxytocin in estrogen-facilitated maternal behaviour in the rat. *Neuroendocrinology* 40: 526–32.

Faiman, C., and Winter, J.S.D. (1971). Diurnal cycles in plasma FSH, testosterone and cortisol in men. *Journal of Clinical Endocrinology* 33: 186–92.

Falahati-Nini, A., Riggs, B.L., Atkinson, E.J., O'Fallon, W.M., Eastell, R., and Khosla, S. (2000). Relative contributions of testosterone and estrogen in regulating bone resorption and formation in normal elderly men. *Journal of Clinical Investigation* 106: 1553–60.

Falkenstein, E., Tillmann, H.-C., Christ, M., Feuring, M., and Wehling, M. (2000). Multiple actions of steroid hormones – a focus on rapid, nongenomic effects. *Pharmacological Review* 52: 513–55.

Falter, C.M., Arroyo, M., and Davis, G.J. (2006). Testosterone: activation or organization of spatial cognition? *Biological Psychology* 73: 132–40.

Farrell, S.F., and McGuinness, M.Y. (2003). Effects of pubertal anabolic-androgenic steroid (AAS) administration on reproductive and aggressive behaviours in male rats. *Behavioral Neuroscience* 117: 904–11.

Feder, H.H. (1981). Estrous cyclicity in mammals. In N.T. Adler (ed.), *Neuroendocrinology of Reproduction*. New York: Plenum Press, pp. 279–348.

Feder, H.H., Storey, A., Goodwin, D., Reboulleau, C., and Silver, R. (1977). Testosterone and '5α-dihydrotestosterone' levels in peripheral plasma of male and female ring doves (*Streptopelia risoria*) during the reproductive cycle. *Biology of Reproduction* 16: 666–77.

Feinberg, D.R., Jones, B.C., Law-Smith, M.J., Moore, F.R., Debruine, L.M., Cornwell, R.E., Hillier, S.G., and Perrett, D.I. (2005). Menstrual cycle, trait estrogen level, and masculinity preferences in the human voice. *Hormones and Behavior* 49: 215–22.

Feldman, M.P., and MacCulloch, M.J. (1971). *Homosexual Behaviour: Therapy and Assessment*. Oxford: Pergamon Press.

Ferguson, J.N., Young, L.J., Hearn, E.F., Matzuk, M.M., Insel, T.R., and Winslow, J.T. (2000). Social amnesia in mice lacking the oxytocin gene. *Nature Genetics* 25: 284–8.

Fernández-Guasti, A., Kruijver, F.P.M., Fodor, M., and Swaab, D.F. (2000). Sex differences in the distribution of androgen receptors in the human hypothalamus. *Journal of Comparative Neurology* 425: 422–35.

Ferris, C.F., and Delville, Y. (1994). Vasopressin and serotonin interactions in the control of agonistic behaviour. *Psychoneuroendocrinology* 19: 593–601.

File, S.E., Jarrett, N., Fluck, E., Duffy, R., Casey, K., and Wiseman, H. (2001). Eating soya improves human memory. *Psychopharmacology* 157: 430–6.

Findling, J.W., Aron, D.C., and Tyrrell, J.B. (1997). Glucocorticoid and adrenal androgens. In F.S. Greenspan and G.J. Strewler (eds.), *Basic and Clinical Endocrinology*. Stamford: Appleton and Lange, 5th edition, pp. 317–58.

Finegan, J.-A.K., Nicols, G.A., and Sitarenios, G. (1992). Relations between prenatal testosterone levels and cognitive abilities at 4 years. *Developmental Psychology* 28: 1075–89.

Fink, B., Brookes, H., Neave, N., and Manning, J.T. (2006). Second to fourth digit ratio and numerical competence in children. *Brain and Cognition* 61: 211–18.

Fink, B., Grammer, K., Mitteroecker, P., Gunz, P., Schaefer, K., Bookstein, F.L., and Manning, J.T. (2005). Second to fourth digit ratio and face shape. *Proceedings of the Royal Society of London, B* 272: 1995–2001.

Fink, B., Grammer, K., and Thornhill, R. (2001). Human (*Homo sapiens*) facial attractiveness in relation to skin texture and color. *Journal of Comparative Psychology* 115: 92–9.

Fink, B., Manning, J.T., Neave, N., and Tan, U. (2004). Second to fourth digit ratio and hand skill in Austrian children. *Biological Psychology* 67: 375–84.

Fink, B., Neave, N., Laughton, K., and Manning, J.T. (2006). Second to fourth digit ratio and sensation seeking. *Personality and Individual Differences* 41: 1253–62.

Fink, B., Neave, N., and Manning, J.T. (2003). Second to fourth digit ratio, body mass index, waist-to-hip ratio and waist-to-chest ratio: their relationships in heterosexual men and women. *Annals of Human Biology* 30: 728–38.

Finkelstein, J.W., Susman, E.J., Chinchilli, V.M., D'Arcangelo, M.R., Kunselman, S.J., Schwab, J., Demers, L.M., Liben, L.S., and Kulin, H.E. (1998). Effects of testosterone on self-reported sexual responses and behaviors in hypogonadal adolescents. *Journal of Clinical Endocrinology and Metabolism* 83: 2281–5.

Finkelstein, J.W., Susman, E.J., Chinchilli, V.M., Kunselman, S.J., D'Arcangelo, M.R., Schwab, J., Demers, L.M., Liben, L.S., Lokkingbill, G., and Kulin, H.E. (1997). Estrogen or testosterone increases self-reported aggressive behaviours in hypogonadal adolescents. *Journal of Clinical Endocrinology and Metabolism* 82: 2433–8.

Fisher, H.E. (1998). Lust, attraction, and attachment in mammalian reproduction. *Human Nature* 9: 23–52.

Fisher, H.E., Aron, A., and Brown, L.L. (2005). Romantic love: an fMRI study of a neural mechanism for mate choice. *Journal of Comparative Neurology* 493: 58–62.

  (2006). Romantic love: a mammalian brain system for mate choice. *Philosophical Transactions of the Royal Society, B* 361: 2173–86.

Fitch, R.H., and Denenberg, V.H. (1998). A role for ovarian hormones in sexual differentiation of the brain. *Behavioral and Brain Sciences* 21: 311–52.

Fitch, W.T., and Giedd, J. (1999). Morphology and development of the human vocal tract: a study using magnetic resonance imaging. *Journal of the Acoustical Society of America* 106: 1511–22.

Fite, J.E., and French, J.A. (2000). Pre- and postpartum sex steroids in female marmosets (*Callithrix kuhlii*): is there a link with infant survivorship and maternal behaviour? *Hormones and Behavior* 38: 1–12.

Fite, J.E., French, J.A., Patera, K., Hopkins, E.C., Rukstalis, M., and Ross, C.N. (2005). Elevated urinary testosterone excretion and decreased maternal caregiving effort in marmosets when conception occurs during the period of infant dependence. *Hormones and Behavior* 47: 39–48.

Fitzpatrick, L.A. (2003). Soy isoflavones: hope or hype? *Maturitas* 44 (Suppl. 1): S21–9.

Fleming, A.S. (1986). Psychobiology of rat maternal behaviour. How and where hormones act to promote maternal behaviour at parturition. *Annals of the New York Academy of Science* 474: 234–51.

Fleming, A.S., and Corter, C. (1988). Factors influencing maternal responsiveness in humans: usefulness of an animal model. *Psychoneuroendocrinology* 13: 189–212.

Fleming, A.S., Corter, C., Stallings, J., and Steiner, M. (2002). Testosterone and prolactin are associated with emotional responses to infant cries in new fathers. *Hormones and Behavior* 42: 399–413.

Fleming, A.S., Krieger, H., and Wong P. (1990). Affect and nurturance in first-time mothers: role of psychobiological influences. In B. Lerer and S. Gershon (eds.), *New Directions in Affective Disorders*. New York: Springer-Verlag, pp. 388–92.

Fleming, A.S., Ruble, D., Krieger, H., and Wong, P.Y. (1997). Hormonal and experiential correlates of maternal responsiveness during pregnancy and the puerperium in human mothers. *Hormones and Behavior* 31: 145–58.

Fleming, A.S., Steiner, M., and Anderson, V. (1987). Hormonal and attitudinal correlates of maternal behaviour during the early postpartum period. *Journal of Reproductive and Infant Psychology* 5: 193–205.

Foley, T.P. Jr. (1990). Disorders of the thyroid: medical overview. In C.S. Holmes (ed.), *Psychoneuroendocrinology: Brain, Behaviour and Hormonal Interactions*. New York: Springer Verlag, pp. 261–72.

Fonda, S.J., Bertrand, R., O'Donnell, A., Longcope, C., and McKinlay, J.B. (2005). Age, hormones, and cognitive functioning among middle-aged men: cross-sectional evidence from the Massachusetts male aging study. *Journals of Gerontology Series A: Biological Sciences and Medical Sciences* 60: 385–90.

Forastieri, V., Andrade, C.P., Souza, A.L., Silva, M.S., El-Hani, C.N., Moreira, L.M., Mott, L.R., and Flores, R.Z. (2002). Evidence against a relationship between dermatoglyphic asymmetry and male sexual orientation. *Human Biology* 74: 861–70.

Forget, H., and Cohen, H. (1994). Life after birth: the influence of steroid hormones on cerebral structure and function is not fixed prenatally. *Brain and Cognition* 26: 243–8.

Fox, C.A., Ismail, A.A.A., Love, D.N., Kirkham, K.E., and Loraine, J.A. (1972).

Studies on the relationship between plasma testosterone levels and human sexual activity. *Journal of Endocrinology* 52: 51–8.

Francis, D.D., Young, L.J., Meaney, M.J., and Insel, T.R. (2002). Naturally-occurring differences in maternal care are associated with the expression of oxytocin and vasopressin (V1a) receptors: gender differences. *Journal of Neuroendocrinology* 14: 349–53.

Franco, O.H., Burger, H., Lebrun, C.E.I., Peeters, P.H.M., Lamberts, S.W.J., Grobbee, D.E., and van der Schouw, Y.T. (2005). Higher dietary intake of lignans is associated with better cognitive performance in postmenopausal women. *Journal of Nutrition* 135: 1190–5.

Frank, L.G. (1986). Social organization of the spotted hyaena *Crocuta crocuta*: II. Dominance and reproduction. *Animal Behaviour* 35: 1510–27.

Frankfurt, M., Gould, E., Wooley, C.S., and McEwen, B.S. (1990). Gonadal steroids modify dendritic spine density in ventromedial hypothalamic neurons: a Golgi study in the adult rat. *Neuroendocrinology* 51: 530–5.

Franklyn, J.A. (2000). Metabolic changes in thyrotoxicosis. In L.E. Braverman and R.D. Utiger (eds.), *Werner and Ingbar's the Thyroid: A Fundamental and Clinical Text*. New York: Lippincott, Williams and Wilkins, 8th edition, pp. 667–72.

French, D., Fitzpatrick, D., and Law, O.T. (1972). Operant investigation of mating preferences in female rats. *Journal of Comparative Physiology and Psychology* 81: 226–32.

Freund-Mercier, M.-J., Stoeckel, M.E., Palacios, J.M., Paxos, A., Reichhart, J.M., Porte, A., and Richard, P. (1987). Pharmacological characteristics and anatomical distribution of [³H] oxytocin-binding sites in the Wistar rat brain studied by autoradiography. *Neuroscience* 20: 599–614.

Friedrich, W.N., Grambsch, P., Broughton, D., Kuiper, J., and Beilke, R.L. (1991). Normative sexual behavior in children. *Pediatrics* 88: 456–64.

Fries, A.B., Ziegler, T.E., Kurian, J.R., Jacoris, S., and Pollack, C.D. (2005). Early experience in humans is associated with changes in neuropeptides critical for regulating social behavior. *Proceedings of the National Academy of Science, USA* 102: 17,237–40.

Furnham, A., and Rawles, R. (1988). Spatial ability at different times of day. *Personality and Individual Differences* 9: 937–9.

Fusani, L., Canonine, V., Goymann, W., Wikelski, M., and Hau, M. (2005). Difficulties and special issues associated with field research in behavioural neuroendocrinology. *Hormones and Behavior* 48: 484–91.

Gadea, M., Gomez, C., Gonzalez-Bono, E., Salvador, A., and Espert, R. (2003). Salivary testosterone is related to both handedness and degree of linguistic lateralization in normal women. *Psychoneuroendocrinology* 28: 274–87.

Gaines, M.S., Fugate, C.L., Johnson, M.L., Johnson, D.C., Hisey, J., and Quadagno, D.M. (1985). Manipulation of aggressive behaviour in prairie voles (*Microtus ochrogaster*) implanted with testosterone in silastic tubing. *Canadian Journal of Zoology* 63: 2525–8.

Galea, L.A.M., Kavaliers, M., Ossenkopp, K.P., and Hampson, E. (1995). Gonadal hormone levels and spatial learning performance in the Morris water maze and female meadow voles, *Microtus pennsylvanicus*. *Hormones and Behavior* 29: 106–25.

Gangestad, S.W., Thornhill, R., and Garver, C.E. (2002). Changes in women's sexual interests and their partners' mate-retention tactics across the menstrual cycle: evidence for shifting conflicts of interest. *Proceedings of the Royal Society of London, B* 269: 975–82.

Gard, P. (1998). *Human Endocrinology*. London: Taylor and Francis.

Garn, S.M., Burdi, A.R., Babler, W.J., and Stinson, S. (1975). Early prenatal attainment of adult metacarpal–phalangeal rankings and proportions. *American Journal of Physical Anthropology* 43: 327–32.

Gartrell, N.K., Loriaux, D.L., and Chase, T.N. (1977). Plasma testosterone in homosexual and heterosexual women. *American Journal of Psychiatry* 134: 1117–18.

Gazzaniga, M.S., Ivry, R.B., and Mangun, G.R. (1998). *Cognitive Neuroscience: The Biology of the Mind*. New York: W.W. Norton.

George, R. (1930). Human finger types. *Anatomical Record* 46: 199–204.

Gerall, A., Dunlop, J.L., and Hendricks, S. (1973). Effects of ovarian secretions on female behavioral potentiality in the rat. *Journal of Comparative and Physiological Psychology* 82: 449–65.

Geschwind, N., and Behan, P. (1982). Left-handedness: association with immune disease, migraine, and developmental learning disorder. *Proceedings of the National Academy of Science, USA* 79: 5097–5100.

Geschwind, N., and Galaburda, A.M. (1985a). Cerebral lateralization: biological mechanisms, associations, and pathology: I. A hypothesis and a program for research. *Archives of Neurology* 42: 428–59.

(1985b). Cerebral lateralization: biological mechanisms, associations, and pathology: II. A hypothesis and a program for research. *Archives of Neurology* 42: 521–52.

(1985c). Cerebral lateralization: biological mechanisms, associations, and pathology: III. A hypothesis and a program for research. *Archives of Neurology* 42: 6341–54.

(1987). *Cerebral Lateralization*. Cambridge, MA: MIT Press.

Gibbs, R.B. (1996). Fluctuations in relative levels of choline acetyltransferase mRNA in different regions of the rat basal forebrain across the estrous cycle: effects of estrogen and progesterone. *Journal of Neuroscience* 16: 1049–55.

(2002). Basal forebrain cholinergic neurons are necessary for estrogen to enhance acquisition of a delayed matching-to-position T-maze task. *Hormones and Behavior* 42: 245–57.

(2005). Testosterone and estradiol produce different effects on cognitive performance in male rats. *Hormones and Behavior* 48: 268–77.

Giedd, J.N. (2004). Structural magnetic resonance imaging of the adolescent brain. *Annals of the New York Academy of Science* 1021: 77–85.

Gimerale, F., Strindberg, L., and Wahlberg, I. (1975). Female work capacity during the menstrual cycle. Physiological and psychological reactions. *Scandinavian Journal of Work, Environment and Health* 1: 120–7.

Gimpl, G., and Fahrenholz, F. (2001). The oxytocin receptor system: structure, function and regulation. *Physiological Reviews* 81: 629–83.

Gladue, B.A. (1994). The biopsychology of sexual orientation. *Current Directions in Psychological Science* 3: 150–4.

Gladue, B.A., Green, R., and Hellman, R.E. (1984). Neuroendocrine response to estrogen and sexual orientation. *Science* 225: 1496–9.

Glickman, S.E., Short, R.V., and Renfree, M.B. (2005). Sexual differentiation in three unconventional mammals: spotted hyenas, elephants and tammar wallabies. *Hormones and Behavior* 48: 403–17.

Gobbetti, A., and Zerani, M. (1999). Hormonal and cellular brain mechanisms regulating the amplexus of male and female water frog (*Rana esculenta*). *Journal of Neuroendocrinology* 11: 589–96.

Goldfien, A., and Monroe, S.E. (1997). Ovaries. In F.S. Greenspan and G.J. Strewler (eds.), *Basic and Clinical Endocrinology*. Stamford: Appleton and Lange, 5th edition, pp. 434–86.

Gonzalez-Bono, E., Salvador, A., Serrano, M.A., and Ricarte, J. (1999). Testosterone, cortisol, and mood in a sports team competition. *Hormones and Behavior* 35: 55–62.

Goodfellow, P.N., and Lovell-Badge, R. (1993). SRY and sex determination in mammals. *Annual Review of Genetics* 27: 71–92.

Goodson, J.L. (2005). The vertebrate social behaviour network: evolutionary themes and variations. *Hormones and Behavior* 48: 11–22.

Gooren, L. (1986a). The neuroendocrine response of luteinizing hormone to estrogen administration in heterosexual, homosexual, and transsexual subjects. *Journal of Clinical Endocrinology and Metabolism* 63: 583–8.

(1986b). The neuroendocrine response of luteinizing hormone to estrogen administration in the human is not sex specific but dependent on the hormonal environment. *Journal of Clinical Endocrinology and Metabolism* 63: 589–93.

(1990). The endocrinology of transsexualism: a review and commentary. *Psychoneuroendocrinology* 15: 3–14.

(2006). The biology of human psychosexual differentiation. *Hormones and Behavior* 15: 3–14.

Gordon, H.W., Corbin, E.D., and Lee, P.A. (1986). Changes in specialized cognitive function following changes in hormone levels. *Cortex* 22: 399–415.

Gordon, H.W., and Lee, P.A. (1986). A relationship between gonadotropins and visuospatial function. *Neuropsychologia* 24: 563–76.

Gorski, R.A. (1985). Sexual differentiation of the brain: possible mechanisms and implications. *Canadian Journal of Physiology and Pharmacology* 63: 577–94.

Gorski, R.A., Csernus, V.J., and Jacobson, C.D. (1981). Sexual dimorphism in the preoptic area. In B. Flerko, G. Setalo, and L. Tima (eds.), *Advances in Physiological Sciences*, vol. 15: *Reproduction and Development*. Oxford: Pergamon Press, pp. 121–30.

Gorski, R.A., Gordon, J.H., Shryne, J.E., and Southam, A.M. (1978). Evidence for a morphological sex difference within the medial preoptic area of the rat brain. *Brain Research* 148: 333–46.

Gouchie, C., and Kimura, D. (1991). The relationship between testosterone levels and cognitive ability patterns. *Psychoneuroendocrinology* 16: 323–34.

Gould, E., Allan, M.D., and McEwen, B.S. (1990a). Dendritic spine density of adult hippocampal pyramidal cells is sensitive to thyroid hormone. *Brain Research* 525: 327–9.

Gould, E., Woolley, C.S., Frankfurt, M., and McEwen, B.S. (1990b). Gonadal steroids regulate dendritic spine density in hippocampal pyramidal cells in adulthood. *Journal of Neuroscience* 10: 1286–91.

Gould, S.J. (1981). *The Mismeasure of Man*. Harmondsworth: Penguin.

Goy, R.W., and McEwen, B.S. (1980). *Sexual Differentiation of the Brain*. Cambridge, MA: MIT Press.

Goy, R.W., and Phoenix, C.H. (1971). The effects of testosterone propionate administration before birth on the development of behavior in genetic female rhesus monkeys. In C.H. Sawyer and R.A. Gorski (eds.), *Steroid Hormones and Brain Function*. Berkeley and Los Angeles: University of California Press, pp. 193–202.

Granger, D.A., Schwartz, E.B., Booth, A., and Arentz, M. (1999). Salivary testosterone determination in studies of child health and development. *Hormones and Behavior* 35: 18–27.

Granger, D.A., Shirtcliff, E.A., Zahn-Waxler, C., Usher, B., Klimes-Dougan, B., and Hastings, P. (2003). Salivary testosterone diurnal variation and psychopathology in adolescent males and females: individual differences and developmental effects. *Developmental Psychopathology* 15: 431–49.

Grant, L.D., and Stumpf, W.E. (1975). Hormone uptake sites in relation to CNS biogenic amine systems. In W.E. Stumpf and L.D. Grant (eds.), *Anatomical Neuroendocrinology*. Basel: Karger, pp. 445–63.

Gray, A., Jackson, D.N., and McKinlay, J.B. (1991). The relation between dominance, anger, and hormones in normally aging men: results from the Massachusetts Male Aging Study. *Psychosomatic Medicine* 53: 375–85.

Gray, P.B. (2003). Marriage, parenting and testosterone variation among Kenyan Swahili men. *American Journal of Physical Anthropology* 122: 279–86.

Gray, P.B., Chapman, J.F., Burnham, T.C., McIntyre, M.H., Lipson, S.F., and Ellison, P.T. (2004). Human male pair bonding and testosterone. *Human Nature* 15: 119–31.

Gray, P.B., Kahlenberg, S.M., Barrett, E.S., Lipson, S.F., and Ellison, P.T. (2002). Marriage and fatherhood are associated with lower testosterone in males. *Evolution and Human Behavior* 23: 193–201.

Gray, P.B., Yang, C.-F.J., and Pope, H.G. Jr. (2006). Fathers have lower salivary testosterone levels than unmarried men and married non-fathers in Beijing, China. *Proceedings of the Royal Society of London, B* 273: 333–9.

Green, R. (1985). Gender identity in childhood and later sexual orientation: follow-up of 78 males. *American Journal of Psychiatry* 142: 339–41.

Greenspan, F.S. (1997). The thyroid gland. In F.S. Greenspan and G.J. Strewler (eds.), *Basic and Clinical Endocrinology*. Stamford: Appleton and Lange, 5th edition, pp. 192–262.

Grimes, J.M., Ricci, L.A., and Melloni, R.H. Jr. (2006). Plasticity in anterior hypothalamic vasopressin correlates with aggression during anabolic-androgenic steroid withdrawal in hamsters. *Behavioral Neuroscience* 120: 115–24.

Grimshaw, G.M., Bryden, M.P., and Finegan, J.-A.K. (1995a). Relations between prenatal testosterone and cerebral lateralization in children. *Neuropsychology* 9: 68–79.

Grimshaw, G.M., Sitarenios, G., and Finegan, J.-A.K. (1995b). Mental rotation at 7 years: relations with prenatal testosterone levels and spatial play experiences. *Brain and Cognition* 29: 85–100.

Grumbach, M.M. (2000). Estrogen, bone growth and sex: a sea change in conventional wisdom. *Journal of Pediatric Endocrinology and Metabolism* 13: 1439–55.

Gustafson, M.L., and Donahoe, P.K. (1994). Male sex determination: current concepts of male sexual differentiation. *Annual Review of Medicine* 45: 505–24.

Halari, R., Hines, M., Kumari, V., Mehrotra, R., Wheeler, M., Ng, V., and Sharma, T. (2005). Sex differences and individual differences in cognitive performance and their relationship to endogenous gonadal hormones and gonadotropins. *Behavioral Neuroscience* 119: 104–17.

Hall, J., and Kimura, D. (1994). Dermatoglyphic asymmetry and sexual orientation in men. *Behavioral Neuroscience* 108: 1203–6.

Halpern, D.F. (1998). Recipe for a sexually dimorphic brain: ingredients include ovarian and testicular hormones. *Behavioral and Brain Sciences* 21: 330.

   (2000). *Sex Differences in Cognitive Abilities*. Hillsdale, NJ: Lawrence Erlbaum Associates.

Halpern, D.F., and Tan, U. (2001). Stereotypes and steroids: using a psychobiological model to understand cognitive sex differences. *Brain and Cognition* 45: 392–414.

Halpern, C.T., Udry, J.R., Campbell, B., and Suchindran, C. (1993). Testosterone and pubertal development as predictors of sexual activity: a panel analysis of adolescent males. *Psychosomatic Medicine* 55: 436–47.

   (1994). Relationships between aggression and pubertal increases in testosterone and: a panel analysis of adolescent males. *Social Biology* 40: 8–24.

Hamer, D.H., Hu, S., Magnuson, V.L., Hu, N., and Pattatucci, A.M.L. (1993). A linkage between DNA markers on the X chromosome and male sexual orientation. *Science* 261: 321–7.

Hamilton, J.B., and Gardner, W.U. (1937). Effects in female young born of pregnant rats injected with androgens. *Proceedings of the Society of Experimental Biology and Medicine* 37: 570–2.

Hammock, E.A., and Young, L.J. (2002). Variation in the vasopressin V1a receptor promoter and expression: implications for inter- and intraspecific variation in social behaviour. *European Journal of Neuroscience* 16: 399–402.

   (2006). Oxytocin, vasopressin and pair bonding: implications for autism. *Philosophical Transactions of the Royal Society, B* 361: 2187–98.

Hampson, E. (1990a). Variations in sex-related cognitive abilities across the menstrual cycle. *Brain and Cognition* 14: 26–43.

   (1990b). Estrogen-related variations in human spatial and articulatory motor skill. *Psychoneuroendocrinology* 15: 97–111.

Hampson, E., and Kimura, D. (1988). Reciprocal effects of hormonal fluctuations on human motor and perceptual-spatial skills. *Behavioral Neuroscience* 102: 456–9.

Hansen, S., Ferreira, A., and Selart, M.E. (1985). Behavioral similarities between mother rats and benzodiazepine-treated non-maternal animals. *Psychopharmacology* 86: 344–7.

Hansen, S., Köhler, C., and Ross, S.B. (1982). On the role of the dorsal mesencephalic tegmentum in the control of masculine sexual behaviour in the rat: effects of electrolytic lesions, ibotenic acid and DSP4. *Brain Research* 240: 311–20.

Harding, C.F., Sheridan, K., and Walters, J. (1983). Hormonal specificity and activation of sexual behavior in male zebra finches. *Hormones and Behavior* 17: 111–33.

Harlow, H.F. (1958). The nature of love. *American Psychologist* 25: 673–85.

Harries, M.L.L., Walker, J.M., Williams, D.M., Hawkins, S., and Hughes, I.A. (1997). Changes in the male voice at puberty. *Archives of Disease in Childhood* 77: 445–7.

Harris, J.A. (1999). Review and methodological considerations in research on testosterone and aggression. *Aggression and Violent Behaviour* 4: 273–91.

Harris, J.A., Rushton, J., Hampson, E., and Jackson, D.N. (1996). Salivary testosterone and self-report aggressive and pro-social personality characteristics in men and women. *Aggressive Behavior* 22: 321–31.

Harrison, R.W., and Lippman, S.S. (1989). How steroid hormones work. *Hospital Practice* 24: 63–76.

Hartley, L.R., Lyons, D., and Dunne, M. (1987). Memory and the menstrual cycle. *Ergonomics* 30: 111–20.

Harvey, S.M. (1987). Female sexual behavior: fluctuations during the menstrual cycle. *Journal of Psychosomatic Research* 31: 101–10.

Haselton, M.G., and Gangestad, S.W. (2006). Conditional expression of women's desires and men's mate guarding across the ovulatory cycle. *Hormones and Behavior* 49: 509–18.

Haselton, M.G., Mortezaie, M., Pillsworth, E.G., Bleske-Rechek, A., and Frederick, D.A. (2007). Ovulatory shifts in human female ornamentation: near ovulation, women dress to impress. *Hormones and Behavior* 51: 40–5.

Hau, M., Wikelski, M., Soma, K.S., and Wingfield, J.C. (2000). Testosterone and year-round territorial aggression in a tropical bird. *General and Comparative Endocrinology* 117: 20–33.

Hausmann, M., Slabbekoorn, D., van Goozen, S.H.M., Cohen-Kettenis, P.T., and Güntürkün, O. (2000). Sex hormones affect spatial abilities during the menstrual cycle. *Behavioral Neuroscience* 114: 1245–50.

Hazan, C., and Shaver, P.R. (1987). Romantic love conceptualized as an attachment. *Journal of Personality and Social Psychology* 52: 511–24.

Hazan, C., and Zeifman, D. (1999). Pair-bonds as attachments: evaluating the evidence. In J. Cassidy and P.R. Shaver (eds.), *Handbook of Attachment Theory and Research*. New York: Guilford, pp. 336–54.

Heap, R.B. (1994). Paracrine and autocrine functions of the placenta: a key to the success of viviparity? *Experimental and Clinical Endocrinology* 102: 262–8.

Helleday, J., Edman, G., Ritzen, M., and Siwers, B. (1993). Personality characteristics and platelet MAO activity in women with congenital adrenal hyperplasia (CAH). *Psychoneuroendocrinology* 18: 343–54.

Helleday, J., Siwers, B., Ritzen, M., and Hugdahl, K. (1994). Normal lateralization for handedness and ear advantage in a verbal dichotic listening task in women with congenital adrenal hyperplasia (CAH). *Neuropsychologia* 32: 875–80.

Hellhammer, D.H., Hubert, W., and Schürmeyer, T. (1985). Changes in saliva testosterone after psychological stimulation in men. *Psychoneuroendocrinology* 10: 77–81.

Heller, C.G., Laidlaw, W.M., Harvey, H.T., and Nelson, W.O. (1958). Effects of prog-
    estational compounds on the reproductive processes of the human male.
    *Annals of the New York Academy of Science* 71: 165–72.

Henderson, J. (2005). Ernest Starling and 'hormones': an historical commentary.
    *Journal of Endocrinology* 184: 5–10.

Henderson, V.W., Watt, L., and Buckwalter, J.G. (1996). Cognitive skills associated
    with estrogen replacement therapy in women with Alzheimer's disease.
    *Psychoneuroendocrinology* 21: 421–31.

Henningsson, S., Westberg, L., Nilsson, S., Lundström, B., Ekselius, L., Bodlund, O.,
    Lindström, E., Hellstrand, M., Rosmond, R., Eriksson, E., and Landén,
    M. (2005). Sex steroid-related genes and male-to-female transsexualism.
    *Psychoneuroendocrinology* 30: 657–64.

Herdt, G.H. (1997). *Same Sex, Different Cultures*. Boulder, CO: Westview Press.

Herdt, G.H., and Davidson, J. (1988). The Sambia 'turnim-man': sociocultural and
    clinical aspects of gender formation in male pseudohermaphrodites with
    5-alpha-reductase deficiency in Papua New Guinea. *Archives of Sexual
    Behavior* 17: 33–56.

Hermans, E.J., Putman, P., and van Honk, J. (2006). Testosterone administration
    reduces empathetic behavior: a facial mimicry study. *Psychoneuro-
    endocrinology* 31: 859–66.

Hier, D.B., and Crowley, W.F. (1982). Spatial ability in androgen-deficient men. *New
    England Journal of Medicine* 306: 1202–5.

Higley, J.D., Mehlman, P.T., Poland, R.E., Taub, D.M., Vickers, J., Suomi, S.J., and
    Linnoila, M. (1996). CSF testosterone and 5-HIAA correlates with different
    types of aggressive behaviors. *Biological Psychiatry* 40: 1067–82.

Higley, J.D., Mehlman, P.T., Taub, D.M., Higley, S.B., Suomi, S.J., Vickers, J.H., and
    Linnoila, M. (1992). Cerebrospinal fluid monoamine and adrenal correlates
    of aggression in free-ranging rhesus monkeys. *Archives of General
    Psychiatry* 49: 436–41.

Hines, M. (1991). Gonadal hormones and human cognitive development. In
    J. Balthazart (ed.), *Hormones, Brain and Behaviour in Vertebrates*. Basel:
    Karger, pp. 51–63.

Hines, M., Allen, L.S., and Gorski, R.A. (1992). Sex differences in subregions of the
    medial nucleus of the amygdala and the bed nucleus of the stria terminalis
    of the rat. *Brain Research* 8: 321–6.

Hines, M., Golombok, S., Rust, J., Johnston, K.J., Golding, J., and the ALSPAC
    Study Team (2002a). Testosterone during pregnancy and gender role
    behavior of preschool children: a longitudinal, population study. *Child
    Development* 73: 1678–87.

Hines, M., Johnston, K.J., Golombok, S., Rust, J., Stevens, M., Golding, J., and the
    ALSPAC Study Team (2002b). Prenatal stress and gender role behaviour in
    girls and boys: a longitudinal, population study. *Hormones and Behavior* 42:
    126–34.

Hines, M., and Shipley, C. (1984). Prenatal exposure to diethylstilbestrol (DES) and
    the development of sexually dimorphic cognitive abilities and cerebral lat-
    eralization. *Developmental Psychology* 20: 81–94.

Hiort, O., and Zitzmann, M. (2004). Androgen receptor: pathophysiology. In
    E. Nieschlag, H.M. Behre and S. Nieschlag (eds.), *Testosterone: Action,
    Deficiency, Substitution*. Cambridge: Cambridge University Press, pp. 93–124.

Ho, H.Z., Gilger, J.W., and Brink, T.M. (1986). Effects of menstrual cycle on spatial information processes. *Perceptual and Motor Skills* 63: 743–51.

Hogervorst, E., Williams, J., Budge, M., Riedel, W., and Jolles, J. (2000). The nature of the effect of female gonadal hormone replacement therapy on cognitive function in post-menopausal women: a meta-analysis. *Neuroscience* 101: 485–512.

Hollander, E., Bartz, J., Chaplin, W., Phillips, A., Sumner, J., Soorya, L., Anagnostou, E., and Wasserman, S. (2007). Oxytocin increases retention of social cognition in autism. *Biological Psychiatry* 61: 498–503.

Hollien, H., Green, R., and Massey, K. (1994). Longitudinal research on adolescent voice change in males. *Journal of the Acoustical Society of America* 96: 2646–54.

Holman, S.D., and Goy, R.W. (1980). Behavioral and mammary responses of adult female rhesus monkeys to strange infants. *Hormones and Behavior* 14: 348–57.

(1995). Experiential and hormonal correlates of care-giving in rhesus macaques. In C.R. Pryce, R.D. Martin and D. Skuse (eds.), *Motherhood in Human and Nonhuman Primates*. Basel: Karger, pp. 87–93.

Holt, S.B. (1968). *The Genetics of Dermal Ridges*. Springfield, IL: Charles C. Thomas.

Hönekopp, J., Voracek, M., and Manning, J.T. (2006). 2nd to 4th digit ratio (2D:4D) and number of sex partners: evidence for effects of prenatal testosterone in men. *Psychoneuroendocrinology* 31: 30–7.

Hooven, C.K., Chabris, C.F., Ellison, P.T., and Kosslyn, S.M. (2004). The relationship of male testosterone to components of mental rotation. *Neuropsychologia* 42: 782–90.

House, J.S., Landis, K.R., and Umberson, D. (1988). Social relationships and health. *Science* 241: 540–5.

Hu, S., Pattatucci, A.M.L., Patterson, C., Li, L., Fulker, D.W., Cherny, S.S., Kruglyak, L., and Hamer, D.H. (1995). Linkage between sexual orientation and chromosome Xq28 in males but not females. *Nature Genetics* 11: 248–56.

Hunter, B.S., Shraer, R., Landers, D.M., Buskirk, E.R., and Harris, D.Y. (1979). The effects of total oestrogen concentration and menstrual-cycle phase on reaction time performance. *Ergonomics* 22: 263–8.

Hutt, S.J., Frank, G., Mychaliw, W., and Hughes, M. (1980). Perceptual-motor performance during the menstrual cycle. *Hormones and Behavior* 14: 116–25.

Hyde, J.S. (1986). Gender differences in aggression. In J.S. Hyde and M.C. Linn (eds.), *The Psychology of Gender: Advances through Meta-Analysis*. Baltimore: Johns Hopkins University Press.

Hyde, J.S., and Linn, M. (1988). Gender differences in verbal ability: a meta-analysis. *Psychological Bulletin* 104: 53–69.

Imperato-McGinley, J., Guerrero, L., Gautier, T., and Peterson, R.E. (1974). Steroid 5 alpha-reductase deficiency in man: an inherited form of male pseudohermaphroditism. *Science* 186: 1213–15.

Imperato-McGinley, J., Pichardo, M., Gautier, T., Voyer, D., and Bryden, M.P. (1991). Cognitive abilities in androgen-insensitive subjects: comparison with control males and females from the same kindred. *Clinical Endocrinology* 34: 341–7.

Iñiguez, M.A., Rodriguez-Peña, A., Ibarrola, N., Aguilera, M., Muñoz, A., and Bernal, J. (1993). Thyroid hormone regulation of RC3, a brain-specific gene encoding a protein kinase C substrate. *Endocrinology* 133: 467–73.

Insel, T.R., Preston, S., and Winslow, J.T. (1995). Mating in the monogamous male: behavioral consequences. *Physiology and Behavior* 57: 615–27.

Insel, T.R., and Winslow, J.T. (1991). Central administration of oxytocin modulates the infant rat's response to social isolation. *European Journal of Pharmacology* 203: 149–52.

Insel, T.R., Winslow, J.T., Wang, Z., and Young, L.J. (1998). Oxytocin, vasopressin, and the neuroendocrine basis of pair bond formation. *Advances in Experimental Medicine and Biology* 449: 215–24.

Insel, T.R., and Young, L.J. (2000). Neuropeptides and the evolution of social behavior. *Current Opinion in Neurobiology* 10: 784–9.

Ishii, S., and Itoh, M. (1992). Amplexus induces surge of luteinizing hormone in male toads, *Bufo japonicus*. *General and Comparative Endocrinology* 86: 34–41.

Jacobsen, C.D., Csernus, V.J., Shryne, J.E., and Gorski, R.A. (1981). The influence of gonadectomy, androgen exposure, or a gonadal graft in the neonatal rat on the volume of the sexually dimorphic nucleus of the preoptic area. *Journal of Neuroscience* 1: 1142–7.

Jacobsen, C.D., and Gorski, R.A. (1981). Neurogenesis of the sexually dimorphic nucleus of the preoptic area of the rat. *Journal of Comparative Neurology* 196: 519–29.

Jacklin, C.N., Wilcox, K.T., and Maccoby, E.E. (1988). Neonatal sex-steroid hormones and cognitive abilities at six years. *Developmental Psychobiology* 21: 567–74.

James, P.J., and Nyby, J.G. (2002). Testosterone rapidly affects the expression of copulatory behaviour in house mice (*Mus musculus*). *Physiology and Behavior* 75: 287–94.

Jamison, C.S., Meier, R.J., and Campbell, B.C. (1993). Dermatoglyphic asymmetry and testosterone levels in normal males. *American Journal of Physical Anthropology* 90: 185–98.

Janowsky, J.S., Oviatt, S.K., and Orwoll, E.S. (1994). Testosterone influences spatial cognition in older men. *Behavioral Neuroscience* 108: 325–32.

Jasieńska, G., Ziomkiewicz, A., Ellison, P.T., Lipson, S.F., and Thune, I. (2004). Large breast and narrow waist indicate high reproductive potential in women. *Proceedings of the Royal Society of London, B* 271: 1213–17

Jenkins, J.S. (1998). The voice of the castrato. *The Lancet* 351: 1877–80.

Johnson, D.F., and Phoenix, C.H. (1976). Hormonal control of female sexual attractiveness, proceptivity, and receptivity in rhesus monkeys. *Journal of Comparative Physiology and Psychology* 90: 473–83.

Jones, B.C., Little, A.C., Boothroyd, L., DeBruine, L.M., Feinberg, D.R., Law Smith, M.J., Cornwall, R.E., Moore, F.R., and Perrett, D.I. (2005). Commitment to relationships and preferences for femininity and apparent health in faces are strongest on days of the menstrual cycle when progesterone levels are high. *Hormones and Behavior* 48: 283–90.

Jones, B.C., Perrett, D.I., Little, A.C., Boothroyd, L., Cornwell, R.E., Feinberg, D.R., Tiddeman, B.P., Whiten, S., Pitman, R.M., Hillier, S.G., Burt, D.M.,

Stirrat, M.R., Law Smith, M.J., and Moore, F.R. (2004). Menstrual cycle, pregnancy and oral contraceptive use alter attraction to apparent health in faces. *Proceedings of the Royal Society of London, B* 272: 347–54.

Joseph, R., Hess, S., and Birecree, E. (1978). Effects of hormone manipulations and explorations on sex differences in maze learning. *Behavioral Biology* 24: 364–77.

Jost, A. (1970). Hormonal factors in the sex differentiation of the mammalian foetus. *Philosophical Transactions of the Royal Society of London, B* 259: 119–30.

Juárez, J., del Rio Portilla, I., and Corsi-Cabrera, M. (1998). Effects of prenatal testosterone on sex and age differences in behaviour elicited by stimulus pups in the female rat. *Hormones and Behavior* 16: 224–33.

Judd, H.L., and Yen, S.S. (1973). Serum androstenedione and testosterone levels during the menstrual cycle. *Journal of Clinical Endocrinology and Metabolism* 36: 475–81.

Kahane, J.C. (1982). Growth of the human prepubertal and pubertal larynx. *Journal of Speech and Hearing Research* 25: 446–55.

Kampen, D.L., and Sherwin, B.B. (1994). Estrogen use and verbal memory in healthy postmenopausal women. *Obstetrics and Gynecology* 83: 979–83.

Kanner, L. (1943). Autistic disturbances of affective contact. *Nervous Child* 2: 217–50.

Kaplan, M.M., McCann, U.D., Yaskoski, K.A., Larsen, P.R., and Leonard, J.L. (1981). Anatomical distribution of phenolic and tyrosol ring iodothyronine deiodinase in the nervous system of normal and hypothyroid rats. *Endocrinology* 109: 397–402.

Karam, J.H. (1997). Pancreatic hormones and diabetes mellitus. In F.S. Greenspan and G.J. Strewler (eds.), *Basic and Clinical Endocrinology*. Stamford: Appleton and Lange, 5th edition, pp. 595–663.

Kasperk, C., Helmboldt, A., Börksök, I., Heuthe, S., Cloos, O., Niethard, F., and Ziegler, R. (1997). Skeletal site-dependent expression of the androgen receptor in human osteoblastic cell populations. *Calcified Tissue International* 61: 464–73.

Kaufman, J.M., T'Sjoen, G., and Vermeulen, A. (2004). Androgens in male senescence. In E. Nieschlag, H.M. Behre and S. Nieschlag (eds.), *Testosterone: Action, Deficiency, Substitution*. Cambridge: Cambridge University Press, pp. 497–541.

Keenan, P.A., Ezzat, W.H., Ginsburg, K., and Moore, G.J. (2001). Prefrontal cortex as the site of estrogen's effect on cognition. *Psychoneuroendocrinology* 26: 577–90.

Kelso, W.M., Nicholls, M.E.R., Warne, G.L., and Zacharin, M. (2000). Cerebral lateralization and cognitive functioning in patients with congenital adrenal hyperplasia. *Neuropsychology* 14: 370–8.

Kempel, P., Gohlke, B., Klempau, J., Zinsberger, P., Reuter, M., and Hennig, J. (2005). Second-to-fourth digit length, testosterone and spatial ability. *Intelligence* 33: 215–30.

Kern, M.D., and King, J.R. (1972). Testosterone-induced singing in female white-crowned sparrows. *The Condor* 74: 204–9.

Kerr, J.H., and Vanschaik, P. (1995). Effects of game venue and outcome on psychological mood states in rugby. *Personality and Individual Differences* 19: 407–10.

Keverne, E.B. (1999). The vomeronasal organ. *Science* 286: 716–20.

Keverne, E.B., Lévy, F., Poindron, P., and Lindsay, D.R. (1983). Vaginal stimulation: an important determinant of maternal bonding in sheep. *Science* 219: 81–3.

Keyser-Markus, L., Stafisso-Sandoz, G., Gerecke, K., Jasnow, A., Nightingale, L., Lambert, K.G., and Kinsley, C.H. (2001). Alterations in medial preoptic area neurons following pregnancy and pregnancy-like steroidal treatment in the rat. *Brain Research Bulletin* 55: 737–45.

Kim, S.J., Young, L.J., Gonen, D., Veenstra-VanderWeele, J., Courchesne, R., Courchesne, E., Lord, C., Leventhal, B.L., Cook, H.E. Jr., and Insel, T.R. (2001). Transmission disequilibrium testing of arginine vasopressin receptor 1A (AVPR1A) polymorphism in autism. *Molecular Psychiatry* 7: 503–7.

Kimura, D. (2002). Sex hormones influence human cognitive function. *Neuroendocrinology Letters Special Issue*, Suppl. 4: 67–77.

Kimura, D., and Carson, M.W. (1995). Dermatoglyphic asymmetry: relation to sex, handedness and cognitive pattern. *Personality and Individual Differences* 19: 471–8.

Kimura, D., and Hampson, E. (1993). Neural and hormonal mechanisms mediating sex differences in cognition. In P.A. Vernon (eds.), *Biological Approaches to the Study of Human Intelligence*. Norwood, NJ: Ablex, pp. 375–97.

Kinsley, C.H., and Lambert, K.G. (2006). The maternal brain. *Scientific American* January: 58–65.

Kleiman, D.G. (1977). Monogamy in mammals. *Quarterly Review of Biology* 52: 39–69.

Knickmeyer, R., Baron-Cohen, S., Fane, B.A., Wheelwright, S., Mathews, G.A., Conway, G.S., Brook, C.G.D., and Hines, M. (2006). Androgens and autistic traits: a study of individuals with congenital adrenal hyperplasia. *Hormones and Behavior* 50: 148–53.

Knuth, E.D., and Etgen, A.M. (2007). Long-term behavioural consequences of brief, repeated neonatal isolation. *Brain Research* 1128: 139–47.

Koehler, N., Rhodes, G., and Simmons, L.W. (2002). Are human female preferences for symmetrical faces enhanced when conception is likely? *Animal Behaviour* 64: 233–8.

Kolb, B., and Whishaw, I.Q. (2001). *An Introduction to Brain and Behavior*. New York: Worth Publishers.

Komnenich, P., Lane, D.M., Dickey, R.P., and Stone, S.C. (1978). Gonadal hormones and cognitive performance. *Physiological Psychology* 6: 115–20.

Kondo, T., Zakany, J., Innis, J.W., and Duboule, D. (1997). Of fingers, toes and penises. *Nature* 390: 29.

Kosfeld, M., Heinrichs, M., Zak, P.J., Fischbacher, U., and Fehr, E. (2005). Oxytocin increases trust in humans. *Nature* 435: 673–6.

Kouri, E.M., Lukas, S.E., Pope, H.G. Jr., and Oliva, P.S. (1995). Increased aggressive responding in male volunteers following the administration of gradually increasing doses of testosterone cypionate. *Drug and Alcohol Dependence* 40: 73–9.

Kovacs, E.G., MacLusky, N.J., and Leranth, C. (2003). Effects of testosterone on hippocampal CA1 spine synaptic density in the male rat are inhibited by fimbria/fornix transaction. *Neuroscience* 122: 807–10.

Kow, L.-M., and Pfaff, D.W. (1975). Induction of lordosis in female rats: two modes of estrogen action and the effect of adrenalectomy. *Hormones and Behavior* 6: 259–76.

Kraemer, H.C., Becker, H.B., Brodie, H.K.H., Doering, C.H., Moos, R.H., and Hamburg, D.A. (1976). Orgasmic frequency and plasma testosterone levels in normal human males. *Archives of Sexual Behavior* 5: 125–32.

Krehbiel, D., Poindron, P., Lévy, F., and Prud'Homme, M.J. (1987). Peridural anesthesia disturbs maternal behaviour in primiparous and multiparous parturient ewes. *Physiology and Behavior* 40: 463–72.

Kreijkamp-Kaspers, S., Kok, L., Grobbee, D.E., de Haan, E.H.F., Aleman, A., Lampe, J.W., and van der Schouw, Y.T. (2004). Effect of soy protein containing isoflavones on cognitive function, bone mineral density, and plasma lipids in postmenopausal women. *Journal of the American Medical Association* 292: 65–74.

Kretschmann, H.-J., Schleicher, A., Wingert, F., Zilles, K., and Loblich, H.J. (1979). Human brain growth in the 19th and 20th century. *Journal of Neurological Science* 40: 169–88.

Krug, R., Born, J., and Rasch, B. (2006). A 3-day estrogen treatment improves prefrontal cortex-dependent cognitive function in postmenopausal women. *Psychoneuroendocrinology* 31: 965–75.

Krüger, T., Exton, M.S., Pawlak, C., von zur Mühlen, A., Hartmann, U., and Schedlowski, M. (1998). Neuroendocrine and cardiovascular response to sexual arousal and orgasm in men. *Psychoneuroendocrinology* 23: 401–11.

Kruijver, F.P.M., Fernandez-Guasti, A., Fodor, M., Kraan, E.M., and Swaab, D.F. (2001). Sex differences in androgen receptors of the human mamillary bodies are related to endocrine status rather than to sexual orientation or transsexuality. *Journal of Clinical Endocrinology and Metabolism* 86: 818–27.

Kung, A.W.C. (2003). Androgen and bone mass in men. *Asian Journal of Andrology* 5: 148–54.

Künzl, C., and Sachser, N. (1999). The behavioral endocrinology of domestication: a comparison between the domestic guinea pig (*Cavia apera f. porcellus*) and its wild ancestor, the cavy (*Cavia apera*). *Hormones and Behavior* 35: 28–37.

Kwan, M., Greenleaf, W.J., Mann, J., Crapo, L., and Davidson, J.M. (1983). The nature of androgen action on male sexuality: a combined laboratory–self report study on hypogonadal men. *Journal of Clinical Endocrinology and Metabolism* 57: 557–62.

Lacreuse, A., and Herndon, J.G. (2003). Estradiol selectively affects processing of conspecifics' faces in female rhesus monkeys. *Psychoneuroendocrinology* 28: 885–905.

LaFrance, M., Hecht, M.A., and Paluck, E.L. (2003). The contingent smile: a meta-analysis of sex differences in smiling. *Psychological Bulletin* 129: 305–34.

Lalumière, M.L., Blanchard, R., and Zucker, K.J. (2000). Sexual orientation and handedness in men and women: a meta-analysis. *Psychological Bulletin* 126: 575–92.

Lamb, D. (1984). Anabolic steroids in athletics. *Clinical Pharmacy* 6: 686–92.

Landfield, P.W., Baskin, R.W., and Pitler, T.A. (1981). Brain-aging correlates:

retardation by hormonal-pharmacological treatments. *Science* 214: 581–4.

Law Smith, M.J., Perrett, D.I., Jones, B.C., Cornwell, R.E., Moore, F.R., Feinberg, D.R., Boothroyd, L.G., Durrani, S.J., Stirrat, M.R., Whiten, S., Pitman, R.M., and Hillier, S.G. (2006). Facial appearance is a cue to oestrogen levels in women. *Proceedings of the Royal Society of London, B* 273: 135–40.

Lazar, M.A. (2002). Mechanism of action of hormones that act on nuclear receptors. In P.R. Larsen, H.M. Kronenburg, S. Melmed, and K.S. Polansky (eds.), *Williams Textbook of Endocrinology*, 10th edition. London: Elsevier, pp. 35–44.

Lee, P.A., Jaffe, R.B., and Midgley, A.R. Jr. (1974). Lack of alteration of serum gonadotropins in men and women following sexual intercourse. *American Journal of Obstetrics and Gynecology* 120: 985–7.

Lejeune, C., Robert, J.C., Montamat, S., Floch-Tudal, C., Mazy, F., Wijkhuisen, N., and Froment, H. (1997). Medical-social outcome of 59 infants born to addicted mothers. *Journal de Gynécologie. Obstétrique et Biologie de la Réproduction* 26: 395–404.

Leonard, J.L., Kaplan, M.M., Visser, T.J., Silva, J.E., and Larsen, P.R. (1981). Cerebral cortex responds rapidly to thyroid hormones. *Science* 214: 571–3.

Leranth, C., Petnehazy, O., and MacLusky, N.J. (2003). Gonadal hormones affect spine density in the CA1 hippocampal subfield of male rats. *Journal of Neuroscience* 23: 1588–92.

LeVay, S. (1991). A difference in hypothalamic structure between heterosexual and homosexual men. *Science* 253: 1034–7.

(1993). *The Sexual Brain*. Cambridge, MA: MIT Press.

(1996). *Queer Science: The Use and Abuse of Research into Homosexuality*. Cambridge, MA: MIT Press.

Leveroni, C., and Berenbaum, S.A. (1998). Early androgen effects on interest in infants: evidence from children with congenital adrenal hyperplasia. *Developmental Neuropsychology* 14: 321–40.

Levine, A., Zagoory-Sharon, O., Feldman, R., Lewis, J.G., and Weller, A. (2007). Measuring cortisol in human psychobiological studies. *Physiology and Behavior* 90: 43–53.

Levy, A., Crown, A., and Reid, R. (2003). Endocrine intervention for transsexuals. *Clinical Endocrinology* 59: 409–18.

Lévy, F., Kendrick, K.M., Keverne, E.B., Piketty, Y., and Poindron, P. (1992). Intracerebral oxytocin is important for the onset of maternal behaviour in experienced ewes delivered under peridural anaesthesia. *Behavioral Neuroscience* 106: 427–32.

Levy, J., and Heller, W. (1992). Gender differences in human neuropsychological function. In A.A. Gerell, H. Moltz, and I.L. Ward (eds.), *Handbook of Behavioral Neurobiology*, vol 11: *Sexual Differentiation*. New York: Plenum Press, pp. 245–74.

Lewis, D.W., and Diamond, M.C. (1995). The influence of gonadal steroids on the asymmetry of the cerebral cortex. In R.J. Davidson and K. Hugdahl (eds.), *Brain Asymmetry*. Cambridge, MA: MIT Press, pp. 31–49.

Lim, M.M., Hammock, E.A.D., and Young, L.J. (2004a). The role of vasopressin in the genetic and neural regulation of monogamy. *Journal of Neuroendo-crinology* 16: 325–32.

Lim, M.M., Murphy, A.Z., and Young, L.J. (2004b). Ventral striatopallidal oxytocin and vasopressin V1a receptors in the monogamous prairie vole (*Microtus ochrogaster*). *Journal of Comparative Neurology* 468: 555–70.

Lim, M.M., Wang, Z., Olazábal, D.E., Ren, X., Terwilliger, E.F., and Young, L.J. (2004c). Enhanced partner preference in a promiscuous species by manipulating the expression of a single gene. *Nature* 429: 754–7.

Lim, M.M., and Young, L.J. (2004). Vasopressin-dependent neural circuits underlying pair bond formation in the monogamous prairie vole. *Neuroscience* 128: 35–45.

Lincoln, G.A., Guinness, F., and Short, R.V. (1972). The way in which testosterone controls the social and sexual behavior of the red deer stag (*Cervus elaphus*). *Hormones and Behavior* 3: 375–96.

Lindeque, M., Skinner, J.D., and Millar, R.P. (1986). Adrenal and gonadal contribution to circulating androgens in spotted hyaenas (*Crocuta crocuta*) as revealed by LHRH, HcG and ACTH stimulation. *Journal of Reproduction and Fertility* 78: 211–17.

Lingappa, V.R., and Mellon, S.H. (2001). *Basic and Clinical Endocrinology*. New York: McGraw Hill.

Lippa, R.A. (2003). Are 2D:4D finger length ratios related to sexual orientation? Yes for men, no for women. *Journal of Personality and Social Psychology* 85: 179–88.

Lipson, S.F., and Ellison, P.T. (1989). Development of protocols for the application of salivary steroid analyses to field conditions. *American Journal of Human Biology* 1: 249–55.

Lloyd, J.A. (1971). Weights of testes, thymi and accessory reproductive glands in relation to rank in paired and grouped housed mice (*Mus musculus*). *Proceedings of the Society for Experimental Biology and Medicine* 137: 19–22.

Lonstein, J.S., and De Vries, G.J. (1999). Sex differences in the parental behaviour of adult virgin prairie voles: independence from gonadal hormones and vasopressin. *Journal of Neuroendocrinology* 11: 441–9.

Loraine, J.A., Ismail, A.A.A., Adamopoulos, D., and Dove, G.A. (1970). Endocrine function in male and female homosexuals. *British Medical Journal* 14th Nov: 406–9.

Low, B.S. (2000). *Why Sex Matters*. Princeton, NJ: Princeton University Press.

Lubinski, D., Tellegen, A., and Butcher, J.N. (1983). Masculinity, femininity, and androgyny viewed and assessed as distinct concepts. *Journal of Personality and Social Psychology* 44: 428–39.

Lucky, A.W. (1995). Hormonal correlates of acne and hirsutism. *American Journal of Medicine* 98: 89–94.

Luecken, L.J., and Lemery, K.S. (2004). Early caregiving and physiological stress responses. *Clinical Psychology Review* 24: 171–91.

Luine, V., Attalla, S., Mohan, G., Costa, A., and Frankfurt, M. (2006). Dietary phytoestrogens enhance spatial memory and spine density in the hippocampus and prefrontal cortex of ovariectomised rats. *Brain Research* 1126: 183–7.

Lutchmaya, S., Baron-Cohen, S., and Raggatt, P. (2002a). Foetal testosterone and eye contact in 12-month-old human infants. *Infant Behavior and Development* 25: 327–35.

(2002b). Foetal testosterone and vocabulary size in 18- and 24-month old infants. *Infant Behavior and Development* 24: 418–24.

Lutchmaya, S., Baron-Cohen, S., Raggatt, P., Knickmeyer, R., and Manning, J.T. (2004). 2nd to 4th digit ratios, fetal testosterone and estradiol. *Early Human Development* 77: 23–8.

Luxen, M.F., and Buunk, B.P. (2005). Second-to-fourth digit ratio related to verbal and numerical intelligence and the Big Five. *Personality and Individual Differences* 39: 959–66.

Macchi, M.M., and Bruce, J.N. (2004). Human pineal physiology and functional significance of melatonin. *Frontiers in Neuroendocrinology* 25: 177–95.

MacLean, P.D. (1949). Psychosomatic disease and the 'visceral brain': recent developments bearing on the Papez theory of emotion. *Psychosomatic Medicine* 11: 338–53.

MacLusky, N.J., and Naftolin, F. (1981). Sexual differentiation of the central nervous system. *Science* 211: 1294–1302.

Macri, S., and Wörbel, H. (2007). Effects of variation in postnatal maternal environment on maternal behaviour and fear and stress responses in rats. *Animal Behaviour* 73: 171–84.

Macrides, F., Bartke, A., and Dalterio, S. (1975). Strange females increase plasma testosterone levels in male mice. *Science* 189: 1104–6.

Maestripieri, D. (1999). The biology of human parenting: insights from nonhuman primates. *Neuroscience and Biobehavioral Reviews* 23: 43–9.

Maestripieri, D., and Megna, N.L. (2000). Hormones and behavior in rhesus macaque abusive and nonabusive mothers, 2. Mother–infant interactions. *Physiology and Behavior* 71: 43–9.

Maestripieri, D., and Zehr, J.L. (1998). Maternal responsiveness increases during pregnancy and after estrogen treatment in macaques. *Hormones and Behavior* 34: 223–30.

Magee, J.C., and Johnston, D.A. (1997). A synaptically controlled, associative signal for Hebbian plasticity in hippocampal neurons. *Science* 275: 209–13.

Mall, F.P. (1909). On several anatomical characters of the human brain, said to vary according to race and sex, with special reference to the weight of the frontal lobe. *American Journal of Anatomy* 9: 1–32.

Maney, D.L., Cho, E., and Goode, C.T. (2006). Estrogen-dependent selectivity of genomic responses to birdsong. *European Journal of Neuroscience* 23: 1523–9.

Manning, J.T. (2002). *Digit Ratio: A Pointer to Fertility, Behavior and Health*. New Brunswick, NJ: Rutgers University Press.

Manning, J.T., Baron-Cohen, S., Wheelwright, S., and Sanders, G. (2001). The 2nd to 4th digit ratio and autism. *Developmental Medicine and Child Neurology* 43: 160–4.

Manning, J.T., Bundred, P.E., Newton, D.J., and Flanagan, B.F. (2003). The second to fourth digit ratio and variation in the androgen receptor gene. *Evolution and Human Behavior* 24: 399–405.

Manning, J.T., Fink, B., Neave, N., and Caswell, N. (2005). Photocopies yield lower digit ratios (2D:4D) than direct finger measurements. *Archives of Sexual Behavior* 34: 329–33.

Manning, J.T., Scutt, D., Wilson, J., and Lewis-Jones, D.J. (1998). The ratio of 2nd to 4th digit length: a predictor of sperm numbers and concentrations of testosterone, luteinizing hormone and oestrogen. *Human Reproduction* 13: 3000–4.

Manning, J.T., and Taylor, R.P. (2001). 2nd to 4th digit ratio and male ability in sport: implications for sexual selection in humans. *Evolution and Human Behavior* 22: 61–9.

Manning, J.T., Trivers, R.L., Singh, D., and Thornhill, R. (1999). The mystery of female beauty. *Nature* 399: 214–15.

Manning, J.T., Trivers, R.L., Thornhill, R., and Singh, D. (2000). The 2nd:4th digit ratio and asymmetry of hand performance in Jamaican children. *Laterality* 5: 121–32.

Mantella, R.C., Vollmer, R.R., Li, X., and Amico, J.A. (2003). Female oxytocin-deficient mice display enhanced anxiety-related behavior. *Endocrinology* 144: 2291–6.

Maras, A., Laucht, M., Gerdes, D., Wilhelm, C., Lewicka, S., Haak, D., Malisova, L., and Schmidt, M.H. (2003). Association of testosterone and dihydrotestosterone with externalizing behaviour in adolescent boys and girls. *Psychoneuroendocrinology* 28: 932–40.

Marazziti, D., Akiskal, H.S., Rossi, A., and Cassano, G.B. (1999). Alteration of the platelet serotonin transporter in romantic love. *Psychological Medicine* 29: 741–5.

Marazziti, D., and Canale, D. (2004). Hormonal changes when falling in love. *Psychoneuroendocrinology* 29: 931–6.

Martel, F.L., Nevison, C.M., Rayment, F.D., Simpson, M.J., and Keverne, E.B. (1993). Opioid receptor reduces affect and social grooming in rhesus monkeys. *Psychoneuroendocrinology* 18: 307–21.

Martel, F.L., Nevison, C.M., Simpson, M.J., and Keverne, E.B. (1995). Effects of opioid receptor blockade on the social behaviour of rhesus monkeys living in large family groups. *Developmental Psychobiology* 28: 71–84.

Martin, C.R. (1985). *Endocrine Physiology*. Oxford: Oxford University Press.

Martin-Soelch, C., Leenders, K.L., Chevalley, A.F., Missimer, J., Kunig, G., Magyar, S., Mino, A., and Schultz, W. (2001). Reward mechanisms in the brain and their role in dependence: evidence from neurophysiological and neuroimaging studies. *Brain Research Reviews* 36: 139–49.

Martinez, M., Salvador, A.S., and Vicente, M. (1994). Behavioral changes over several successive encounters between male mice: effects of type of 'standard opponent'. *Aggressive Behaviour* 20: 441–51.

Martínez-Sanchis, S., Salvador, A., Moya-Albiol, L., González-Bono, E., and Simón, V.M. (1998). Effects of chronic treatment with testosterone propionate on aggression and hormonal levels in intact male mice. *Psychoneuroendocrinology* 23: 275–93.

Maruniak, J., and Bronson, F. (1976). Gonadotropic responses of male mice to female urine. *Endocrinology* 99: 963–9.

Mas, M. (1995). Neurobiological correlates of masculine sexual behaviour. *Neuroscience and Biobehavioral Reviews* 19: 261–77.

Mason, W.A., and Mendoza, S.P. (1998). Generic aspects of primate attachments: parent's offspring and mates. *Psychoneuroendocrinology* 23: 765–78.

Matteo S., and Rissman, E.F. (1984). Increased sexual activity during the midcycle portion of the human menstrual cycle. *Hormones and Behavior* 18: 249–55.

Matuszczyk, J.V., and Larsson, K. (1994). Experience modulates the influence of gonadal hormones on sexual orientation of male rats. *Physiology and Behavior* 55: 527–31.

Mayo, A., Macintyre, H., Wallace, A.M., and Ahmed, S.F. (2004). Transdermal testosterone application: pharmacokinetics and effects on pubertal status, short-term growth, and bone turnover. *Journal of Clinical Endocrinology and Metabolism* 89: 681–7.

Mazur, A. (1985). A biosocial model of status in face-to-face primate groups. *Social Forces* 64: 377–402.

(1995). Biosocial models of deviant behaviour among male army veterans. *Biological Psychology* 41: 313–33.

Mazur, A., and Booth, A. (1998). Testosterone and dominance in men. *Behavioral and Brain Sciences* 21: 353–97.

Mazur, A., and Lamb, T.A. (1980). Testosterone, status and mood in human males. *Hormones and Behavior* 14: 171–93.

Mazur, A., and Michalek, J. (1998). Marriage, divorce, and male testosterone. *Social Forces* 77: 315–30.

Mazur, A., Susman, E.J., and Edelbrock, S. (1997). Sex differences in testosterone response to a video game contest. *Evolution and Human Behavior* 18: 317–26.

McCarthy, M.M., and Konkle, A.T.M. (2005). When is a sex difference not a sex difference? *Frontiers in Neuroendocrinology* 26: 85–102.

McCarthy, M.M., and Pfaus, J.G. (1996). Steroid modulation of neurotransmitter function to alter female reproductive behavior. *Trends in Endocrinology and Metabolism* 7: 327–33.

McCauley, E., Kay, T., Ito, J., and Treder, R. (1987). The Turner syndrome: cognitive deficits, affective discrimination, and behavior problems. *Child Development* 58: 464–73.

McCormack, C.M., Kehoe, P., and Kovacs, S. (1998). Corticosterone release in response to repeated, short episodes of neonatal isolation: evidence of sensitization. *International Journal of Developmental Neuroscience* 16: 175–85.

McEwen, B.S. (1976). Interactions between hormones and nerve tissue. *Scientific American* 235 (July): 48–58.

(1981). Neural gonadal steroid actions. *Science* 211: 1303–11.

(1988). Glucocorticoid receptors in the brain. *Hospital Practice* 23 (15th August): 107–21.

McEwen, B.S., and Alves, S.E. (1999). Estrogen actions in the central nervous system. *Endocrine Reviews* 20: 279–307.

McEwen, B.S., Biegon, A., Rainbow, T., Paden, C., Snyder, L., and De Groff, D. (1981). In K. Fuxe, J.-A. Gustafsson, and L. Wetterberg (eds.), *Steroid Hormone Regulation of the Brain*. Oxford: Pergamon, pp. 15–29.

McEwen, B.S., Davis, P.G., Parsons, B., and Pfaff, D.W. (1979). The brain as a target for steroid hormone action. *Annual Review of Neuroscience* 2: 65–112.

McEwen, B.S., de Kloet, E.R., and Rostene, W. (1986). Adrenal steroid receptors and actions in the nervous system. *Physiological Reviews* 66: 1121–88.

McFadden, D. (2000). Masculinizing effects on otoacoustic emissions and auditory evoked potentials in women using oral contraceptives. *Hearing Research* 142: 23–33.

(2002). Masculinization effects in the auditory system. *Archives of Sexual Behavior* 31: 99–111.

McFadden, D., and Shubel, E. (2002). Relative lengths of fingers and toes in human males and females. *Hormones and Behavior* 42: 492–500.

McGeer, P.L., Eccles, J.C., and McGeer, E.G. (1987). *Molecular Neurobiology of the Mammalian Brain,* 2nd edition. New York: Plenum Press.

McGuire, E.J., Courneya, R.S., Widmeyer, W.N., and Carron, A.V. (1992). Aggression as a potential mediator of the home advantage in professional ice hockey. *Journal of Sport and Exercise Psychology* 14: 148–58.

McGuire, L.S., Ryan, K.O., and Omenn, G.S. (1975). Congenital adrenal hyperplasia. II. Cognitive and behavioral studies. *Behavior Genetics* 5: 175–88.

McIntyre, M.H. (2006). The use of digit ratios as markers for perinatal androgen action. *Reproductive Biology and Endocrinology* 4: 1–9.

McIntyre, M.H., Barrett, E.S., McDermott, R., Johnson, D.D.P., Cowden, J., and Rosen, S.P. (2007). Finger length ratio (2D:4D) and sex differences in aggression during a simulated war game. *Personality and Individual Differences* 42: 755–64.

McIntyre, M.H., Gangestad, S.W., Gray, P.B., Chapman, J.F., Burnham, T.C., O'Rourke, M.T., and Thornhill, R. (2006). Romantic involvement often reduces men's testosterone levels – but not always: the moderating role of extrapair sexual interest. *Journal of Personality and Social Psychology* 91: 642–51.

McIntyre, M.H., Lipson, S.F., and Ellison, P.T. (2003). Effects of developmental and adult androgens on male abdominal adiposity. *American Journal of Human Biology* 15: 662–6.

McKeever, W.F., and Deyo, R.A. (1990). Testosterone, dihydrotestosterone, and spatial task performance of males. *Bulletin of the Psychonomic Society* 28: 305–8.

McPhaul, M.J., and Griffin, J.E. (1999). Male pseudohermaphroditism caused by mutations of the human androgen receptor. *Journal of Clinical Endocrinology and Metabolism* 84: 3435–41.

Medvei, V.C. (1993). *The History of Clinical Endocrinology: A Comprehensive Account of Endocrinology from Earliest Times to the Present Day.* Carnforth: Parthenon Press.

Meek, L.R., Schulz, K.L., and Keith, C.A. (2006). Effects of prenatal stress on sexual partner preference in mice. *Physiology and Behavior* 89: 133–8.

Mehta, P.H., and Josephs, R.A. (2006). Testosterone changes after losing predicts the decision to compete again. *Hormones and Behavior* 50: 684–92.

Meinlschmidt, G., and Heim, C. (2007). Sensitivity to intranasal oxytocin in adult men with early parental separation. *Biological Psychiatry* 61: 1109–11.

Meisel, R.L., and Sachs, B. (1994). The physiology of male reproduction. In E. Knobil and J.D. Neill (eds.), *The Physiology of Reproduction,* vol. 2. New York: Raven Press, pp. 3–105.

Melis, M.R., Argiolas, A., and Gessa, G.L. (1986). Oxytocin-induced penile erection and yawning: site of action in the brain. *Brain Research* 398: 259–65.

Melo, K.F.S., Mendonca, B.B., Billerbeck, E.C., Costa, E.M.F., Inácio, M., Silva, F.A.Q., Leal, A.M.O., Latronico, A.C., and Arnhold, I.J.P. (2003). Clinical, hormonal, behavioural, and genetic characteristics of androgen insensitivity syndrome in a Brazilian cohort: five novel mutations in the androgen receptor gene. *Journal of Endocrinology and Metabolism* 88: 3241–50.

Menard, C.S., and Dohanich, G.P. (1994). Estrogen dependence of cholinergic systems that regulate lordosis in cycling female rats. *Pharmacology, Biochemistry and Behavior* 48: 417–21.

Mendel, C.M. (1989). The Free Hormone Hypothesis: a physiologically based mathematical model. *Endocrine Reviews* 10: 232–74.

Mendonca, B.B. (2003). Male pseudohermaphroditism due to 5 alpha-reductase deficiency: outcome of a Brazilian cohort. *Endocrinologist* 13: 201–4.

Meston, C.M., and Frohlich, P.F. (2000). The neurobiology of sexual function. *Archives of General Psychiatry* 57: 1012–30.

Meyer, G., Ferres-Torres, R., and Mas, M. (1978). The effects of puberty and castration on hippocampal dendritic spines of mice. A Golgi study. *Brain Research* 155: 108–12.

Meyer, W.J. III., Finkelstein, J.W., Stuart, C.A., Webb, A., Smith, E.R., Payer, A.F., and Walker, P.A. (1981). Physical and hormonal evaluation of transsexual patients during hormonal therapy. *Archives of Sexual Behavior* 10: 347–56.

Meyer, W.J. III., Webb, A., Stuart, C.A., Finkelstein, J.W., Lawrence, B., and Walker, P.A. (1986). Physical and hormonal evaluation of transsexual patients: a longitudinal study. *Archives of Sexual Behavior* 15: 121–38.

Meyer-Bahlburg, H.F.L. (1979). Sex hormones and female homosexuality: a critical examination. *Archives of Sexual Behavior* 8: 101–19.

  (1999). Gender assignment and reassignment in 46,XY pseudohermaphroditism and related conditions. *Journal of Clinical Endocrinology and Metabolism* 84: 3455–8.

  (2002). Gender assignment and reassignment in intersexuality: controversies, data, and guidelines for research. *Advances in Experimental Medicine and Biology* 511: 199–223.

Meyer-Bahlburg, H.F.L., Baker, S.W., Dolezal, C., Carlson, A.D., Obeid, J.S., and New, M.I. (2003). Long-term outcome in congenital adrenal hyperplasia: gender and sexuality. *Endocrinologist* 13: 227–32.

Meyer-Bahlburg, H.F.L., Bruder, G.E., Feldman, J.F., Ehrhardt, A.A., Healey, J.M., and Bell, J. (1985). Cognitive abilities and hemispheric lateralization in females following idiopathic precocious puberty. *Developmental Psychology* 21: 878–87.

Michael, R.P., Bonsall, R.W., and Rees, H.D. (1987). Sites at which testosterone may act as an estrogen in the brain of the male primate. *Neuroendocrinology* 46: 511–21.

Michael, R.P., Rees, H.D., and Bonsall, R.W. (1989). Sites in the male primate brain at which testosterone acts as an androgen. *Brain Research* 502: 11–20.

Migeon, C.J., and Wisniewski, A.B. (1998). Sexual differentiation: from genes to gender. *Hormone Research* 50: 245–51.

Mikhail, M.S., Youchah, J., DeVore, N., Ho, G.Y., and Anyaegbunam, A. (1995). Decreased maternal–fetal attachment in methadone-maintained pregnant women: a preliminary study. *Journal of the Association for Academic Minority Physicians* 6: 112–14.

Miles, C., Green, R., and Hines, M. (2006). Estrogen treatment effects on cognition, memory and mood in male-to-female transsexuals. *Hormones and Behavior* 50: 708–17.

Miles, C., Green, R., Sanders, G., and Hines, M. (1998). Estrogen and memory in a transsexual population. *Hormones and Behavior* 34: 199–208.

Miller, J.F.A.P. (2002). The discovery of thymus function and of thymus-derived lymphocytes. *Immunological Reviews* 185: 7–14.

Miller, K.K. (2001). Androgen deficiency in women. *Journal of Clinical Endocrinology and Metabolism* 86: 2395–401.

Modahl, C., Green, L.A., Fein, D., Morris, M., Waterhouse, L., Feinstein, C., and Levin, H. (1998). Plasma oxytocin levels in autistic children. *Biological Psychiatry* 43: 270–7.

Moffat, S.D., and Hampson, E. (1996). Salivary testosterone levels in left- and right-handed adults. *Neuropsychologia* 34: 225–33.

Molenda-Figueira, H.A., Williams, C.A., Griffin, A.L., Rutledge, E.M., Blaustein, J.D., and Tetel, M.J. (2006). Nuclear receptor coactivators function in estrogen receptor- and progestin receptor-dependent aspects of sexual behaviour in female rats. *Hormones and Behavior* 50: 383–92.

Møller, A.P. (1998). Developmental instability as a general measure of stress. *Advances in the Study of Behavior* 27: 181–213.

Monaghan, E.P., and Glickman, S.E. (1992). Hormones and aggressive behavior. In J.B. Becker, S.M. Breedlove, and D. Crews (eds.), *Behavioral Endocrinology*. Cambridge, MA: MIT Press, pp. 261–85.

Money, J. (1970). Use of an androgen-depleting hormone in the treatment of male sex offenders. *Journal of Sex Research* 6: 165–72.

  (1973). Turner's syndrome and parietal lobe functions. *Cortex* 9: 387–96.

  (1975). Ablatio penis: normal male infant sex-reassigned as a girl. *Archives of Sexual Behavior* 4: 65–71.

  (1981). The development of sexuality and eroticism in human kind. *Quarterly Review of Biology* 56: 379–404.

Money, J., Schwartz, M., and Lewis, V.G. (1984). Adult erotosexual status and fetal hormonal masculinization and demasculinization: 46, XX congenital virilizing adrenal hyperplasia and 46, XY androgen-insensitivity syndrome compared. *Psychoneuroendocrinology* 9: 405–14.

Moore, F.L., Boyd, S.K., and Kelley, D.B. (2005). Historical perspective: hormonal regulation of behaviors in amphibians. *Hormones and Behavior* 48: 373–83.

Morris, J.A., Gobrogge, K.L., Jordan, C.L., and Breedlove, S.M. (2004). Brain aromatase: dyed-in-the-wool homosexuality. *Endocrinology* 145: 475–7.

Morris, R.G.M. (1984). Developments of a water-maze procedure for studying spatial learning in the rat. *Journal of Neuroscience Methods* 11: 47–60.

Morris, R.G.M., Anderson, E., Lynch, G.S., and Baudry, M. (1986). Selective impairment of learning and blockade of long-term potentiation by an N-methyl-D-aspartate receptor antagonist, AP5. *Nature* 319: 774–6.

Mortlock, D.P., and Innis, J.W. (1997). Mutation of *Hoxa13* in hand-foot-genital syndrome. *Nature Genetics* 15: 179–80.

Moss, R.L. (1979). Actions of hypothalamic-hypophysiotropic hormones on the brain. *Annual Review of Physiology* 41: 617–31.

Mougeot, F., Dawson, A., Redpath, S.M., and Leckie, F. (2005). Testosterone and autumn territorial behavior in male red grouse. *Hormones and Behavior* 47: 576–84.

Moyer, K.E. (1968). Kinds of aggression and their physiological basis. *Communications in Behavioral Biology* 2A: 65–87.

Mueller, N. (1977). Control of sex differences in the plumage of the house sparrow, *Passer domesticus. Journal of Experimental Zoology* 202: 45–8.

Müller, M.J. (1994). Salivary testosterone and simple reaction time parameters. *Neuropsychobiology* 30: 173–7.

Muller, M.N., and Wrangham, R.W. (2004). Dominance, aggression and testosterone in wild chimpanzees: a test of the 'challenge hypothesis'. *Animal Behaviour* 67: 113–23.

Mulnard, R.A., Cotman, C.W., Kawas, C., van Dyck, C.H., Sano, M., Doody, R., Koss, E., Pfeiffer, E., Jin, S., Gamst, A., Grundman, M., Thomas, R., and Thal, L.J. (2000). Estrogen replacement therapy for treatment of mild to moderate Alzheimer's disease. *Journal of the American Medical Association* 28: 1007–15.

Murphy, M.R. (1973). Effects of female hamster vaginal discharge on the behaviour of male hamsters. *Behavioral Biology* 9: 367–75.

Musatov, S., Chen, W., Pfaff, D.W., Kaplitt, M.G., and Ogawa, S. (2006). RNAi-mediated silencing of estrogen receptor α in the ventromedial nucleus of the hypothalamus abolishes female sexual behaviors. *Proceedings of the National Academy of Science, USA* 103: 10,456–60.

Mustanski, B.S., Bailey, J.M., and Kaspar, S. (2002). Dermatoglyphics, handedness, sex and sexual orientation. *Archives of Sexual Behavior* 31: 113–22.

Myers, L.S., Dixen, J., Morrissette, J., Carmichael, M., and Davidson, J.M. (1990). Effects of estrogen, androgen, and progestin in sexual psychophysiology in postmenopausal women. *Journal of Clinical Endocrinology and Metabolism* 70: 1124–31.

Naftolin, F. (1981). Understanding the bases of sex differences. *Science* 211: 1263–4.

Naftolin, F., Ryan, K.J., Davies, I.J., Reddy, V.V., Flores, F., Petro, Z., Kuhn, M., White, R.J., Takaoka, Y., and Wolin, L. (1975). The formation of estrogens by central neuroendocrine tissues. *Recent Progress in Hormone Research* 31: 295–319.

Nass, R., and Baker, S. (1991). Learning disabilities in children with congenital adrenal hyperplasia. *Journal of Child Neurology* 6: 306–12.

Neave, N., Laing, S., Fink, B., and Manning, J.T. (2003). Second to fourth digit ratio, testosterone and perceived male dominance. *Proceedings of the Royal Society of London, B* 270: 2167–72.

Neave, N., Menaged, M., and Weightman, D. (1999). Sex differences in cognition: the role of testosterone and sexual orientation. *Brain and Cognition* 41: 245–62.

Neave, N., and Wolfson, S. (2003). Testosterone, territoriality and the 'home advantage'. *Physiology and Behavior* 78: 269–75.

(2004). The home advantage: psychological and physiological factors in soccer. In D. Lavalle, J. Thatcher, and M.V. Jones (eds.), *Coping and Emotion in Sport*. New York: Nova Science Publishers Inc.

Netley, C., and Rovet, J. (1982). Atypical hemispheric lateralization in Turner syndrome subjects. *Cortex* 18: 377–84.

Neumann, I.D., Torner, L., and Wigger, A. (2000). Brain oxytocin: differential inhibition of neuroendocrine stress responses and anxiety-related behaviour in virgin, pregnant, and lactating rats. *Neuroscience* 95: 567–75.

Newman, M.L., Sellers, J.G., and Josephs, R.A. (2005). Testosterone, cognition, and social status. *Hormones and Behavior* 47: 205–11.

Nielson, J., and Pelsen, B. (1987). Follow-up 20 years later of 34 Klinefelter males with karotype 47XXY and 16 hypogonadal males with karotype 46XY. *American Journal of Human Genetics* 77: 188–92.

Nieschlag, E. (1974). Circadian rhythm of plasma testosterone. In J. Aschoff, F. Ceresa, and F. Halberg (eds.), *Chronobiological Aspects of Endocrinology*. Symposia Medica Hoechst 9. New York: Schattauer, pp. 116–28.

Nissen, E., Uvnäs-Moberg, K., Svensson, K., Stock, S., Widstrom, A.M., and Winberg, J. (1996). Different patterns of oxytocin, prolactin but not cortisol release during breastfeeding in women delivered by caesarean section or by the vaginal route. *Early Human Development* 45: 103–18.

Noda, K., Chang, H-P., Takahashi, I., Kinoshita, Z., and Kawamoto, T. (1994). Effects of the anabolic steroid nandrolone phenylproprionate on craniofacial growth in rats. *Journal of Morphology* 220: 25–33.

Norman, A.W., and Litwack, G. (1987). *Hormones*. London: Academic Press.

Nottebohm, F. (1970). Ontogeny of bird song. *Science* 167: 950–6.

(1981). A brain for all seasons: cyclical anatomical changes in song control nuclei of the canary brain. *Science* 214: 1368–70.

Nottebohm, F., and Arnold, A.P. (1976). Sexual dimorphism in vocal control areas of the songbird brain. *Science* 194: 211–13.

Nunes, S., Fite, J.E., Patera, K.J., and French, J.A. (2001). Interactions among paternal behaviour, steroid hormones, and parental experience in male marmosets (*Callithrix kuhlii*). *Hormones and Behavior* 39: 70–82.

Nunez, J. (1984). Effects of thyroid hormones during brain differentiation. *Molecular and Cellular Endocrinology* 37: 125–32.

Nunez, J.L., Sodhi, J.M., and Juraska, J.M. (2002). Ovarian hormones after postnatal day 20 reduce neuron number in the rat primary visual cortex. *Journal of Neuroscience* 52: 312–21.

Nyborg, H. (1983). Spatial ability in men and women: review and theory. *Advances in Behavior Research and Therapy* 5: 89–140.

Oatridge, A., Barnard, M.L., Puri, B.K., Taylor-Robinson, S.D., Hajnal, J.V., Saeed, N., and Bydder, G.M. (2002). Changes in brain size with treatment in patients with hyper- or hypothyroidism. *American Journal of Neuroradiology* 23: 1539–44.

Obrzut, J.E., and Atkinson, M.H. (1993). Relations among learning disorders, handedness, and immune disease. *Journal of Clinical and Experimental Neuropsychology* 15: 86.

O'Carroll, R.E. (1984). Androgen administration to hypogonadal and eugonadal men – effects on measures of sensation seeking, personality and spatial ability. *Personality and Individual Differences* 5: 595–8.

O'Connor, D.B., Archer, J., Hair, W.M., and Wu, F.C.W. (2001). Activational effects of testosterone on cognitive function in men. *Neuropsychologia* 39: 1385–94.

   (2002). Exogenous testosterone, aggression, and mood in eugonadal and hypogonadal men. *Physiology and Behavior* 75: 557–66.

O'Connor, D.B., Archer, J., and Wu, F.C.W. (2004). Effects of testosterone on mood, aggression, and sexual behaviour in young men: a double-blind, placebo-controlled, cross-over study. *Journal of Clinical Endocrinology and Metabolism* 89: 2837–45.

O'Hara, R., Schröder, C.M., Bloss, C., Bailey, A.M., Alyeshmerni, A.M., Mumenthaler, M.S., Friedman, L.F., and Yesavage, J.A. (2005). Hormone replacement therapy and longitudinal cognitive performance in post-menopausal women. *American Journal of Geriatric Psychiatry* 13: 1107–10.

Ogawa, S., Washburn, T.F., Taylor, J., Lubahn, D.B., Korach, K.S., and Pfaff, D.W. (1998). Modification of testosterone-dependent behaviours by estrogen receptor-α gene disruption in male mice. *Endocrinology* 139: 5058–69.

Ökten, A., Kalyoncu, M., and Yari, N. (2002). The ratio of second- and fourth-digit lengths and congenital adrenal hyperplasia due to 21-hydroxylase deficiency. *Early Human Development* 70: 47–54.

Oliveira, R.F., Carneiro, L.A., and Cánario, A.V.M. (2005). No hormonal response in tied fights. *Nature* 437: 207.

Olton, D.S., and Samuelson, R.J. (1976). Remembrance of places passed: spatial memory in rats. *Journal of Experimental Psychology: Animal Behavior Processes* 2: 97–116.

Olweus, D., Mattsson, A., Schalling, D., and Low, H. (1980). Testosterone, aggression, physical, and personality dimensions in normal adolescent males. *Psychosomatic Medicine* 42: 253–69.

   (1988). Circulating testosterone levels in and aggression in normal adolescent males. *Psychosomatic Medicine* 50: 261–72.

Oñate, S.A., Tsai, S.Y., Tsai, M.J., and O'Malley, B.W. (1995). Sequence and characterization of a coactivator for the steroid hormone receptor superfamily. *Science* 270: 1354–7.

Orsini, J. (1981). Hypothalamic neurons responsive to increased plasma level of testosterone in the male rat. *Brain Research* 212: 489–93.

Ostrowski, N.L. (1998). Oxytocin receptor mRNA expression in the rat brain: implications for behavioral integration and reproductive success. *Psychoneuroendocrinology* 23: 989–1004.

Oyegbile, T.O., and Marler, C.A. (2005). Winning fights elevates testosterone levels in California mice and enhances future ability to win fights. *Hormones and Behavior* 48: 259–67.

Ozisik, G., Achermann, J.C., Meeks, J.J., and Jameson, J.L. (2003). SF1 in the development of the adrenal gland and gonads. *Hormone Research* 59 (Suppl. 1): 94–8.

Pajer, K., Tabbah, R., Gardner, W., Rubin, R.T., Czambel, R.K., and Wang, Y. (2006). Adrenal androgen and gonadal hormone levels in adolescent girls with conduct disorder. *Psychoneuroendocrinology* 31: 1245–56.

Panskepp, J., Nelson, E., and Bekkedal, M. (1997). Brain systems for the mediation of social separation-distress and social reward. *Annals of the New York Academy of Science* 807: 78–100.

Pappas, C.T.E., Diamond, M.C., and Johnson, R.E. (1979). Morphological changes in the cerebral cortex of rats with altered levels of ovarian hormones. *Behavioral and Neural Biology* 26: 298–310.

Papez, J.W. (1937). A proposed mechanism of emotion. *Archives of Neurology and Psychiatry* 38: 725–44.

Pavlidis, K., McCauley, E., and Sybert, V.P. (1995). Psychosocial and sexual functioning in women with Turner syndrome. *Clinical Genetics* 47: 85–9.

Pedersen, C.A. (1997). Oxytocin control of maternal behaviour. Regulation by sex steroids and offspring stimuli. *Annals of the New York Academy of Science* 807: 126–45.

Pennington, B.F., Heaton, R.K., Karzmark, P., Pendleton, M.G., Lehman, R., and Shucard, D.W. (1985). The neuropsychological phenotype in Turner syndrome. *Cortex* 21: 391–404.

Penrose, L.S. (1967). Finger-print pattern and the sex chromosomes. *Lancet* 1: 298–300.

Penton-Voak, I.S., and Perrett, D.I. (2000). Female preference for male faces changes cyclically: further evidence. *Evolution and Human Behavior* 21: 39–48.

Penton-Voak, I.S., Perrett, D.I., Castles, D.L., Kobayashi, T., Burt, D.M., Murray, L.K., and Minamisawa, R. (1999). Menstrual cycle alters face preference. *Nature* 399: 741–2.

Perelle, I.B., and Ehrman, L. (1994). An international study of human handedness. *Behavior Genetics* 24: 217–27.

Perlman, S.M. (1973). Cognitive abilities of children with hormone abnormalities: screening by psychoeducational tests. *Journal of Learning Disabilities* 6: 21–9.

Pert, C.B., Snowman, A.M., and Snyder, S.H. (1974). Localization of opiate receptor binding in presynaptic membranes of rat brain. *Brain Research* 70: 184–8.

Petersen, A.C. (1976). Physical androgyny and cognitive functioning in adolescence. *Developmental Psychology* 12: 524–33.

Pfaff, D.W. (1966). Morphological changes in the brains of adult male rats after neonatal castration. *Journal of Endocrinology* 36: 415–16.

Pfaff, D.W., Diakow, C., Montgomery, M., and Jenkins, F.A. (1978). X-ray cinematographic analysis of lordosis in female rats. *Journal of Comparative Physiology and Psychology* 92: 937–41.

Pfaff, D.W., Gerlach, J.L., McEwen, B.S., Ferin, M., Carmel, P., and Zimmerman, E.A. (1976). Autoradiographic localization of hormone-concentrating cells in the brain of the female rhesus monkey. *Journal of Comparative Neurology* 170: 279–94.

Pfaff, D.W., and McEwen, B.S. (1983). Actions of estrogens and progestins on nerve cells. *Science* 219: 808–14.

Pfaff, D.W., and Pfaffmann, C. (1969). Olfactory and hormonal influences on the basal forebrain of the male rat. *Brain Research* 539: 94–102.

Pfaff, D.W., Silva, M.T.A., and Weiss, J.M. (1971). Telemetered recording of hormone effects on hippocampal neurons. *Science* 172: 394–5.

Pfaus, J.G. (1996). Homologies of animal and human sexual behaviors. *Hormones and Behavior* 30: 187–200.

Pfeiffer, C.A. (1936). Sexual differences of the hypophyses and their determination by the gonads. *American Journal of Anatomy* 58: 195–225.

Pfeiffer, C.A., and Johnston, R.E. (1992). Socially stimulated androgen surges in male hamsters: the roles of vaginal secretions, behavioural interactions, and housing conditions. *Hormones and Behavior* 26: 283–93.

Phelps, V.R. (1952). Relative index finger length as a sex-influenced trait in man. *American Journal of Human Genetics* 4: 72–89.

Phillips, S.M., and Sherwin, B.B. (1992). Variations in memory functions and sex steroid hormones across the menstrual cycle. *Psychoneuroendocrinology* 17: 497–506.

Phillips, S.M., and Silverman, I. (1997). Differences in the relationship of menstrual cycle phase to spatial performance on two- and three-dimensional tasks. *Hormones and Behavior* 17: 167–75.

Phoenix, C.H., Goy, R.W., Gerall, A.A., and Young, W.C. (1959). Organizing action of prenatally administered testosterone propionate on the tissues mediating mating behavior in the female guinea pig. *Endocrinology* 65: 369–82.

Pinel, J.P.J. (2006). *Biopsychology*, 6th edition. New York: Pearson Education Inc.

Pitkow, L.J., Sharer, C.A., Ren, X., Insel, T.R., Terwilliger, E.F., and Young, L.J. (2001). Facilitation of affiliation and pair-bond formation by vasopressin receptor gene transfer into the ventral forebrain of a monogamous vole. *Journal of Neuroscience* 21: 7392–6.

Plante, E., Boliek, C., Binkiewicz, A., and Erly, W.K. (1996). Elevated androgen, brain development and language/learning disabilities in children with congenital adrenal hyperplasia. *Developmental Medicine and Child Neurology* 38: 423–37.

Pol, H.E.H., Cohen-Kettenis, P.T., van Haren, N.E.M., Peper, J.S., Brans, R.G.H., Cahn, W., Schnack, H.G., Gooren, L.G.J., and Kahn, R.S. (2006). Changing your sex changes your brain: influences of testosterone and estrogen on adult human brain structure. *European Journal of Endocrinology* 155: S107–14.

Poulin, M., O'Connell, R.L., and Freeman, L.M. (2004). Picture recall skills correlate with 2D:4D ratio in women but not men. *Evolution and Human Behavior* 25: 174–81.

Pruessner, J.C., Wolf, O.T., Hellhammer, D.H., Buske-Kirschbaum, A., von Auer, K., Jobst, S., Kaspers, F., and Kirschbaum, C. (1997). Free cortisol levels after awakening: a reliable biological marker for the assessment of adrenocortical activity. *Life Sciences* 61: 2539–49.

Pryce, C.R., Abbott, D.H., Hodges, J.H., and Martin, R.D. (1988). Maternal behaviour is related to prepartum urinary estradiol levels in red-bellied tamarind monkeys. *Physiology and Behavior* 44: 717–26.

Pryce, C.R., Döbelli, M., and Martin, R.D. (1993). Effects of sex steroids on maternal motivation in the common marmoset (*Callithrix jachus*): development and application of an operant system with maternal reinforcement. *Journal of Comparative Psychology* 10: 353–67.

Putz, D.A., Gaulin, S.J.C., Sporter, R.J., and McBurney, D.H. (2004). Sex hormones and finger length. What does 2D:4D indicate? *Evolution and Human Behavior* 25: 182–99.

Quadagno, D.M., Briscoe, R., and Quadagno, J.S. (1977). Effect of perinatal gonadal hormones on selected nonsexual behavior patterns: a critical assessment of the non-human and human literature. *Psychological Bulletin* 84: 62–80.

Rabinowicz, T., Dean, D.E., Petetot, J.M.-C., and de Courten-Myers, G.M. (1999). Gender differences in the human cerebral cortex: more neurons in males; more processes in females. *Journal of Child Neurology* 14: 98–107.

Raboch, J., Kobilkova, J., Raboch, J., and Stârka, L. (1985). Sexual life of women with Stein-Leventhal syndrome. *Archives of Sexual Behaviour* 14: 263–70.

Rahman, Q. (2005a). Fluctuating asymmetry, second to fourth finger length ratios and human sexual orientation. *Psychoneuroendocrinology* 30: 382–91.

(2005b). The neurodevelopment of human sexual orientation. *Neuroscience and Biobehavioral Reviews* 29: 1057–66.

Rahman, Q., and Wilson, G.D. (2003a). Born gay? The psychobiology of human sexual orientation. *Personality and Individual Differences* 34: 1337–82.

(2003b). Sexual orientation and the 2nd to 4th finger length ratio: evidence for organizing effects of sex hormones or developmental instability? *Psychoneuroendocrinology* 28: 288–303.

Rahman, Q., Wilson, G.D., and Abrahams, S. (2004). Biosocial factors, sexual orientation and neurocognitive functioning. *Psychoneuroendocrinology* 29: 867–81.

Raisman, G., and Field, P.M. (1971). Sexual dimorphism in the preoptic area of the rat. *Science* 173: 20–2.

Rami, A., Rabie, A., and Patel, A.J. (1986). Thyroid hormone and development of the rat hippocampus: morphological alterations in granule and pyramidal cells. *Neuroscience* 19: 1217–26.

Rammsayer, T.H., and Troche, S.J. (2007). Sexual dimorphism in second-to-fourth digit ratio and its relation to gender-role orientation in males and females. *Personality and Individual Differences* 42: 911–20.

Rasmussen, A.K. (2000). Cytokine actions on the thyroid gland. *Danish Medical Bulletin* 47: 94–114.

Reburn, C.J., and Wynne-Edwards, K.E. (1999). Hormonal changes in males of a naturally biparental and a uniparental mammal. *Hormones and Behavior* 35: 163–76.

Regan, P.C. (1996). Rhythms of desire: the association between menstrual cycle phases and female sexual desire. *Canadian Journal of Human Sexuality* 5: 145–57.

Reid, S.N.M., and Juraska, J.M. (1992). Sex differences in the gross size of the rat neocortex. *Journal of Comparative Neurology* 321: 442–7.

Reinisch, J.M., and Sanders, S.A. (1992). Effects of prenatal exposure to diethylstilbestrol (DES) on hemispheric laterality and spatial ability in human males. *Hormones and Behavior* 26: 62–75.

Resnick, S.M., Berenbaum, S.A., Gottesman, I.I., and Bouchard, T.J. Jr. (1986). Early hormonal influences on cognitive functioning in congenital adrenal hyperplasia. *Developmental Psychology* 22: 191–8.

Resnick, S.M., Gottesman, I.I., and McGue, M. (1993). Sensation seeking in opposite-sex twins: an effect of prenatal hormones? *Behavior Genetics* 23: 323–9.

Riad-Fahmy, D., Read, G.F., Joyce, B.G., and Walker, R.F. (1981). Steroid immunoassays in endocrinology. In A. Voller, A. Bartlett, and D. Bidwell (eds.), *Immunoassays for the 80's*. Lancaster: MTP Press, pp. 205–62.

Rice, G., Anderson, C., Risch, N., and Ebers, G. (1999). Male homosexuality: absence of linkage to microsatellite markers at Xq28. *Science* 284: 665–7.

Richardson, J.T.E. (1989). Student learning and the menstrual cycle: premenstrual symptoms and approaches to studying. *Educational Psychology* 9: 215–38.

(1991). Cognition, memory, and the menstrual cycle. *European Bulletin of Cognitive Psychology* 11: 3–26.

Riddle, O., Bates, R.W., and Lahr, E.L. (1935). Prolactin induces broodiness in fowl. *American Journal of Physiology* 111: 352–60.

Riedel, G., Platt, B., and Micheau, J. (2003). Glutamate receptor function in learning and memory. *Behavioral Brain Research* 140: 1–47.

Rissman, E.F., Early, A.H., Taylor, J.A., Korach, K.S., and Lubahn, D.B. (1997). Estrogen receptors are essential for female sexual receptivity. *Endocrinology* 138: 507–10.

Roberts, S.C., Havlicek, J., Flegr, J., Hruskova, M., Little, A.C., Jones, B.C., Perrett, D.I., and Petrie, M. (2004). Female facial attractiveness increases during the fertile phase of the menstrual cycle. *Proceedings of the Royal Society of London, B (Suppl.)* 271: S270–2.

Robinson, S.J., and Manning, J.T. (2000). The ratio of the 2nd to 4th digit length and male homosexuality. *Evolution and Human Behavior* 21: 333–45.

Rode, C., Wagner, M., and Güntürkün, O. (1995). Menstrual cycle affects functional cerebral asymmetries. *Neuropsychologia* 33: 855–65.

Rohwer, S., and Rohwer, F.C. (1978). Status signalling in Harris' sparrows: experimental deceptions achieved. *Animal Behaviour* 26: 1012–22.

Romero, L.M., Soma, K.K., O'Reilly, K.M., Suydam, R., and Wingfield, J.C. (1998). Hormones and territorial behaviour during breeding in snow buntings (*Plectrophenax nivalis*): an arctic-breeding songbird. *Hormones and Behavior* 33: 40–7.

Rommerts, F.F.G. (2004). Testosterone: an overview of biosynthesis, transport, metabolism and non-genomic actions. In E. Nieschlag, H.M. Behre and S. Nieschlag (eds.), *Testosterone: Action, Deficiency, Substitution.* Cambridge: Cambridge University Press, pp. 1–37.

Roney, J.R., and Maestripieri, D. (2004). Relative digit lengths predict men's behavior and attractiveness during social interactions with women. *Human Nature* 15: 271–82.

Roney, J.R., Mahler, S.V., and Maestripieri, D. (2003). Behavioural and hormonal responses of men to brief interactions with women. *Evolution and Human Behavior* 24: 365–75.

Roof, R.L., and Havens, M.D. (1992). Testosterone improves maze performance and induces development of a male hippocampus in females. *Brain Research* 572: 310–13.

Rose, R.M., Gordon, T.P., and Bernstein, I.S. (1972). Plasma testosterone levels the male rhesus: influences of sexual and social stimuli. *Science* 178: 643–5.

Roselli, C.E., Abdelgadir, S.E., and Resko, J.A. (1997). Regulation of aromatase gene expression in the adult rat brain. *Brain Research Bulletin* 44: 351–7.

Roselli, C.E., Larkin, K., Resko, J.A., Stellflug, J.N., and Stormshak, F. (2004). The volume of a sexually dimorphic nucleus in the ovine medial preoptic area/anterior hypothalamus varies with sexual partner preference. *Endocrinology* 145: 478–83.

Rosen, G.D., Berrebi, A.S., Yutzey, D.A., and Denenberg, V.H. (1984). Prenatal testosterone causes shifts of asymmetry in neonatal tail posture of the rat. *Developmental Brain Research* 9: 99–101.

Rosen, G.D., Sherman, G.F., and Galaburda, A.M. (1991). Ontogenesis of cortical asymmetry: a [H$^3$] thymidine study. *Neuroscience* 7: 3198–206.

Rosen, J.B. (2006). Translational research: parallels of human and animal research in biological psychology. *Biological Psychology* 73: 1–2.

Rosenberg, L., and Park, S. (2002). Verbal and spatial functions across the menstrual cycle in healthy young women. *Psychoneuroendocrinology* 27: 835–41.

Rosenblitt, J.C., Soler, H., Johnson, S.E., and Quadagno, D.M. (2001). Sensation seeking and hormones in men and women: exploring the link. *Hormones and Behavior* 40: 396–402.

Rosenzweig, M.R., Breedlove, S.M., and Leiman, A.L. (2002). *Biological Psychology*, 3rd edition. Sunderland, MA: Sinauer.

Roth, G.S. (1979). Hormone receptor changes during adulthood and senescence: significance for aging research. *Federation Proceedings* 38: 1910–14.

Rothchild, A.J., Langlais, P.J., Schatzberg, A.F., Walsh, F.X., Cole, J.O., and Bird, E.D. (1984). Dexemethasone increases plasma free dopamine in man. *Journal of Psychological Research* 18: 217–23.

Rovet, J., and Netley, C. (1982). Processing deficits in Turner's syndrome. *Developmental Psychology* 18: 77–94.

Rovet, J.F., Netley, C., Keenan, M., Bailey, J., and Stewart, D. (1996). The psychoeducational profile of boys with Klinefelter syndrome. *Journal of Learning Disabilities* 29: 180–96.

Rowe, P.H., Lincoln, G.A., Racey, P.A., Lehane, J., Stephenson, M.J., Shenton, J.C., and Glover, T.D. (1974). Temporal variations of testosterone levels in the peripheral blood plasma of men. *Journal of Endocrinology* 61: 63–73.

Rowell, T.E. (1972). Female reproductive cycles and social behaviour in primates. *Advances in the Study of Behavior* 4: 69–105.

Rowland, I.R., Wiseman, H., Sanders, T.A., Adlercreutz, H., and Bowey, E.A. (2000). Interindividual variation in metabolism of soy isoflavones and lignans: influence of habitual diet on equal production by the gut microflora. *Nutrition and Cancer* 36: 27–32.

Rozanov, C.B., and Dratman, M.B. (1996). Immunohistochemical mapping of brain triiodothyronine reveals prominent localization in central noradrenergic systems. *Neuroscience* 74: 897–915.

Rupprecht, R. (2003). Neuroactive steroids: mechanisms of action and neuropsychopharmacological properties. *Psychoneuroendocrinology* 28: 139–68.

Rupprecht, R., and Holsboer, F. (1999). Neuroactive steroids: mechanisms of action and neuropsychopharmacological properties. *Trends in Neurosciences* 22: 410–16.

Russell, D.C. (2006). Raise your hand if you think I am attractive: second and fourth digit ratio as a predictor of self- and other-ratings of attractiveness. *Personality and Individual Differences* 40: 997–1005.

Russell, D.W., and Wilson, J.D. (1994). Two genes/ two enzymes. *Annual Review of Biochemistry* 63: 25–61.

Sachs, B.D., and Leipheimer, R.E. (1988). Rapid effects of testosterone on striate muscle activity in rats. *Neuroendocrinology* 48: 453–8.

Salminen, E., Portin, R., Korpela, J., Backman, H., Parvinen, L.-M., Helenius, H., and Nurmi, M. (2003). Androgen deprivation and cognition in prostate cancer. *British Journal of Cancer* 89: 971–6.

Salminen, E., Portin, R., Koskinen, A., Helenius, H., and Nurmi, M. (2004). Associations between serum testosterone fall and cognitive function in prostate cancer patients. *Clinical Cancer Research* 10: 7575–82.

Salamone, J.D., Correa, M., Mingote, S.M., and Weber, S.M. (2005). Beyond the reward hypothesis: alternative functions of nucleus accumbens dopamine. *Current Opinion in Pharmacology* 5: 34–41.

Salonia, A., Nappi, R.E., Pontillo, M., Daverio, R., Smeraldi, A., Briganti, A., Fabbri, F., Zanni, G., Rigatti, P., and Montorsi, F. (2005). Menstrual cycle-related changes in plasma oxytocin are relevant to normal sexual function in healthy women. *Hormones and Behavior* 47: 164–9.

Salvador, A., Simon, V.M., Suay, F., and Llorens, L. (1987). Testosterone and cortisol responses to competitive fighting in human males: a pilot study. *Aggressive Behavior* 13: 9–13.

Salvador, A., Suay, F., Martinez-Sanchis, S., Simon, V.M., and Brain, P.F. (1999). Correlating testosterone and fighting in male participants in judo contests. *Physiology and Behavior* 68: 205–9.

Sanders, D., and Bancroft, J. (1982). Hormones and the sexuality of women – the menstrual cycle. *Clinical Endocrinology and Metabolism* 11: 639–59.

Sandstrom, N.J., Kim, J.H., and Wasserman, M.A. (2006). Testosterone modulates performance on a spatial working memory task in male rats. *Hormones and Behavior* 50: 18–26.

Sandstrom, N.J., and Williams, C.L. (2001). Memory retention is modulated by acute estradiol and progesterone replacement. *Behavioral Neuroscience* 115: 384–93.

Sar, M., and Stumpf, W.E. (1975). Distribution of androgen-concentrating neurons in rat brain. In W.E. Stumpf and L.D. Grabt (eds.), *Anatomical Neuroendocrinology*. Basel: Karger, pp. 120–33.

Sassoon, D.A., Gray, G.E., and Kelley, D.B. (1987). Androgen regulation of muscle fiber type in the sexually dimorphic larynx of *Xenopus laevis*. *Journal of Neuroscience* 7: 3198–206.

Schaal, B., Tremblay, R.E., Soussignan, R., and Susman, E.J. (1996). Male testosterone linked to high social dominance but low physical aggression in early adolescence. *Journal of the American Academy of Child and Adolescent Psychiatry* 34: 1322–30.

Schäfer, E.A. (1895). Internal secretions. *Lancet* 10 August: 321–4.

Scher, D., Purcell, D.G., and Caputo, S.J. (1985). Visual acuity at two phases of the menstrual cycle. *Bulletin of the Psychonomic Society* 23: 119–25.

Schlinger, B.A., and Callard, G.V. (1990). Aromatization mediates aggressive behaviour in quail. *General and Comparative Endocrinology* 79: 39–53.

Schlinger, B.A., Soma, K.K., and London, S.E. (2001). Neurosteroids and brain sexual differentiation. *Trends in Neurosciences* 24: 429–31.

Schmidt, G., and Clement, U. (1990). Does peace prevent homosexuality? *Archives of Sexual Behavior* 19: 183–7.

Schneider, H.J., Pickle, J., and Stalla, G.K. (2006). Typical 2nd–4th finger length (2D:4D) ratios in male-to-female transsexuals – possible implications for prenatal androgen exposure. *Psychoneuroendocrinology* 31: 265–9.

Schradin, C., Reeder, D.M., Mendoza, S.P., and Anzenberger, G. (2003). Prolactin and paternal care: comparison of three species of monogamous New World monkeys (*Callicebus cupreus, Callithrix jacchus*, and *Callimico goeldi*). *Journal of Comparative Psychology* 117: 166–75.

Schreiner-Engel, P., Schiavi, R.C., Smith, H., and White, D. (1981). Sexual arousability and the menstrual cycle. *Psychological Medicine* 43: 199–214.

Schulz, K.M., Richardson, H.M., Zehr, J.L., Osetek, A.J., Menard, T.A., and Sisk, C.L. (2004). Gonadal hormones masculinise and defeminise reproductive behaviors during puberty in the male Syrian hamster. *Hormones and Behavior* 45: 242–9.

Scott, S.K., Young, A.W., Calder, A.J., Hellawell, D.J., Aggleton, J.P., and Johnson, M. (1997). Impaired auditory recognition of fear and anger following bilateral amygdale lesions. *Nature* 385: 254–7.

Scoville, W.B., and Milner, B. (1957). Loss of recent memory after bilateral hippocampal lesion. *Journal of Neurology, Neurosurgery and Psychiatry* 20: 11–21.

Seeman, E. (1997). From density to structure: growing up and growing old on the surface of bones. *Journal of Bone and Mineral Research* 12: 509–21.

Seftel, A.D., Mack, R.J., Secrest, A.R., and Smith, T.M. (2004). Restorative increases in serum testosterone levels are significantly correlated to improvements in sexual functioning. *Journal of Andrology* 23: 963–72.

Selmanoff, M.K., Brodkin, L.D., Weiner, R.I., and Siiteri, P.K. (1977). Aromatization and 5α reduction of androgens in discrete hypothalamic and limbic regions of the male and female rat. *Endocrinology* 101: 841–8.

Selye, H. (1942). Correlation between the chemical structure and the pharmacological actions of the steroids. *Endocrinology* 30: 437–53.

Sharp, P.J., Macnamee, M.C., Talbot, R.T., Sterling, R.J., and Hall, T.R. (1984). Aspects of the neuroendocrine control of ovulation and broodiness in the domestic hen. *Journal of Experimental Zoology* 232: 475–83.

Shaywitz, B.A., Shaywitz, S.E., Pugh, K.R., Constable, R.T., Skudlarski, P., Fulbright, R.K., Bronsen, R.A., Fletcher, J.M., Shankweller, D.P., Katz, L., and Gore, J.C. (1995). Sex differences in the functional organization of the brain for language. *Nature* 373: 607–9.

Shepard, R., and Metzler, J. (1971). Mental rotation of three dimensional objects. *Science* 171:701–3.

Sheridan, P.J. (1979). The nucleus interstitialis striae terminalis and the nucleus amygdaloideus medialis: prime targets for androgen in the rat forebrain. *Endocrinology* 104: 130–6.

  (1983). Androgen receptors in the brain: what are we measuring? *Endocrine Reviews* 4: 171–8.

Sherwin, B.B. (1988). Estrogen and/or androgen replacement therapy and cognitive functioning in surgically menopausal women. *Psychoneuroendocrinology* 13: 345–57.

  (1991). The impact of different doses of estrogen and progestin on mood and sexual behavior in postmenopausal women. *Journal of Clinical Endocrinology and Metabolism* 72: 336–43.

Sherwin, B.B., Gelfand, M.M., and Brender, W. (1985). Androgen enhances sexual motivation in females: a prospective, crossover study of sex steroid administration in the surgical menopause. *Psychosomatic Medicine* 47: 339–51.

Sherwin, B.B., and Phillips, S. (1990). Estrogen and cognitive functioning in surgically menopausal women. *Annals of the New York Academy of Science* 592: 474–5.

Shifren, J.L., Braunstein, G.D., Simon, J.A., Casson, P.R., Buster, J.E., Redmond, G.P., Burki, R.E., Ginsburg, E.S., Rosen, R.C., Leiblum, S.R., Caramelli, K.E., and Mazer, N.A. (2000). Transdermal testosterone treatment in women with impaired sexual function after oophorectomy. *New England Journal of Medicine* 343: 682–8.

Shirtcliff, E.A., Granger, D.A., and Likos, A. (2002). Gender differences in the validity of testosterone measured in saliva by immunoassay. *Hormones and Behavior* 42: 62–9.

Shirtcliff, E.A., Granger, D.A., Schwartz, E., and Curran, M.J. (2001). Use of salivary biomarkers in biobehavioral research: cotton-based sample collection methods can interfere with salivary immunoassay results. *Psychoneuroendocrinology* 26: 165–73.

Shute, V., Pellegrino, J.W., Hubert, L., and Reynolds, R.W. (1983). The relationship between androgen levels and human spatial abilities. *Bulletin of the Psychonomic Society* 21: 465–8.

Silbert, A., Wolff, P.H., and Lilienthal, J. (1977). Spatial and temporal processing in patients with Turner's syndrome. *Behavior Genetics* 7: 11–21.

Silva, J.E. (2000). Catecholamines and the sympathoadrenal system in thyrotoxicosis. In L.E. Braverman and R.D. Utiger (eds.), *Werner and Ingbar's the Thyroid: A Fundamental and Clinical Text*. New York: Lippincott, Williams and Wilkins, 8th edition, pp. 642–51.

Silver, R. (1978). The parental behaviour of ring doves. *American Scientist* 66: 209–15.

Silverman, I., Kastuk, D., Choi, J., and Phillips, K. (1999). Testosterone levels and spatial ability in men. *Psychoneuroendocrinology* 24: 813–22.

Silverman, I., and Phillips, K. (1993). Effects of estrogen changes during the menstrual cycle on spatial performance. *Ethology and Sociobiology* 14: 257–70.

Simon, N.G., and Whalen, R.E. (1986). Hormonal regulation of aggression: evidence for a relationship among genotype, receptor binding, and behavioural sensitivity to androgen and estrogen. *Aggressive Behavior* 12: 255–66.

Simpson, K. (2001). The role of testosterone in aggression. *McGill Journal of Medicine* 6: 32–40.

Sinforiani, E., Livieri, C., Mauri, M., Bisio, P., Chiesa, L., and Martelli, A. (1994). Cognitive and neuroradiological findings in congenital adrenal hyperplasia. *Psychoneuroendocrinology* 19: 55–64.

Singh, D. (1993). Body shape and women's attractiveness: the critical role of the waist-to-hip ratio. *Human Nature* 4: 297–321.

Singh, D., and Bronstad, P.M. (2001). Female body odour is a potential cue to ovulation. *Proceedings of the Royal Society of London, B* 268: 797–801.

Sisk, C.L., and Zehr, J.L. (2005). Pubertal hormones organize the adolescent brain and behavior. *Frontiers in Neuroendocrinology* 26: 163–74.

Skuse, D.H., James, R.S., Bishop, D.V.M., Coppin, B., Dalton, P., Aamodt-Leeper, G., Bacarese-Hamilton, M., Creswell, C., McGurk, R., and Jacobs, P.A. (1997). Evidence from Turner's syndrome of an imprinted X-linked locus affecting cognitive function. *Nature* 387: 705–8.

Slabbekoorn, D., van Goozen, S.H.M., Megens, J., Gooren, L.J.G., and Cohen-Kettenis, P.T. (1999). Activating effects of cross-sex hormones on cognitive functioning: a study of short-term and long-term hormone effects in transsexuals. *Psychoneuroendocrinology* 24: 423–47.

Slabbekoorn, D., van Goozen, S.H.M., Sanders, G., Gooren, L.J.G., and Cohen-Kettenis, P.T. (2000). The dermatoglyphic characteristics of transsexuals: is there evidence for an organizing effect of sex hormones? *Psychoneuroendocrinology* 25: 365–75.

Slijper, F.M.E. (1984). Androgens and gender role behaviour in girls with congenital adrenal hyperplasia (CAH). In G.J. De Vries, J.P.C. De Bruin, H.B.M. Uylings, and M.A.Corner (eds.), *Progress in Brain Research*, vol. 61. Amsterdam: Elsevier, pp. 417–22.

Slob, A.K., Bax, C.M., Hop, W.C.J., Rowland, D.L., and van der Werff ten Bosch, J.J. (1996). Sexual arousability and the menstrual cycle. *Psychoneuroendocrinology* 21: 545–58.

Slob, A.K., Ernste, M., and van der Werff ten Bosch, J.J. (1991). Menstrual cycle phase and sexual arousability in women. *Archives of Sexual Behavior* 20: 567–77.

Smith, C.D., and Ain, K.B. (1995). Brain metabolism in hypothyroidism studies with $^{31}$P magnetic-resonance spectroscopy. *The Lancet* 345: 619–20.

Smith, E.R., Damassa, D.A., and Davidson, J.M. (1977). Plasma testosterone and sexual behaviour following intracerebral implantation of testosterone propionate in the castrated male rat. *Hormones and Behavior* 8: 77–87.

Smith, L.C., Raouf, S.A., Brown, M.B., Wingfield, J.C., and Brown, C.R. (2005). Testosterone and group size in cliff swallows: testing the 'challenge hypothesis' in a colonial bird. *Hormones and Behavior* 47: 76–82.

Snowden, C.T., Ziegler, T.E., Schultz-Darken, N.J., and Ferris, C.F. (2006). Social odours, sexual arousal and pair-bonding in primates. *Philosophical Transactions of the Royal Society, B* 361: 2079–89.

Solís-Ortiz, S., Ramos, J., Arce, C., Guevara, M.A., and Corsi-Cabrera, M. (1994). EEG oscillations during menstrual cycle. *International Journal of Neuroscience* 76: 279–92.

Soloff, M.S., Morrsion, M.J., and Swartz, T.L. (1972). A comparison of the estrone-estradiol-binding proteins in the plasmas of prepubertal and pregnant rats. *Steroids* 20: 597–608.

Soltis, J., Wegner, F.H., and Newman, J.D. (2005). Urinary prolactin is correlated with mothering and allo-mothering in squirrel monkeys. *Physiology and Behavior* 84: 295–301.

Soma, K.K., Sullivan, K., and Wingfield, J. (1999). Combined aromatase inhibitor and antiandrogen treatment decreases territorial aggression in a wild songbird during the nonbreeding season. *General and Comparative Endocrinology* 115: 442–53.

Sommer, B. (1972). Menstrual cycle changes and intellectual performance. *Psychosomatic Medicine* 34: 263–9.

(1992). Cognitive performance and the menstrual cycle. In J.T.E. Richardson (ed.), *Cognition and the Menstrual Cycle*. London: Springer-Verlag, pp. 39–66.

Speiser, P.W., and White, P.C. (2003). Congenital adrenal hyperplasia. *New England Journal of Medicine* 349: 776–88.

Spielberger, C.D. (1972). Anxiety as an emotional state. In C.D. Spielberger (eds.), *Anxiety: Current Trends in Theory and Research*, vol. 1. New York: Academic Press, pp. 23–49.

Springer, S.P., and Deutsch, G. (1993). *Left Brain, Right Brain*. New York: W.H. Freeman and Co.

Squire, L.R. (1992). Memory and the hippocampus: a synthesis of findings with rats, monkeys, and humans. *Psychological Review* 2: 195–231.

Squire, L.R., Ojemann, J.G., Miezin, F.M., Petersen, S.E., Videen, T.O., and Raichle, M.E. (1992). Activation of the hippocampus in normal humans: a functional anatomical study of memory. *Proceedings of the National Academy of Science USA* 89: 1837–41.

Steimer, T., and Hutchison, J.B. (1981). Androgen increases formation of behaviourally effective oestrogen in dove brain. *Nature* 292: 345–7.

Stern, J.M. (1989). Maternal behaviour: sensory, hormonal, and neural determinants. In F.R. Bush and S. Levine (eds.), *Psychoendocrinology*. New York: Academic Press, pp. 103–226.

Stern, J.M., and Eisenfeld, A.J. (1971). Distribution and metabolism of 3H-testosterone in castrated male rats: effects of cyproterone, progesterone and unlabeled testosterone. *Endocrinology* 88: 1117–25.

Stewart, J., and Kolb, B. (1988). The effects of neonatal gonadectomy and prenatal stress on cortical thickness and asymmetry in rats. *Behavioral and Neural Biology* 49: 344–60.

Stoléru, S.G., Ennaji, A., Cournot, A., and Spira, A. (1993). LH pulsatile secretion and testosterone blood levels are influenced by sexual arousal in human males. *Psychoneuroendocrinology* 18: 205–18.

Storey, A.E., Walsh, C.J., Quinton, R.L., and Wynne-Edwards, K.E. (2000). Hormonal correlates of paternal responsiveness in new and expectant fathers. *Evolution and Human Behavior* 21: 79–95.

Strauss, R.H., Ligett, J.E., and Lanesse, R.R. (1985). Anabolic steroid use and perceived effects in 10 weight trained women. *Journal of the American Medical Association* 253: 2871–3.

Styne, D. (1997). Puberty. In F.S. Greenspan and G.J. Strewler (eds.), *Basic and Clinical Endocrinology*. Stamford: Appleton and Lange, 5th edition, pp. 521–47.

Svare, B., and Kinsley, C.H. (1987). Hormones and sex related behavior: a comparative analysis. In K. Kelley (ed.), *Females, Males and Sexuality: Theories and Research*. Albany, NY: SUNY Press, pp. 13–58.

Swaab, D.F., and Fliers, E. (1985). A sexually dimorphic nucleus in the human brain. *Science* 228: 1112–15.

Swaab, D.F., Gooren, L.J.G., and Hofman. M.A. (1992). The human hypothalamus in relation to gender and sexual orientation. In D.F. Swaab, M.A. Hofman, M. Mirmiran, R. Ravid and F.W. van Leeuwen (eds.), *Progress in Brain Research*, vol. 93. Amsterdam: Elsevier, pp. 205–19.

Swaab, D.F., and Hofman, M.A. (1984). Sexual differentiation of the human brain. A historical perspective. In G.J. De Vries, J.P.C. De Bruin, H.B.M. Uylings, and M.A. Corner (eds.), *Progress in Brain Research*, vol. 61. Amsterdam: Elsevier, pp. 361–74.

Symons, D. (1979). *The Evolution of Human Sexuality*. Oxford: Oxford University Press.

Tan, Ü. (1990). Relationship of testosterone and hand preference in right-handed young visuomotor adults. *International Journal of Neuroscience* 53: 157–65.

(1991a). Serum testosterone levels in male and female subjects with standard and anomalous dominance. *International Journal of Neuroscience* 58: 211–14.

(1991b). The relationship between serum testosterone and visuomotor learning in hand skill in right handed young men. *International Journal of Neuroscience* 56: 19–24.

Tausk, M. (1984). Androgens and anabolic steroids. In M.J. Parnham and J Bruinvels (eds.), *Discoveries in Pharmacology*, vol. 2. Amsterdam: Elsevier Science, pp. 307–20.

Taylor, S.E., Klein, L.C., Lewis, B.P., Gruenewald, T.L., Gurung, R.A.R., and Updegraff, J.A. (2000). Biobehavioral responses to stress in females: tend-and-befriend, not fight-or-flight. *Psychological Review* 107: 411–29.

Thackare, H., Nicholson, H.D., and Whittington, K. (2006). Oxytocin – its role in male reproduction and new potential therapeutic uses. *Human Reproduction Update* 12: 437–48.

Thilers, P.P., MacDonald, S.W.S., and Herlitz, A. (2006). The association between endogenous free testosterone and cognitive performance: a population-based study in 35 to 90 year-old men and women. *Psychoneuroendocrinology* 31: 565–76.

Tinbergen, N. (1951). *The Study of Instinct*. Oxford: Clarendon Press.

Toda, K., Saibara, T., Okada, S., Onishi, Y., and Shizuta, A. (2001). A loss of aggressive behaviour and its reinstatement by oestrogen in mice lacking the aromatase gene (Cyp 19). *Journal of Endocrinology* 168: 217–20.

Trainor, B.C., Kyomen, H.H., and Marler, C.A. (2006). Estrogenic encounters: how interactions between aromatase and the environment modulate aggression. *Frontiers in Neuroendocrinology* 27: 170–9.

Trainor, B.C., and Marler, C.A. (2001). Testosterone promotes paternal behaviour in a monogamous mammal via conversion to oestrogen. *Proceedings of the Royal Society of London, B* 269: 823–9.

Travison, T.G., Morley, J.E., Araujo, A.B., O'Donnell, A.B., and McKinlay, J.B. (2006). The relationship between libido and testosterone levels in aging men. *Journal of Clinical Endocrinology and Metabolism* 91: 2509–13.

Tremblay, R.E., Schaal, B., Boulerice, B., Arseneault, L., Soussignan, R.G., Paquette, D., and Laurent, D. (1998). Testosterone, physical aggression, dominance, and physical development in early adolescence. *International Journal of Behavioral Development* 22: 753–77.

Tsutsui, K., and Ishii, S. (1981). Effects of sex steroids on aggressive behavior of adult male Japanese quail. *General and Comparative Endocrinology* 44: 480–6.

Tulpe, I.A., and Torchinov, E.A. (2000). The castrati ('Skoptsy') sect in Russia:

history, teaching and religious practice. *International Journal of Transpersonal Studies* 19: 77–87.

Turner, H.H. (1938). A syndrome of infantilism, congenital webbed neck and cubitus valgus. *Endocrinology* 23: 566–78.

Twigg, D.G., Popolow, H.B., and Gerall, A.A. (1978). Medial preoptic lesions and male sexual behavior: age and environmental interactions. *Science* 200: 1414–15.

Udry, J. (1990). Biosocial models of adolescent behaviour problems. *Social Biology* 37: 1–10.

Udry, J.R., Billy, J.O.G., Morris, N.M., Groff, T.R., and Raj, M.H. (1985). Serum androgenic hormones motivate sexual behavior in adolescent boys. *Fertility and Sterility* 43: 90–4.

Udry, J.R., Morris, N.M., and Kovenock, J. (1995). Androgen effects on women's gendered behavior. *Journal of Biosocial Science* 27: 359–68.

Uvnäs-Moberg, K. (1997). Physiological and endocrine effects of social contact. *Annals of the New York Academy of Science* 807: 146–63.

(1998). Oxytocin may mediate the benefits of positive social interactions and emotions. *Psychoneuroendocrinology* 23: 819–35.

Vague, J., Meignen, J.M., and Negrin, J.F. (1984). Effects of testosterone and estrogens on deltoid and trochanter adipocytes in two cases of transsexualism. *Hormone Metabolic Research* 16: 380–1.

van Anders, S.M., Hamilton, L.D., and Watson, N.V. (2007a). Multiple partners are associated with higher testosterone in North American men and women. *Hormones and Behavior* 51: 454–9.

van Anders, S.M., Hamilton, L.D., Schmidt, N., and Watson, N.V. (2007b). Associations between testosterone secretion and sexual activity in women. *Hormones and Behavior* 51: 477–82.

van Anders, S.M., and Hampson, E. (2005). Testing the prenatal androgen hypothesis: measuring digit ratios, sexual orientation, and spatial abilities in adults. *Hormones and Behavior* 47: 92–8.

van Anders, S.M., and Watson, N.V. (2006a). Social neuroendocrinology. Effects of social contexts and behaviors on sex steroids in humans. *Human Nature* 17: 212–37.

(2006b). Relationship status and testosterone in North American heterosexual and non-heterosexual men and women: cross-sectional and longitudinal data. *Psychoneuroendocrinology* 31: 715–23.

(2007a). Testosterone levels in women and men who are single, in long-distance relationships, or same-city relationships. *Hormones and Behavior* 51: 286–91.

(2007b). Effects of ability- and chance-determined competition outcome on testosterone. *Physiology and Behavior* 90: 634–42.

van Bokhoven, I., van Goozen, S.H.M., van Engeland, H., Schaal, B., Arseneault, L., Séguin, J.R., Assaad, J.-M., Nagin, D.S., Vitaro, F., and Tremblay, R.E. (2006). Salivary testosterone and aggression, delinquency, and social dominance in a population-based longitudinal study of adolescent males. *Hormones and Behavior* 50: 118–25.

van den Berghe, P.L., and Frost, P. (1986). Skin colour preference, sexual dimorphism and sexual selection: a case of gene-culture co-evolution? *Ethnic and Racial Studies* 9: 87–118.

van Goozen, S.H.M., Cohen-Kettenis, P.T., Gooren, L.J.G., Frijda, N.H., and van de Poll, N.E. (1994). Activating effects of androgens on cognitive performance: causal evidence in a group of female-to-male transsexuals. *Neuropsychologia* 32: 1153–7.

van Goozen, S.H.M., Cohen-Kettenis, P.T., Gooren, L.J.G., Frijda, N.H., and van de Poll, N.E. (1995). Gender differences in behaviour: activating effects of cross-sex hormones. *Psychoneuroendocrinology* 20: 343–63.

van Goozen, S.H.M., Wiegant, V.M., Endert, E., Helmond, F.A., and Van de Poll, N.E. (1997). Psychoendocrinological assessment of the menstrual cycle: the relationship between hormones, sexuality and mood. *Archives of Sexual Behavior* 26: 359–82.

van Honk, J., Tuiten, A., Hermans, E., Putman, P., Koppaschaar, H., Thijssen, J., Verbaten, R., and van Doornen, L. (2001). A single administration of testosterone induces cardiac accelerative responses to angry faces in healthy young volunteers. *Behavioral Neuroscience* 115: 238–42.

van Honk, J., Tuiten, A., Verbaten, R., van den Hout, M., Koppaschaar, H., Thijssen, J., and de Haan, E. (1999). Correlations among salivary testosterone, mood, and selective attention to threat in humans. *Hormones and Behavior* 36: 17–24.

van Kesteren, P.J., Gooren, L.J., and Megens, J.A. (1996). An epidemiological and demographic study of transsexuals in the Netherlands. *Archives of Sexual Behavior* 25: 589–600.

van Seters, A.P., and Slob, A.K. (1988). Mutually gratifying heterosexual relationship with micropenis of husband. *Journal of Sex and Marital Therapy* 14: 98–107.

Veldhuis, J.D., King, J.C., Urban, R.J., Rogol, A.D., Evans, W.S., Kolp, S.A., and Johnson, M.L. (1987). Operating characteristics of the male hypothalamo–pituitary–gonadal axis: pulsatile release of testosterone and follicle-stimulating hormone and their temporal coupling with luteinising hormone. *Journal of Clinical Endocrinology and Metabolism* 65: 929–41.

Verdonck, A., Gaethofs, M., Carels, C., and de Zegher, F. (1999). Effect of low-dose testosterone treatment on craniofacial growth in boys with delayed puberty. *European Journal of Orthodontics* 21: 137–43.

Vermeulen, A., Goemaere, S., and Kaufman, J.M. (1999). Testosterone, body composition and aging. *Journal of Endocrinological Investigation* 22: 110–16.

Vermeulen, A., and Verdonck, L. (1976). Plasma androgen levels during the menstrual cycle. *American Journal of Obstetrics and Gynecology* 125: 491–4.

Vermeulen, A., Verdonck, L., and Kaufman, J.M. (1999). A critical evaluation of simple methods for the estimation of free testosterone in serum. *Journal of Clinical Endocrinology and Metabolism* 84: 3666–72.

Vittek, J., L'Hommedieu, D.G., Gordon, G.G., Rappaport, S.C., and Southren, A.L. (1985). Direct radioimmunoassay (RIA) of salivary testosterone: correlations with free and total serum testosterone. *Life Sciences* 37: 711–16.

Vogel, W., Broverman, D.M., Klaiber, E.L., Abraham, G., and Cone, F.L. (1971). Effects of testosterone infusions upon EEG's of normal male adults. *Electroencephalography and Clinical Neurophysiology* 31: 400–3.

Vom Saal, F. (1989). Sexual differentiation in litter-bearing mammals: influence of sex of adjacent fetuses in utero. *Journal of Animal Science* 67: 1824–40.

Vom Saal, F., and Bronson, F.H. (1978). In utero proximity of female mouse fetuses to males: effect on reproductive performance during later life. *Biology of Reproduction* 19: 842–53.

(1980). Sexual characteristics of adult female mice are correlated with their blood testosterone levels during prenatal development. *Science* 208: 597–9.

Voracek, M., Manning, J.T., and Dressler, S.G. (2007). Repeatability and intraobserver error of digit ratio (2D:4D) measurements made by experts. *American Journal of Human Biology* 19: 142–6.

Voyer, D. (1996). On the magnitude of laterality effects and sex differences in functional lateralities. *Laterality* 1: 51–83.

Voyer, D., Voyer, S., and Bryden, M. (1995). Magnitude of sex differences in spatial abilities: a meta-analysis and consideration of critical variables. *Psychological Bulletin* 117: 250–70.

Vrbancic, M.I., and Mosley, J.L. (1988). Sex-related differences in hemispheric lateralization: a function of physical maturation. *Developmental Neuropsychology* 4: 151–67.

Vuorenkoski, V., Lenko, H.L., Tjernlund, P., Vuorenkoski, L., and Perheentupa, J. (1978). Fundamental voice frequency during normal and abnormal growth and after androgen treatment. *Archives of Disease in Childhood* 53: 201–9.

Waber, D.P. (1977). Sex differences in mental abilities, hemispheric lateralization, and rate of physical growth at maturation. *Developmental Psychology* 13: 29–38.

(1979). Neuropsychological aspects of Turner's syndrome. *Developmental Medicine and Child Neurology* 21: 58–70.

Waber, D.P., Mann, M.B., Merols, J., and Moylan, P.M. (1985). Physical maturation rate and cognitive performance in early adolescence: a longitudinal examination. *Developmental Psychology* 21: 666–81.

Wagner, C.K. (2006). The many faces of progesterone: a role in adult and developing male brain. *Frontiers in Neuroendocrinology* 27: 40–59.

Wagner, J.D., Flinn, M.V., and England, B.G. (2002). Hormonal responses to competition among male coalitions. *Evolution and Human Behavior* 23: 437–42.

Wallen, K. (1990). Desire and ability: hormones and the regulation of female sexual behaviour. *Neuroscience and Biobehavioral Reviews* 14: 233–41.

Wallen, K., Mann, D.R., Davis-DaSilva, M., Gaventa, S., Lovejoy, J.C., and Collins, D.C. (1986). Chronic gonadotropin-releasing hormone agonist treatment suppresses ovulation and sexual behaviour in group-living female rhesus monkeys. *Physiology and Behavior* 36: 369–75.

Wallen, K., Winston, L.A., Gaventa, S., Davis-DaSilva, M., and Collins, D.C. (1984). Periovulatory changes in female sexual behaviour and patterns of ovarian steroid secretion in group-living rhesus monkeys. *Hormones and Behavior* 18: 431–50.

Walsh, R.N., Budtz-Olsen, I., Leader, C., and Cummins, R.A. (1981). The menstrual cycle, personality, and academic performance. *Archives of General Psychiatry* 38: 219–21.

Wang, C., Swerdloff, R.S., Iranmanesh, A., Dobs, A., Snyder, P.J., Cunningham, G., Matsumoto, A.M., Weber, T., and Berman, N. (2000). Transdermal testosterone gel improves sexual function, mood, muscle strength, and body composition in hypogonadal men. *Journal of Clinical Endocrinology and Metabolism* 85: 2839–53.

(2001). Effects of transdermal testosterone gel on bone turnover markers and bone mineral density in hypogonadal men. *Clinical Endocrinology* 54: 739–50.

Ward, I.L. (1972). Prenatal stress feminizes and demasculinizes the behaviour of males. *Science* 175: 82–4.

(1984). The prenatal stress syndrome: current status. *Psychoneuroendocrinology* 9: 3–11.

Ward, I.L., and Weisz, J. (1980). Maternal stress alters plasma testosterone in fetal males. *Science* 207: 328–9.

Watkins, J.C., and Jane, D.E. (2006). The glutamate story. *British Journal of Pharmacology* 147 (Suppl.): S100–8.

Watson, M. (1877). On the female generative organs of *Hyaena crocuta. Proceedings of the Zoological Society of London* 24: 369–78.

Watson, P.J., and Thornhill, R. (1994). Fluctuating asymmetry and sexual selection. *Trends in Ecology and Evolution* 9: 21–5.

Wehling. M. (1997). Specific, nongenomic actions of steroid hormones. *Annual Review of Physiology* 59: 369–93.

Weiland, N.G. (1992). Estradiol selectively regulates agonist binding sites on the N-methyl-D-aspartate receptor complex in the CA1 region of the hippocampus. *Endocrinology* 131: 662–8.

Weinberg, S.M., Scott, N.M., Neiswanger, K., and Marazita, M.L. (2005). Intraobserver error associated with measurements of the hand. *American Journal of Human Biology* 17: 368–71.

Wesson, D.W., and McGuinness, M.Y. (2006). Stacking anabolic androgenic steroids (AAS) during puberty in rats: a neuroendocrine and behavioural assessment. *Pharmacology, Biochemistry and Behavior* 83: 410–19.

Whalen, R.E. (1974). Estrogen-progesterone induction of mating in female rats. *Hormones and Behavior* 5: 157–62.

Whembolua, G.-L.S., Granger, D.A., Singer, S., Kivlighan, K.T., and Marguin, J.A. (2006). Bacteria in the oral mucosa and its effects on the measurement of cortisol, dehydroepiandrosterone, and testosterone in saliva. *Hormones and Behavior* 49: 478–83.

Wickham, M. (1958). The effects of the menstrual cycle on test performance. *British Journal of Psychology* 49: 34–41.

Wilczynski, W., Lynch, K.S., and O'Bryant, E.L. (2005). Current research in amphibians: studies integrating endocrinology, behavior, and neurobiology. *Hormones and Behavior* 48: 440–50.

Williams, C.L., Barnett, A.M., and Meck, W.H. (1990). Organizational effects of early gonadal secretions on sexual differentiation in spatial memory. *Behavioural Neuroscience* 104: 84–97.

Williams, J.H.G., Greenhalgh, K.D., and Manning, J.T. (2003). Second to fourth finger ratio and possible precursors of developmental psychopathology in preschool children. *Early Human Development* 72: 57–65.

Williams, J.R., Catania, K.C., and Carter, C.S. (1994). Development of partner preferences in female prairie voles (*Microtus ochrogaster*): the role of social and sexual experience. *Hormones and Behavior* 26: 339–49.

Williams, J.R., Insel, T.R., Harbaugh, C.R., and Carter, C.S. (1994). Oxytocin administered centrally facilitates formation of a partner preference in female prairie voles (*Microtus ochrogaster*). *Journal of Neuroendocrinology* 6: 247–50.

Williams, R.W., and Herrup, K. (1988). The control of neuron number. *Annual Review of Neuroscience* 11: 423–53.

Williams, T.J., Pepitone, M.E., Christensen, S.E., Cooke, B.M., Huberman, A.D., Breedlove, N.J., Breedlove, T.J., Jordan, C.L., and Breedlove, S.M. (2000). Finger-length ratios and sexual orientation. *Nature* 404: 455–6.

Wilson, J.D. (1999). The role of androgens in male gender role behaviour. *Endocrine Reviews* 20: 726–37.

(2005). The evolution of endocrinology. Plenary lecture at the 12th International Congress of Endocrinology, Lisbon, Portugal, 31 August 2004. *Clinical Endocrinology* 62: 389–96.

Wilson, M., and Daly, M. (1985). Competitiveness, risk-taking and violence: the young male syndrome. *Ethology and Sociobiology* 6: 59–73.

Wilson, M.E., Gordon, T.P., and Collins, D.C. (1982). Variation in ovarian steroids associated with the annual mating period in female rhesus (*Macaca mulatta*). *Biology of Reproduction* 27: 530–9.

Wingfield, J.C. (1984). Androgens and mating systems: testosterone-induced polygyny in normally monogamous birds. *Auk* 101: 665–71.

(1985). Short-term changes in plasma levels of hormones during establishment and defence of a breeding territory in male song sparrows, *Melospiza melodia*. *Hormones and Behavior* 19: 174–87.

(1994). Regulation of territorial behavior in the sedentary song sparrow, *Melospiza melodia morphina*. *Hormones and Behavior* 28: 1–15.

(2005). Historical contributions of research on birds to behavioral neuroendocrinology. *Hormones and Behavior* 48: 395–402.

Wingfield, J.C., Ball, G.F., Duffy, A.M., Hegner, R.E., and Ramenofsky, M. (1987). Testosterone and aggression in birds. *American Scientist* 75: 602–8.

Wingfield, J.C., Hegner, R.E., Dufty, A.M., and Ball, G.F. (1990). The 'challenge hypothesis': theoretical implications for patterns of testosterone secretion, mating systems, and breeding strategies. *American Naturalist* 136: 829–46.

Wingfield, J.C., Jacobs, J.D., Tramontin, A.D., Perfito, N., Meddle, S., Maney, D.L., and Soma, K. (2000). Toward an ecological basis of hormone–behavior interactions in reproduction in birds. In K. Whalen and J.E. Schneider (eds.), *Reproduction in Context: Social and Environmental Influences on Reproductive Physiology and Human Behavior*. Cambridge, MA: MIT Press, pp. 85–128.

Wingfield, J.C., and Wada, M. (1989). Changes in plasma levels of testosterone during male–male interactions in the song sparrow, *Melospiza melodia*: time course and specificity of response. *Journal of Comparative Physiology, A* 166: 189–94.

Winslow, J.T., Hastings, N., Carter, C.S., Harbaugh, C.R., and Insel, T.R. (1993). A role for central vasopressin in pair bonding in monogamous prairie voles. *Nature* 365: 545–8.

Winslow, J.T., and Insel, T.R. (1993). Effects of central vasopressin administration to infant rats. *European Journal of Pharmacology* 233: 101–7.

Wirth, M.M., and Schultheiss, O.C. (2007). Basal testosterone moderates responses to anger faces in humans. *Physiology and Behavior* 90: 496–505.

Wisniewski, A.B. (1998). Sexually-dimorphic patterns of cortical asymmetry, and the role for sex steroid hormones in determining cortical patterns of lateralization. *Psychoneuroendocrinology* 23: 519–47.

Witelson, S.F. (1991). Neural sexual mosaicism: sexual differentiation of the human tempero-parietal region for functional asymmetry. *Psychoneuroendocrinology* 16: 131–54.

Witelson, S.F., and Nowakowski, R.S. (1991). Left out axons make men right: a hypothesis for the origin of handedness and functional asymmetry. *Neuropsychologia* 27: 1207–19.

Wolf, O.T., and Kirschbaum, C. (2002). Endogenous estradiol and testosterone levels are associated with cognitive performance in older women and men. *Hormones and Behavior* 41: 259–66.

Wooley, C.S., and McEwen, B.S. (1992). Estradiol mediates fluctuation in hippocampal synapse density during the estrous cycle in the adult rat. *Journal of Neuroscience* 12: 2549–54.

Wooley, C.S., Weiland, N.G., McEwen, B.S., and Schwartzkronin, P.A. (1997). Estradiol increases the sensitivity of hippocampal CA1 pyramidal cells to NMDA receptor-mediated synaptic input: correlation with dendritic spine density. *Journal of Neuroscience* 17: 1838–59.

Wu, S., Jia, M., Ruan, Y., Liu, J., Guo, Y., Shuang, M., Gong, X., Zhang, Y., Yang, X., and Zhang, D. (2005). Positive association of the oxytocin receptor gene (OXTR) with autism in the Chinese Han population. *Biological Psychiatry* 58: 74–7.

Yang, C.F., Hooven, C.K., Boynes, M., Gray, P.B., and Pope, H.G. Jr. (2007). Testosterone levels and mental rotation performance in Chinese men. *Hormones and Behavior* 51: 373–8.

Young, L.J., Lim, M.M., Gingrich, B., and Insel, T.R. (2001). Cellular mechanisms of social attachment. *Hormones and Behavior* 40: 133–8.

Young, L.J., Nilsen, R., Waymire, K.G., MacGregor, G.R., and Insel, T.R. (1999). Increased affiliative response to vasopressin in mice expressing the vasopressin receptor from a monogamous vole. *Nature* 400: 766–8.

Young, W.C., Goy, R.W., and Phoenix, C.H. (1965). Hormones and sexual behavior. In J. Money (ed.), *Sex Research, New Developments*. New York: Holt.

Zaastra, B.M., Seidell, J.C., Van Noord, P.A.H., te Velde, E.R., Habbema, J.D.F., Vrieswijk, B., and Karbaat, J. (1993). Fat and female fecundity: prospective study of effect of body fat distribution on conception rates. *British Medical Journal* 306: 484–7.

Zak, P.J., Kurzban, R., and Matzner, W.T. (2005). Oxytocin is associated with human trustworthiness. *Hormones and Behavior* 48: 522–7.

Zehr, J.L., Maestripieri, D., and Wallen, K. (1998). Estradiol increases female sexual initiation independent of male responsiveness in rhesus monkeys. *Hormones and Behavior* 33: 95–103.

Zhou, J.-N., Hofman, M.A., Gooren, L.J.G., and Swaab, D.F. (1995). A sex difference in the human brain and its relation to transsexuality. *Nature* 378: 68–70.

Ziegler, T.E., Epple, G., Snowdon, C.T., Porter, T.A., Belcher, A., and Kuederling, I. (1993). Detection of the chemical signals of ovulation in the cotton-top tamarin, *Saguinus oedipus*. *Animal Behaviour* 45: 313–22.

Ziegler, T.E., and Snowdon, C.T. (2000). Preparental hormone levels and parenting experience in male cotton-top tamarins, *Saguinus oedipus. Hormones and Behavior* 38: 159–67.

Ziegler, T.E., Wegner, F.H., and Snowdon, C.T. (1996). Hormonal responses to parental and nonparental conditions in male cotton-top tamarins, *Saguinus oedipus*, a New World primate. *Hormones and Behavior* 30: 287–97.

Zimmerman, E., and Parlee, M.B. (1973). Behavioural changes associated with the menstrual cycle: an experimental investigation. *Journal of Applied Social Psychology* 3: 335–44.

Zitzmann, M., and Nieschlag, E. (2004). Androgens and bone metabolism. In E. Nieschlag, H.M. Behre and S. Nieschlag (eds.), *Testosterone: Action, DeWciency, Substitution*. Cambridge: Cambridge University Press, pp. 233–54.

Zuckerman, M. (1979). *Sensation Seeking: Beyond the Optimal Level of Arousal*. Hillsdale, NJ: Erlbaum.

Zuger, B. (1984). Early effeminate behaviour in boys: outcome and significance for homosexuality. *Journal of Nervous and Mental Disease* 172: 90–7.

# Index

acetylcholine (ACh), 24
  cholinergic drugs and sexual behaviour, 165
  cholinergic pathways, 20, 251
  general information on, 17–18
  influence of estradiol on ACh production, 251
  influence on dendritic spine density, 250–1
  influence on hormone release, 82
  synthesis of, 16
Addison's disease, see adrenal glands
adenosine triphosphate (ATP), 11, 14
adrenal glands, 38–9
  Addison's disease, 39
  adrenal cortex, 38–9
   androstenedione production from the, 102
   dehydroepiandrosterone production from the, 102
   estrogen production from the, 96
   testosterone production from the, 27
   see also corticoids, steroid hormones
  adrenal medulla
   blood pressure, 23
   release of catecholamines from the, 26
   release of monoamines from the, 39
   see also adrenaline/epinephrine, noradrenaline/norepinephrine
  adrenarche, 102
  Cushing's disease, 33, 39
adrenaline (epinephrine)
  effect on heartbeat of, 16
  effects on sexual behaviour of, 127
  general information on, 18, 26
  relationship with the thyroid hormones of, 76, 81–2, 83
  release by the adrenal medulla of, 39
adrenocorticotropic hormone (ACTH)
  cellular activity in the hippocampus, 80–1
  in CAH , 109, 258
  production in the adrenal glands of, 39
  stimulation by CRH, 31, 33–4
  synthesis from prohormones, 30
aggression, see behaviour
alpha-fetoprotein (AFP), role in sex determination of, 92
amplexus, 53

amygdala
  androgen receptors in the, 73–4
  connections with the bed nucleus of the stria terminalis, 141
  connections with the olfactory system, 160–1, 194
  effects on maternal behaviours of the, 206
  estrogen receptors in the, 72
  general information on, 5, 6
  glucocorticoid receptors in the, 75
  oxytocin receptors in the, 189, 206
  progesterone receptors in the, 73
  role in social processing of the, 6, 245
  thyroid hormone receptors in the, 76
androgens
  androgen insensitivity syndrome (AIS)
   effects on cognitive ability, 259
   effects on gender identity, 114, 120
   general information on, 113
  androstenedione, 26–7
   association with gender identity of, 99
   castration and replacement of, 67
   concentration in spotted hyena, 94
   conversion to estrone, 72
   conversion to testosterone, 29, *2.2*
   levels during the menopause of, 28, 187
   levels in transsexuals of, 122
   production in the testes of, 41
   relationship with cognitive ability, 256
   role in homosexuality of, 128
   salivary sampling problems in the measurement of, 45
   secretion of during puberty, 102
   sexual receptivity, 185
  androsterone, 26
   castration and replacement, 67
  dehydroepiandrosterone (DHEA), 26
   as a neurosteroid, 29
   measurement issues, 46
   relationship to dominance of, 243
   secretion from adrenal cortex of, 102
   synthesis, *2.2*
  dehydroepiandrosterone sulfate (DHEAS),
   levels in transsexuals of, 122
   secretion from adrenal cortex of, 102

androgens (*cont.*)
  dihydrotestosterone (DHT), 26
    effects on aggressive behaviours of, 232, 236
    effects on sexual behaviours of, 163
    effects on sexual differentiation of, 90, 117
    synthesis of, 27, 30, 117, 159, *2.2*
  testosterone
    binding to SHBG of, 25
    diurnal fluctuations in, 41, 46
    effects on EEG pattern of, 78
    effects on skin condition of, 180
    influence of thyroid hormones on, 83
    levels of in females, 27
    levels of in left-handers, 47
    measurements of circulating levels of, 43–7
    production of, 27, 41, 62, 89–90
    relationship with cognitive ability
      in animals, 25153
      in humans
        evidence from clinical syndromes, 257–61
        evidence from digit ratio studies, 253–6
        evidence from foetal sampling, 256–7
        evidence from reduction studies, 281–2
        evidence from supplementation studies, 272–5, 279–80
        relationship with  circulating levels, 261–5
    relationship with dermotoglyphic characteristics, 58
    relationship with finger length ratios, 59–60
    role of in aggression
      in animals, 65, 218, 225–33
      in humans, 201, 233–47
    role of in AIS, 113
    role of in amplexus, 53
    role of in attachment behaviours, 201
    role of in CAH, 109–11
    role of in cerebral lateralisation, 143, 144–5, 147–9, 150–3
    role of in competitive behaviours, 53,
    role of in IHH, 115
    role of in Klinefelter syndrome, 114–15
    role of in maternal behaviours, 213–14
    role of in paternal behaviours,
      in animals, 213, 217–20
      in humans, 220–3
    role of in pheromones, 51
    role of in relationship status, 201–4
    role of in sexual behaviours
      in birds, 67
      in humans, 170–9, 184–8, 201–4
      in primates, 167,
      in rodents, 63, 77, 91, 158–63,
    role of in sexual differentiation, 43, 51, 90–1, 97
      in avian song centres, 57, 136
      in gender role, 99–102, 111–15, 120–1
      in homosexuals, 126, 127, 129, 131, 133, 142

    in human brain regions, 74, 150–3
    in hyenas, 94
    at puberty, 102–8
    in rodents, 56, 137–8, 144
    in transsexuals, 122, 123
    role of in social behaviours, 197–9,
    seasonal variations in, 47
    synthesis and conversion of, 26–7, 29, 30, 72–4, 89, 92, 117, 144, 217, *2.2*
antidiuretic hormone, see vasopressin
arginine vasopressin, see vasopressin
aromatase, 27, 92
  aromatase regulation, 72
  in bone tissue, 104–5
  in homosexuality, 138
  in transsexuals, 123
aromatisation,
  in the activation of sexual behaviours, 159–60, 161–2
  in avian parental behaviours, 217
  catecholamine action on, 72
  cerebral asymmetry and, 144
  estrogen receptors, 73, 92
  in homosexuality, 134
  hypothalamus and sex differences, 144
  process of, 27, 72, 92, 2.2
attachment bonds, see behaviour

basal ganglia, 5, 7
behaviour
  aggressive behaviours
    anabolic androgenic steroids (AAS), 229–30, 243
    ARKO animals and aggression, 233
    challenge hypothesis in animals, 225–33
    challenge hypothesis in humans, 234–45
    characteristics of aggression, 224–5
    castration as aggression reduction, 225
    competitive aggression, 241–3
    definition in animals, 224
    definition in humans, 233–4
    dominance, 243–5
    ERKO animals and aggression, 233
    finger lenth ratio and, 246–7
    home advantage in sport, 240–1
    loser effect in animals, 232
    loser effect in humans, 237–9
    personality factors in, 245
    puberty in animals, 230
    puberty in humans, 234–7
    reproductive effort, 218
    role of estradiol/aromatase, 232
    role of vasopressin, 230, 232
    seasonal variations in , 226, 229
    territorial aggression, 55, 65, 224, 229
    testosterone supplementation, 229–30, 242–3

winner effect in animals, 230–2
winner effect in humans, 237–41
amygdala and social behaviours, 6
attachment behaviours
  definition, 192–3
  in monkeys, 65
  offspring–parent attachment, 204–6
    role of oxytocin in, 205–6
    role of stress in, 205
  parent–offspring attachment in animals
    maternal behaviours in birds, 207–8
      prolactin and broodiness, 208
    maternal behaviour in mammals, 208–17
      mPOA alterations in, 211
      role of endogenous opioids in, 213
      role of lactation in, 210
      role of oxytocin in, 209–10, 213
      role of prolactin in, 207–8
      role of steroid hormones in, 211–13
  parental bonds in humans,
    evidence from CAH females, 214
    relationship with steroid hormones, 214–16
    role of endogenous opioids in, 216
  paternal behaviour in birds, 217
    role of steroid hormones in, 217
  paternal behaviours in humans, 220–222
    role of prolactin in, 222
    role of steroid hormones in, 221–2
  paternal behaviour in primates, 219–20
    role of prolactin in, 219
    role of steroid hormones in, 219–20
  paternal behaviour in rodents, 217–19
    role of steroid hormones in, 217–18
    role of prolactin in, 217
  social bonds in animals, 193–96
    role of oxytocin in, 193–6
    role of pheromones in, 192, 194
    role of progesterone in, 192–3
    role of vasopression in, 194–6
  social bonds in humans, 196–204
    individuals with social deficits, 196–7
      role of oxytocin in, 197
      role of testosterone in, 197–8
      role of vasopressin in, 197
    heterosexual attraction
      emotion of love, 200–1
      hormone profiles during love, 201
      oxytocin and trustworthiness, 199–200
      role of empathy in, 198–9
      testosterone and relationship commitment, 202–4, 229
      testosterone and smiling, 199
reproductive/sexual behaviours, 154–90
  brain regions associated with sexual behaviours, 137–9, 160
  categorising sexual behaviours in humans, 124, 168–70, 179–80

categorising sexual behaviours in primates, 166–8
categorising sexual behaviours in rodents, 155–8,
individual difference in sexual behaviours, 161–3
in ERKO mice, 162, 164–5
role of neurotransmitters in, 160, 165–6
role of the olfactory system in, 157, 158, 160
role of oxytocin in, 189–90
steroid hormones and sexual behaviours, 23, 27, 28, 33, 71, 158–61, 162–8
  associations with fluctuating hormone levels,
  in human females, 183–4
  in human males, 176–7
  in primates, 166–8
  attractivity in human females, 180–1
  castration and replacement studies, 63, 66–7, 86, 91, 158–9, 161, 167–8, 228
  chemical castration in human males, 174–5
  effect of social context, 51
  evidence from digit ratio studies, 177
  HRT studies, 188–9
  proceptivity in human females, 181–4
  receptivity in human females, 184–7
  role of steroid hormone receptors, 73–4, 162, 165
  testosterone administration studies, 170–5
    in elderly males, 175
    in hypogonadal males, 170–2
    in normal males, 172–5
  sexual behaviour and hormone levels, 177–9
  sexual behaviour in the menopause, 187–9
behavioural endocrinology,
  background and history, 48–51
  comparative studies, 64–6
  definitions of behaviour, 53–5
  establishing relationships between hormones and behaviour, 66–8
  hormone–behaviour interactions, 51–2,
  measuring hormone levels,
    bioassay, 24, 43, 207–8
    circulating hormone measurement, 43–7
    dermotoglyphic patterns, 58
    finger length ratio, 59–61
      historical background, 59
      in aggression, 246–7
      in attractiveness, 177
      in autism, 198
      in CAH, 110–11
      in cognitive ability, 253–6
      in dominance, 246
      in hand skill, 151
      in homosexuals, 131, 134
      measurement issues of, 61
      and number of sex partners, 177

behavioural endocrinology (*cont.*)
    as a proxy marker for hormone exposure,
      59–61
    in relation to body morphology, 103, 106
    in relation to gender role, 101–2
    in transsexuals, 123
    organisational versus activational hypothesis,
      56–63
    radioimmunoassay (RIA), 44, 46

castration
  castrati, 22, 86–7
  chemical castration, 174
  hormone replacement and aggressive
    behaviours following, 225–8
  hormone replacement and cognition
    following, 252–3
  hormone replacement and parental
    behaviours following, 218
  hormone replacement and sexual behaviours
    following, 63, 66, 67, 91, 96, 159, 161
  organisational versus activational debate, 62
  physical effects of, 22, 86, 105
  sexual dimorphism following, 136, 141
  Skoptsy sect, 87
catecholamines, 18, 25–6, 72
  relationship with adrenal hormones, 82
  relationship with thyroid hormones, 81
cerebral cortex, see nervous system
cerebral lateralisation,
  callosal hypothesis, 151–3
  cerebral asymmetry in humans, 142–4
  changes during the menstrual cycle in, 146–7,
    272
  changes during puberty in, 145–6
  cortical asymmetry in rats, 144
  dichotic listening in DES-exposed individuals,
    145, 261
  dichotic listening method, 143
  GBG model, 147–53
  hormones and cerebral asymmetry, 144–53
  lateralisation in CAH, 145, 258
  lateralisation in Turner's syndrome, 145
  sex differences in cortical activation, 143
  testosterone and lateralisation,
    circulating testosterone and handedness, 150
    prenatal testosterone and degree of
      lateralisation for subitising, 256
    prenatal testosterone and lateralisation,
      150–1
choline acetyltransferase (ChAT), 251
chromosomes
  autosomal chromosomes, 10
  sex chromosomes, 10
  sex chromosomes and sexual differentiation,
    88, 90, 118, 120
  Turner's syndrome, 259–60

cognition
  definition of, 248–9, 266
  effects of hormone reduction on, 281–2
  human sex differences in, 249
  maze learning tasks
    Morris maze, 250, 251, 253
    radial-arm maze, 250–1, 253
    T-maze, 252
  mental rotation test (MRT), 254, 255, 257,
    259, 261–5, 270–1, 274, 277
  numerical, 255–6
  rodent sex differences in, 249–53
  role of steroid hormones,
    animal evidence, 249–53
    circulating hormones and cognition,
      DHT, 261–3
      estrogens/progestins, 265–72
      gonadotropins, 262, 271
      testosterone, 261–5
    correlations with foetal blood samples, 256–7
    evidence from clinical samples,
      AIS, 259
      CAH, 258–9
      DES exposed individuals, 260–1
      IHH, 272–3
      Turner's syndrome, 259–60
    evidence from digit ratio, 253–6
    supplementation evidence,
      HRT in the elderly,
        females, 275–9
        males, 279–80
        phytoestrogens, 280–1
      hypogonadal males, 272–4
      in transsexuals, 274–5
communication systems, 8
congenital adrenal hyperplasia (CAH)
  autism, 198
  cerebral lateralisation, 145, 258
  cognitive performance, 258
  gender identity, 111–13, 120
  general information on, 109–10
  parental behaviours, 214
  2D:4D ratio in, 60, 110–11
corpus callosum, 3, 6
  racial differences in size and shape in, 152
  role in cerebral lateralisation, 152
  sex differences in size and shape in, 152–3
corpus luteum, 28, 35, 40, 275
corticoids
  definition of, 28
  glucocorticoids
    corticosterone, 28, 74–5, 80, 158, 205
    cortisol, 28
      adrenal hormone receptors and, 75
      calculation of free cortisol, 45
      diurnal pattern of, 28, 34, 46–7
      measurement by RIA, 44

production by the adrenal cortex, 38
relationships with aggressive behaviours,
    235, 238, 239, 242, 244–5, 247
relationships with attachment behaviours,
    201, 205–6
relationships with parental behaviours, 212,
    215–17, 219–21
relationships with sexual behaviours, 170
role of in CAH, 109
role of in Cushing's disease, 33, 39
mineralocorticoids, 29
functions of aldosterone, 29
influence of ACTH on, 33–4
receptors for, 70, 74–5
treatment in CAH, 110
corticotropin-releasing hormone (CRH), 31,
    33–34
couvade, see parental behaviours in humans
cretinism, see thyroid gland
crop sac, 49, 68, 207–8
Cushing's disease, see adrenal glands

daidzein, see phytoestrogens
deoxyribonucleic acid (DNA)
chemical bases, 10–11
hormone receptors, 70, 74, 123
dermatoglyphic measures, 58
in transsexuals, 132
diabetes, see pancreas
dopamine (DA)
in aggressive behaviours, 232
aromatase regulation, 72
effect on vasopressin release of, 82
in the formation of pair bonds, 195, 201, 208,
    222, 223
general information on, 18, 21
influence of the glucocorticoids on, 82
influence of thyroid hormones on, 81
influence on sexual behaviours of, 160–1, 165–6
production in adrenal medulla, 39
regulation of hypothalamic hormones, 35
relationship with estrogen receptors, 81
synthesis of adrenaline/noradrenaline, 26

eicosanoids, 25
electroencephalogram (EEG), 78
recordings during the menstrual cycle, 78
endogenous opioids,
in parental behaviours, 209, 213, 216–17, 223
epinephrine, see adrenaline
estrogens
effects on bone formation of, 104–5
effects in transsexuals of, 103,
effects on hypothalamic–pituitary–gonadal
    axis of, 128–9
effects on nervous system of, 77, 250–1
effects on other hormones of, 35, 250–1

effects on oxytocin receptors of, 193
effects on vocal characteristics, 108
estrogen synthase, see aromatase
diethylstilbestrol (DES), 138, 145, 260–1
estradiol
effects of thyroid hormones on, 83
effects on cerebral lateralisation of, 144, 146,
effects on the GABAergic system of, 81
effects on the nervous sytem of, 79–81, 250–1
measurement of, 44–7
production and synthesis of, 27–30, 41, 72–3,
    2.2
receptors for, 73–4
role in aggressive behaviour of, 227, 232, 247
role in cognitive ability,
in animals, 251–3
in humans
    evidence from supplementation studies,
        275, 277–8, 280
    relationship with circulating levels, 257,
        263, 267, 270–1, 279–80
role in digit ratio of, 60
role in parental behaviours of
in animals, 211–12, 218–20
in humans, 215, 217, 221
role in sexual behaviours of
in animals, 52, 67, 92, 158–61, 164–8
in humans, 172–4, 179, 184, 186, 188
role in sexual differentiation of, 95, 115,
    133–4, 144
role in social behaviours of, 192
estrone, 28, 41, 72, 128, 278
general information on, 28
in Turner's syndrome, 116, 145
production and synthesis and of, 28, 34,
    39–40, 62, 2.2
receptors for, 70–4, 81, 92, 141
role at puberty, 102, 104
role in aggressive behaviours, 227, 229, 232–3
role in cognitive ability
in animals, 252
in humans
    evidence from digit ratios, 254
    evidence from supplementation studies,
        275–9, 280–1
    evidence from Turner's syndrome, 259–61
    relationship with circulating levels, 263,
        265–73
role in digit ratios, 59–60
role in parental behaviours
in animals, 207–9, 212, 218
role in sexual behaviours
in animals, 67, 77, 92, 159–65, 167–8
in humans, 180–1, 184, 187–9
role in sexual differentiation, 56–7, 90–2, 94–8,
    104–5, 120, 134, 138, 141–2, 144
role in transsexualism, 123

estrus
  anestrus state, 157, 163
  effects of dopamine on, 165
  hormones and estrus, 77, 79, 163, 164, 211,
      252
  neuronal activation during, 77
  parental behaviour and, 218
  sexual behaviours during, 163–5, 167, 168–9,
      172, 180, 185, 193, 228
  synaptic density during, 79

free hormone hypothesis, 45

gamma-aminobutyric acid (GABA), 19
  estradiol and the GABAergic system, 81
  GABA receptors, 19
    neurosteroids, 29
    influence of progesterone, 73
  GABAergic projections, 251
  influence on pituitary hormones, 35
genistein, see phytoestrogens
glia, 9
glutamate, 19
  hippocampal function and, 79–80
  receptors for, 19
goitre, see thyroid gland
gonadotropins
  effects on vocal parameters, 108
  follicle stimulating hormone (FSH)
    associations with cognitive performance, 262,
        271
    control by GnRH, 31
    levels during menopause of, 275
    levels during romantic attraction of, 201
    regulation of gonadal hormone production
        of, 34–5, 40–1, 42
    role in human menstrual cycle of, 40
    role in puberty of, 62–3, 102
    role in rodent estrus cycle of, 163
  influences of clasping behaviours in
      amphibians, 53
  luteinising hormone (LH)
    associations with cognitive performance, 262,
        271
    control by GnRH, 31
    levels in males viewing pornography, 178
    pheromonal influences on, 158, 192
    regulation of gonadal hormone production
        of, 34–5, 42
    role in broodiness of, 208
    role in human menstrual cycle of, 40, 44
    role in puberty of, 62–3, 102
    role in rodent estrus cycle of, 163
    role in testosterone fluctuation on, 41
    role of steroids in LH release, 35
    surge in response to estrogen in homosexual
        males, 129

see also idiopathic hypogonadotropic
    hypogonadism
gonadotropin-releasing hormone (GnRH)
  agonist and antagonist effects on testosterone
      of, 172–3
  agonists and ovulation prevention, 167
  effects during puberty of, 62, 102
  effects of urinary pheromones on, 158
  negative feedback loop of, 42
  synthesis and actions of, 31, 35, 163
Graves' disease, 37
growth hormone (GH), 31
  actions of, 32, 34, 102
  effects on bone tissue of, 104
  inhibitory action of eicosanoids on release of,
      30
  peptide hormones, 26
  treatment in Turner's syndrome, 116
growth hormone-inhibiting hormone (GH-IH),
    see somatostatin
growth hormone-releasing hormone (GH-RH),
    31

hermaphrodite, see intersex
hippocampus
  adrenal hormone receptors in, 75
  alterations during puberty of, 62, 63
  androgen hormone receptors in, 73
  aromatisation within, 72
  description and location of, 5, 6
  hormonal effects in, 77, 78–82, 97, 251, 253,
      269, 281
  role in learning and memory, 5, 6, 250, 253,
      269
  thyroid hormone receptors in, 76
homosexuality
  abdominal adiposity in, 104
  androgen receptor expression in, 74
  animal models of, 127–8
  in CAH females, 113
  cognitive performance in, 254
  confusion with transsexuality, 122
  developmental instability in, 132
  dimorphism in CNS structures in, 141–2
  finger length ratios in, 131–2
  gender nonconformity in, 124–5
  genetic factors in, 124–5
  hormonal theories of, 125–34
  incidence in the population, 123–4
  role of aromatisation, 138
  steroid hormone levels in, 126, 203
hormone replacement therapy (HRT), cognitive
    effects of, 275–81
hormones
  amino acid hormones, 25–6
  definition of, 24–5, 2.1
  glycoproteins, 34–5

historical background of research on, 22–4
hormone receptor complex, 41, 70,
hormone regulation, 42–3, *2.4*
lipids, 30
measurement of, 43–7, 71–2
neurological effects of, 70–1, 76–84
peptide hormones, 26
pheromones, 25, 51, 158, 160, 192
prohormones, 25
releasing hormones, 31–3, *2.3*
tropic hormones, 33–4
see also steroid hormones; thyroid hormones
human chorionic gonadotropin, 44
hydrocortisone, see cortisol
hypothalamus
    aggressive behaviours and, 230, 232
    androgen receptors in, 73
    aromatisation in, 72, 74, 134
    connectivity of, 5, 6, 7
    estradiol effects on GAD in, 81
    estrogen receptors in, 72
    estrus cycle relationships, 77, 81
    glucocorticoid receptors in, 75
    hormones secreted by, 31–3, 35, *2.3*
    IHH, see idiopathic hypergonadotropic
        hypogonadism
    influence on menstrual cycle by, 40
    influence on puberty of, 63, 102
    influence on steroid production of, 41
    medial preoptic area (mPOA)
        estrogenic effects on, 77
        interstitial nuclei of, 142
        oxytocin receptors in, 206
        role in sexual behaviours of, 71, 126, 160,
            165, 190, 211
        steroid receptors in, 72, 73, 74, 162, 210
    neurotransmitter pathways, 20
    paraventricular nuclei, 31–3
        adrenal hormone receptors in, 76
        maternal care and, 206
        oxytocin production in, 189, 193
        vasopressin production in, 193
    progesterone receptors, 73
    relationships with the pituitary gland, 31–5,
        40, 42, 52, 62–3, *2.3*
    serotonergic effects in, 82
    sex differences in, 97, 137–9, 142
    sexual behaviours and, 134, 160
    sexual determination and, 87, 89
    suprachiasmatic nucleus (SCN), 36
    thyroid hormone receptors in, 76

idiopathic hypogonadotropic hypogonadism
    (IHH)
    cognitive performance in, 272–3
    gender identity in, 115
    general information on, 115

role of gonadotropins in, 115, 272
vocal characteristics, 108
indoleamines, 18–19
    amino acid hormones and, 25
    see also melatonin; serotonin
intersex, 89, 118, 120–1
ionotropic receptors
    for acetylcholine, 18
    characteristics of, 17
    for GABA, 19
    for glutamate, 19, 79

Kallmann's syndrome
    general information on, 115
    gender identity in, 115, 120
Klinefelter's syndrome (46XXY)
    general information on, 114–15
    gender identity, 115, 120

lignans, see phytoestrogens
limbic system
    attachment bond formation and, 223
    components and functions of, 5
    connectivity of, 5, 20
    glucocorticoid inhibition of steroid hormone
        activity within, 71
    links with neuropeptides, 35
    role in motivation and reward, 195
lipids, 17, 30
long-term potentiation (LTP), 79–80
lordosis
    definition of, 91, 156
    effects of androgens on, 91, 92
    effects of cholinergic antagonists on, 165
    effects of estradiol/estrogen on, 164–5
    effects of maternal stress on offspring lordosis,
        127
    effects of oxytocin on, 190
    effects of progesterone on, 164
    effects of serotonin on, 166
    as a measurement of sexual receptivity, 158
    pheromone effects on, 51
luteinising hormone releasing hormone (LH-RH)
    effects on broodiness of, 208
    effects of pheromones on, 192
luteotropin, see prolactin

maternal behaviour, see behaviour
medial preoptic area, see hypothalamus
melatonin
    effects on LH and FSH, 44
    production and synthesis of, 26, 35–6
menopause
    alteration in sexual behaviours during, 187–8
    alteration in steroid hormone levels during,
        28, 108, 187, 275
    cognitive effects of, 276–7, 281

menstrual cycle
  body scent during, 181
  cerebral lateralisation during, 146
  EEG recordings during, 78
  fluctuations in cognitive processing during,
    265–72
  fluctuations in oxytocin levels during, 190
  fluctations in steroid hormone levels during,
    27–8, 34, 40, 47
  perceptual changes during, 57
  premenstrual syndrome/tension (PMS/T), 268
  sexual behaviours during, 168, 179, 182–3,
    185–7
  skin colour changes during, 180
  vocal characteristics during, 108
metabotropic receptors
  acetylcholine, 18
  adrenergic system, 83
  characteristics of, 18
  GABA, 19
  glutamate, 19
  similarity with hormonal effects, 69
monoamine oxidase (MAO), 269
monoamines, 18–19
  adrenal medulla release of, 39

neuroanatomical directions, 1
neurohypophysis, see pituitary gland
neurons
  action potential within, 14–15
  chemical events within, 13–14
  electrical events within, 12–13
  communication between, 16–17
  structure of, 9–12
neurosteroids, 29, 73, 77, 96, 158
neurotransmitters, 17–20
nervous system
  autonomic nervous system (ANS), 2, 1.1
  basal ganglia, 7
  brain organization, 2–8, 1.2, 1.3
  central nervous system (CNS), 1–2, 1.1
  cerebral cortex, 3–6
  definition of, 1–2
  diencephalon, 7, 1.3
  forebrain, 3–7
  functions of the lobes, 4–6
  hindbrain, 9
  limbic system, 7
  midbrain, 8
  organization of the nervous system, 1–2, 1.1,
    1.2
  peripheral nervous system (PNS), 1–2, 1.1
  somatic nervous system (SNS), 1, 1.1
  telencephalon, 3–7, 1.3
nonapeptide, see oxytocin
noradrenaline,
  effects on aromatisation of, 72

effects on cognition of, 269
effects on oxytocin and vasopressin of, 82
effects on sexual behaviour of, 158, 165, 179
effects on social bond formation of, 192
general information on, 18, 26
relationship with the thyroid hormones, 76,
  81–3
release by the adrenal medulla of, 39
norepinephrine, see noradrenaline
orchidectomy, orchiectomy, see castration
organizational versus activational hypothesis
  re-evaluation of the theory, 61–3
  standard assumption, 56–61
organotherapy, 22–4, 275–6
orgasm, 169–70
  oxytocin levels during, 189–90, 194
  prolactin levels during, 179
  testosterone levels during, 176
ovariectomy
  effect on cognitive performance of, 252–3,
    281
  effect on cortical thickness of, 144
  effect on dendritic spine density of, 79, 97
  effect on GABA of, 81
  effect on neuronal activation of, 77
  effect on parental behaviours of, 207, 211
  effect on sexual behaviours of, 67, 97, 158–9,
    163–4, 165, 167, 168
  effect on sexual differentiation of, 96
  effect on social behaviours of, 194
  use in estrogen-binding studies of, 72
oxytocin
  definition of, 26, 189
  effects of, 189
  influence of acetylcholine on, 82
  influence of soy isoflavones on, 280
  levels during orgasm, 189–90, 194
  receptor binding in the CNS, 193–4
  role in sexual behaviours of, 189–90
  role in social bonding in animals of, 193–6,
    205–6, 209–10, 213, 222–3
  role in social bonding in humans of, 197,
    199–200, 206, 216, 222–3

pancreas, 37–8
  diabetes, 37–8
  insulin and down regulation, 42
  insulin and glucose, 38
  insulin-like growth factor (IGF-1), 34
  insulin secretion and function, 23, 25, 26, 32,
    37
Pap test, 50, 163
Papez circuit, see limbic system
parental behaviour, see behaviour
paternal behaviour, see behaviour
peptides, 20, 25
  corticotrophin-related peptides, 33–4

neuropeptides, 25, 35
pancreatic polypeptides, 37–8
peptide hormones, 26; see also oxytocin and
    vasopressin
polypeptide hormones, 26, 41
phytoestrogens, soy isoflavones and cognition,
    280–1
pituitary gland, 7, 33
  androgen receptors within, 73
  effects of tumours within, 39
  estrogen receptors within, 72
  glucocorticoid receptors within, 75
  hormones produced within, 30, 33–5, 82, 189,
      193, 207
  progesterone receptors within, 73
  relationship with the adrenal glands, 66
  relationship with the gonads, 39–41, 173
  relationship with the hypothalamus, 30–5, 42,
      52, 223
  relationship with the pineal gland, 36
  relationship with the thyroid gland, 36, 48, 83
  response to estrogens, 128–9
  role during puberty, 62–3, 102
  role during the menopause, 275
  sexual dimorphism within the, 139
progestins, 28
  progesterone, 28
    and cognition, 252–3, 267, 269–72, 275, 278
    and dendritic spine density, 79–80, 97
    effects on hypothalamic nuclei of, 97
    effects on mPOA neurons of, 210
    effects on parental behaviours of, 192–3,
        207, 209, 211–12, 215
    effects on sexual behaviours of, 28, 73, 77,
        158, 162–8, 174, 179, 183–6, 188–9
    effects on vocal characteristics of, 108
    and facial preferences, 183
    influence of genistein on, 280
    measurement in saliva of, 46
    menstrual cycle fluctuations in, 34–5, 146
    neurosteroids effects on, 29
    production by the corpus luteum of, 28, 35,
        40, 275
    receptor action of, 70, 71
    receptor localisation of, 73
    role in sexual differentiation, 98
    role in the menopause, 187
    ovarian production of, 39–40
    and skin colour, 180
    testicular production of, 40
    and waist-to-hip ratio, 180
polycystic ovary syndrome (PCOS), see
    transsexuality
prolactin
  association with broodiness, 208
  association with parental behaviours, 217,
      219–21

association with orgasm, 179
effects of gonadal steroids on, 34
effects of serotonin on, 208
effects of TRH on, 35
functions of, 34, 49, 68, 207–8
influence of lactation on, 210, 216
up-regulation and, 42
pseudohermaphroditism, 117
  gender identity in, 117–18
puberty
  aggression during, 230, 231–7, 246, 265
  androgen surge in males at, 27
  breast development in males at, 114
  castration studies and, 66, 86, 97, 159, 225, 251
  changes in the male larynx during, 57
  CNS changes in, 62–3
  delay of, 63, 105–6, 114–16, 171, 172, 176–7,
      259, 272–3
  endocrine activity during, 63, 89, 98, 102–3
  female menstrual cycle at, 40
  secondary sexual characteristics in animals at,
      49
  sex differences in maturation at, 146
  sexual behaviours during, 170, 176–7,
  sexual differentiation at, 102–8, 261
    body morphology, 103–4
    bone metabolism, 104–6
    vocal characteristics, 106–8
  Tanner stages of, 103, 107
  virilisation at puberty in
      pseudohermaphroditism, 117, 120

ribonucleic acid (RNA), 10
  messenger RNA (mRNA), 34, 74, 76, 138

salivary sampling, see hormones
second to fourth finger length ratio (2D:4D),
    see behavioural endocrinology
serotonin
  effects on lordosis, 166
  influence of glucocorticoids on, 82
  general information on, 19, 26
  melatonin synthesis, 35
  relationship with estrogen receptors, 81
  role in aggression of, 228, 232
  role in broodiness and maternal behaviours,
      208, 223
sex determination
  in AIS, 113
  animal models of, 90–5
  in CAH, 109–11
  in enzyme deficiency syndromes, 117
  genetic basis of, 88–9, 95–6
  historical background, 86–7
  in homosexuals, 123–5
  hormonal effects on, 89–99
  hormonal models of, 98

sex determination (*cont.*)
  in IHH, 115
  in Klinefelter's syndrome, 114–15
  role of AFP in, 92
  in transsexuals, 121–3
  in Turner's syndrome, 116
  types of, 87–8
sex differentiation
  during puberty, 102–8
  in body shape, 103–4
  in bone metabolism, 104–6
  in the voice, 106–8
  in avian song centres, 135–6
  in cognition, 248–9
    evidence from animal studies, 249–51
    spatial ability in humans, 254–5
    from AIS individuals, 258
    from CAH girls, 258
    from DES-exposed children, 260–1
    from Turner girls, 259–60
  in gender role, 99–102
    androgens and gender role, 102–3
    definition, 85, 99
    gender identity in AIS, 114, 120, 259
    gender identity in CAH, 111–13, 120
    gender identity in enzyme deficiency
        syndromes, 117–18
    gender identity in homosexuals, 123–5, 133–4
    gender identity in Klinefelter's syndrome,
        114–15, 120
    gender identity in John/Joan case, 118–19,
        120–1
    gender identity in transsexuals, 121
    gender role identity in IHH, 115
    gender role identity in Turner's syndrome, 117
    maternal stress and gender role, 99–101
    2D:4D ratio and gender role, 102
    gender role reassignment, 110
  in human brain,
    brain size, 139–41
    cerebral asymmetry, 142–53
      evidence from dichotic task, 143
      evidence from menstrual cycle studies,
          146–7
      evidence from MRI, 143
      evidence from prenatal studies, 144–5
      evidence from pubertal maturation, 146
      in CAH females, 145
      the callosal theory, 151–3
      the GBG model, 147–53
    hypothalamus, 141–2
    in rodent cortex, 144
    in rodent hypothalamus, 137–8
    in rodent tail bias, 144
    in sheep hypothalamus, 138
sex hormone binding globulin (SHBG), 26,
    100, 185, 187

sexual behaviours, see behaviour
social bonds, see attachment behaviours
somatomammotropins, 34
somatostatin (SOM), 32–3
somatotropin, see growth hormone
steroid hormones, 26–9, 2.2
  detection by autoradiography, 71–2
  neurosteroids, 29–30, 79–80, 99, 163
  receptor binding, 72–4
  see also androgens; estrogens; glucocorticoids;
      mineralocorticoids; neurosteroids;
      progestins
suprachiasmatic nucleus, see hypothalamus
synapse
  chemical events at the, 16
  general information on, 12–13
  long-term potentiation at the, 79

thalamus
  androgen receptors within the, 73
  location of the, 6, 31
  projections to the, 20
  relationship to the hypothalamus, 30
  structure of the, 7
  thyroid hormone action in the, 76
thyroid hormones
  functions of, 27, 36–7
  role in brain development of, 80, 82–3
  role in goitre of, 36, 48
  manufacture, release and transport of,
      36–7
  receptor binding of, 76
  regulation of, 42–3, 2.4
  relationships with adreneregic system, 76
  role in cretinism, 37, 48
  thyroxine (T$_4$), 26, 36–7, 76
  triiodothyronine (T$_3$), 26, 34, 36–7
thyroid stimulating hormone (TSH), 32, 34–5,
    42, 43, 48
thyrotropin, see thyroid stimulating hormone
thyrotropin-releasing hormone (TRH), 32,
    34–5, 42
transsexuality
  alterations in brain volume in, 141
  androgen receptors in, 74
  body fat distribution in, 103
  definition of, 121–2
  dermotoglyphic characteristics in, 123
  digit ratio in, 123
  estrogen treatment in male–female
      transsexuals, 103
  gender dysphoria in, 113, 121
  hormone administration and cognition in,
      274–5
  incidence of PCOS in, 122
  LH response in, 129
  receptor polymorphisms in, 123

Turner's syndrome,
  cerebral lateralisation, 145
  cognitive performance in, 259–60
  gender identity in, 116, 120
  general information on, 116

vasopressin (arginine vasopressin), 25–6
  association with aggressive behaviours, 230, 232
  association with attachment behaviours,
      194–6, 206, 218, 222
  association with autism, 197

association with sexual behaviours, 193
association with social memory, 194
chemical similarity with oxytocin, 189
effect on lactation on production of, 210
functions of, 32
influence of neurotransmitters on, 82
location of receptors for, 193, 195, 201
ventral tegmental area (VTA)
  brain activation during romantic attraction,
      201
  dopaminergic projections, 20